BIOSTATISTICS

BIOSTATISTICS

K.L.A.P. Sarma
Department of Statistics
Sri Krishnadevaraya University
Anantapur-515 003, A.P.

B. Ravindra Reddy
Department of Statistics & Mathematics
S.V. Agricultural College,
Acharya N.G. Ranga Agricultural University
Tirupati–517 502, A.P.

&

T. Pullaiah
Department of Botany,
Sri Krishnadevaraya University
Anantapur-515 003, A.P.

2013

Daya Publishing House®
A Division of Astral International Pvt. Ltd.
New Delhi-110002

ISBN 9789351301189

Published by : **Daya Publishing House**®
A Division of
Astral International Pvt. Ltd.
– ISO 9001:2008 Certified Company –
4760-61/23, Ansari Road, Darya Ganj
New Delhi-110 002
Ph. 011-43549197, 23278134
E-mail: info@astralint.com
Website: www.astralint.com

Laser Typesetting : **Classic Computer Services**, Delhi - 110 035

Printed at : **Replika Press Pvt. Ltd.**

PRINTED IN INDIA

PREFACE

Biostatistics is a part of curriculum of M.Phil. and Ph.D. written examination (Research Methdology paper), Post Graduate courses in Agriculture, Veterinary Science, Fishery Science, Medicine, Forestry, Pharmacy, Botany, Zoology, Biochemistry, Microbiology, Biotechnology and Bioinformatics. It is also a part of curriculum in undergraduate courses of Medicine, Agriculture, Veterinary Science, Biotechnology and Bioinformatics. Not many books are available in the market on this subject. This book is answer to this requirement. In fact the idea of writing this book came from the suggestions made by many biological students studying, M.Sc. Zoology, Botany, Microbiology, Biochemistry, Biotechnology and Sericulture. Keeping the needs of students studying above courses, relevant topics were discussed clearly, using less mathematical symbols with many real life examples. Much concentration was made to explain the need, applications of statistical tools and techniques for experimental data.

The book can also be used by research scholars working for their Ph.D., degrees in above fields along with M.B.A., Commerce, Economics, Rural development and engineering. Scholars working in Agriculture, industrial applications, fisheries, market research, share fore casting and forest reseach can use this book as 'hand book' which can give guidance in conducting their respectie experiments. This book covers the syllabus of Biostatistics of all the above mentioned courses. We request the Teachers and students to give suggestions for improvement of the book.

We thank all the teachers for their suggestions and stimulating discussion on the subject.

Anantapur

K.L.A.P. Sarma

B. Ravindra Reddy

T. Pullaiah

ABOUT THE BOOK

The book 'Biostatistics' consists of ten chapters explaining statistical tools used in analyzing biological, biomedical and biochemical experimental data. Statistical tools, techniques and methods are explained with many real life problems and special care is taken to explain mathematical formulae and calculations keeping in view that the readers are non-mathematical students who are not having much mathematical background.

The book mainly concentrates on (1) Collection, classification and tabulation of data, (2) Presentation of Data (both diagrammatic and graphical repreentation) (3) Analysis and (4) Inference (both estimation of parameters and testing of hypotheses). Most popularly used DMR test, by any biological students is also discussed along with its applications. At the end of each chapter, self assessment questions are given. This book can also be used by civil, mechanical, electrical and computer engineers in analyzing their experimental data and to take statistically valid decisions.

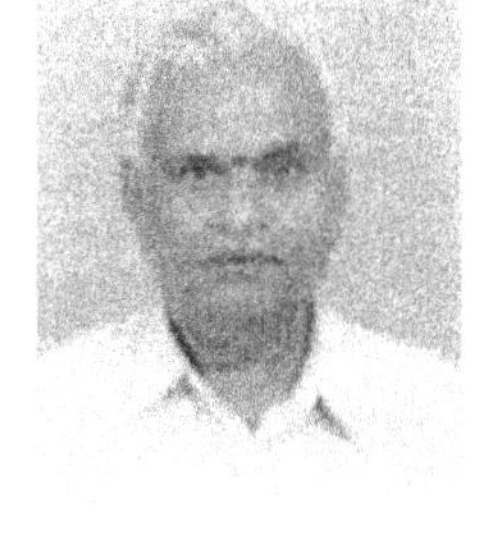

Prof. K.L.A.P Sarma, is working as Professor and Head, Department of Statistics, Sri Krishnadevaraya University, Anantapuram - 515 003 since 1981. Born on 17-5-1953, Prof. Sarma worked as Chairman, BOS for 9 years and having 32 years of teaching experience of Micro-biology and Sericulture coureses. He has guided 8 M.Phil. candidates and 12 Ph.D. candidates successfully and 3 more candidates are presently working for Ph.D. degree.

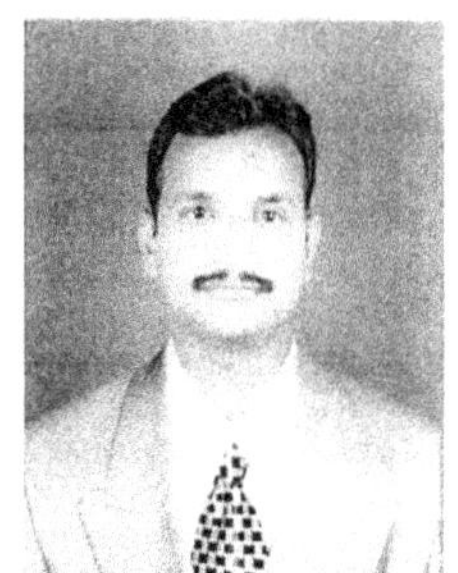

Dr. B. Ravindra Reddy is Assistant Professor of Statistics & Mathematics in the Department of Statistics and Mathematics, S.V. Agricultural College, Acharya N.G. Ranga Agricultural University, Tirupati (A.P) where he has been involved in the activities of teaching and research since 2006.

T. Pullaiah

Dr. T. Pullaiah, Professor, Department of Botany, Sri Krishnadevaraya university, Anantpur. Besides this, he held several positions in the University which include Dean, Head of the Department, Member of Species Survival Commission on International Union for Conservation of Nature (IUCN) and Natural Resources.

CONTENTS

1 INTRODUCTION TO BIOSTATISTICS

1.1 NEED FOR DECISION MAKING (DM)

In recent times, there is a need for taking optimum decisions by every person, starting from a common man in his daily activities to a scientist in his/her scientific enquiries. An able administrator has to take decisions with regards to the well being of his people under his jurisdiction. A student has to take most beneficial decision to choose the appropriate course, suitable to his/her career, or to choose which educational institution providing job oriented courses and so on. Thus, decision making is a routine job of every individual, starting from early morning rising from bed, till return to bed. The decisions should be optimum; that is, they should provide maximum benefit. How to take such optimum decisions? Which is the basic question before every one of us? The procedure followed should be quick, scientific and reliable. Using statistical tools and techniques, one can take such optimum decisions, in a relatively shorter time, using a scientific procedure and the decisions taken are more reliable. Such decisions must have "Statistical Validity". What this statistical validity means? It implies that the decisions taken through this approach are true in 95 cases out of 100 cases (i.e. 95% validity). Sometimes, we can make 99% valid (i.e. 99% validity) decisions.

Usually, decisions are taken based on his/her individual past experience or experience of seniors like parents, teachers or friends, who got some past experience about the problem. This past experience, collected from parents/teachers/senior friends or through observation by him/her is known as 'DATA' in statistics. Data is the foundation for entire statistical analysis and decision making. If data is erroneous, our decisions taken based on such data, also contain errors. Hence, qualitative data is more essential to take more statistically valid decisions.

This can be more clearly explained through the following examples.

Example (1.1.1) : Think that you want to cross a busy road. To do this safely, one must naturally observe the vehicle traffic, speed of the vehicle, distance of the vehicle to the crossing point, where you want to cross and so on. If you conform that you can cross safely, then only you try to cross the road otherwise you wait until the vehicle traffic is clear. Hasty and wrong decisions lead to disaster/ an accident. To take the decision here, what data you are collecting? And what statistical tool you are using? We are observing the speed of the vehicle, (just by looking the vehicle moment) and estimate the time taken to cross the road and so on. All these calculations and estimations and predictions are done in a quick and fast manner in our mind and take the decision. All these are done by experience. Children's mind is not in a position to take decisions in this manner and hence require elders help to cross the road up to a certain age, until they themselves can take decisions.

Example (1.1.2): A district collector wants to vacate people from those places to be affected by a cyclone, located at Bay of Bengal. To do this, it is necessary to collect the data relating to this cyclone like wind speed, its direction, distance from the coast at which it is concentrated, pressure on the sea, temperature of sea surface and so on. Based on the available information meteorology department people can estimate the expected time to cross the coast by the cyclone, so that necessary steps can be taken by the district administration so that losses from the cyclone can be minimized.

Example (1.1.3): A Doctor wants to prescribe the type of treatment to be given to the patient suffering from a cardio vascular disease. Perhaps he/she requires the information of the patient's blood pressure both systolic and diastolic, blood hemoglobin, blood cholesterol, LDL, VLDL, serum cholesterol, serum cretin, blood sugar and so on and can take decision to go for an operation, or treatment through an injection or oral drug or an exercise and so on. The data in this case is to be collected through laboratory tests/clinical tests. Such clinical experimental data is usually known as "clinical data".

Example (1.1.4): A Student studying M.Sc., Zoology wants to infer the effect of a particular drug on male albino rats. Perhaps, he has conducted the experiment on some 12 animals and wants to compare these results with those of 10 control animals, where the drug is not demonstrated. Based on the experimental results by comparing control observations with that of experimental observation the decision is to be taken, whether the drug has any effect on the animals or not?

Example (1.1.5): A Civil Engineer wants to determine the strength of the slab for various combinations of proportions of mixture of steel, cement, metal, water and sand. Which proportion of these can give maximum life/strength to the building under construction? Which sizes of steel beams are to be used? Which company cement is to be used? What should be the budget estimate for a Project under the proposal and so on?

Example (1.1.6): A Company manager wants to take the decision to appoint how many employees to meet the increased demand for the product. What raw material is to be used? When to replace the machinery with new and improved technology? How to utilize maximum capacity of the machines and employees? What policies and what incentives are to be given to the employees? And so on. To take decisions, he may require information about the production time, production cost, and available time of equipments, financial position and idle time of employees and so on.

Above examples from (1.1.1) to (1.1.6), explains the need for DM in different situations by different people. Basic objective of this book is to introduce different statistical tools and techniques to take optimum decisions. Usually decisions are taken in two ways, namely:

Situation – 1: By comparing two or more situations

Situation – 2: By predicting the behavior of the phenomena near future and to take appropriate decisions.

Thus the objective of this book is two-fold, namely, to make familiar the reader about techniques used under above explained two situations, with many real life examples.

From chapter-1 to chapter-5, techniques useful for situation-1 and from chapter-6 to chapter -10 techniques useful for situation-2 are discussed. Now we proceed to concentrate on some basic definitions, terms and methods used in Bio-statistics.

1.2 BASIC CONCEPTS

We frequently use following terms/words throughout this book. These terms/ words require some clarity before reading this book. This is because of the fact that these are used with slightly different meaning in statistics than used in day to day life. Hence, we concentrate on such basic terms and words in the following sub-sections.

1.2.1. Unit/Statistical Unit

The Unit is a basic thing from which the experimenter/researcher collects or measures/observes the required information.

In example (1.1.1) a Vehicle in the traffic at that point, in example (1.1.2.) cyclone concentrated at Bay of Bengal, in example (1.1.3) the patient taking the treatment, in example (1.1.4) the male albino rat on which the experiment is designed, in example (1.1.5) the building/structure under construction and in example (1.1.6) employee working in that company/the person going to get employment in that company will be the statistical unit. Thus statistical unit will be different thing for different decision makers. Statistical unit is called as 'Unit' for brevity sake throughout this book.

1.2.2. Data

Information collected/recorded/observed from units is called "Data".

In the above examples, speed of the vehicle, time required to cross the road, wind speed or direction, pressure on the sea, temperature of the sea surface, blood pressure, blood sugar, serum cholesterol, dosage of the medicine, urine color of the patient, effect of the drug on the rat, strength of the beam or slab, qualifications/ experience of the employee, cost or the age of the machine, time required to produce the product, demand for the product, salary of employees and so on. All these information forms the data that is information relating to the unit under consideration. Data is of two types. Namely: (1) attributes and (2) variables.

1.2.3. Attributes

Quantitative type of information/data, which cannot be measured/expressed in numeric form, but can be comparable, is known as an attribute.

For example, pain, skin color, eye color, sincerity of the employee, beauty of a girl, working efficiency of the employee, reaction to a stimulus treatment such as positive or negative or no reaction, infection present in the patient's body or not? Paint color used for the building, breed of the animal, direction of the wind, machine in working state of repair state, urine color-yellow or pale yellow, blood group of the patient, stomach pain, head ache, smoothness of the finished wall of a building, satisfaction derived after using a product and so on. Note that all these are not expressible in the form of numbers. Such qualities information/data is known as an attribute or qualitative nature data.

1.2.4. Variables

If the information or data is a measurable one, that is we can express the data in numeric form, such information is called "Variables".

For example, height, weight, time, blood glucose in 1ml of blood, Red Blood Cells (RBCs) in a patient blood, body temperature, cost of production of an item are some examples of variables. Similarly, salary/wages to be paid to an employee, wind speed, diameter of a bullet, cost of construction of an building of a structure or a fly over, marks obtained by students in a competitive examination/annual examination of a course, number of study hours per week, content of a chemical in 100 ml of syrup, duration of an experiment, growth rates in male and female children below 1 year, number of customers visited a service counter, number of affected spots on the skin, in a skin diseased patient, number of deaths in an accident, number of accidents, number of print mistakes per page in news papers, number of patients discharged from a hospital on a particular day, number admitted patients into the hospital on a day and so on are some other examples of "Variables". Sometimes these variables also termed as "Random Variables" because they cannot be predicted exactly, in advance. One cannot predict exactly the height/weight of a new born baby, when he/she attains the age of 10 years or 25 years. Similarly, we cannot predict exactly now, the tomorrow's day/night temperature of a town. We can perhaps suggest an interval for the temperature, based on the present day knowledge on the temperature of that town. We briefly call random variable as variable, throughout this book.

Based on the nature of data, Variables are further classified into two categories, namely:

(a) Discrete variables, and

(b) Continuous variables.

1.2.5. Discrete Variables

A discrete random variable is characterized by jumps or gaps between some specific numbers in the values that it can take. It can take some pre-determined values only like $a_1, a_2, a_3, ..., a_n$ and not in between values.

For example, number of births in a hospital on a day will be 25 or 26 or 30 but not 25.285 or 25.628 or 27.378 or 28.956 or 29.825 and so on. Variables having such jumping property from a_i to a_j, are known as discrete variables.

For example, defective spots on skin, number of AIDS patients in a town, number of animals in a lab, number of accidents occurred in a town, during a month or in one year, red blood cells (RBC)/white blood cells (WBC) count, number of students in a class room, number of defective items produced from a machine, print mistakes per page in a book or in a news paper, number of missing/defective/decayed /filled teeth per child in an elementary school/high school, number of tube lights/fans/air conditioners/water coolers in an office, number of affected leaves in a farm due to some disease, number of employees in a firm, number of heart beats per minute and so on.

1.2.6. Continuous Random Variable

If the variable takes any value in a specified relevant interval '*a*' to '*b*' such a variable is known as "Continuous Variable" or "Continuous Random Variable".

For example, birth time, weight of a new born baby, temperature of town, leaf length, area of a room, percentage of marks obtained by students in a class, blood characteristics like glucose levels, cholesterol levels, serum uric acid, LDL, VLDL, and so on. It is important to note that, because of limitations of available measuring instruments, however, observations on continuous variables which are inherently continuous are recorded as if they are discrete, by rounding off to the nearest decimal point or digit. For example, marks of students "rounded off" to nearest integer 65 or 82 or 43 instead of awarding 64.82 or 82.227 or 42.89 respectively. This does not mean that marks in the examination are discrete variables. In this connection, in some situations, variables takes values like 0, 0.5, 1.0, 1.5, 2.00, 2.5, 3.00 but the variable under consideration is a discrete variable. We should not conclude that discrete variables should take only integer values like 0, 1, 2, 3, ... *n*. For example, in insects or birds wings and legs will be in pairs as follows:

Number of wings:	0	2	4	6	8
Number of legs:	2	4	6	8	10

The ratio of wings to legs takes the values 0, 0.2 (2/10) 0.25(2/8), 0.33(2/6), 0.4(4/10), 0.5(2/4 or 4/8) 0.6 (6/10) , 0.66(4/6), 0.75(6/8), 0.8(8/10), 1.0 (2/2 or 4/4 or 6/6 or 8/8),1.33 (8/6), 1.5 (6/4), 2(4/2 or 8/4), 3 (6/2), 4 (8/2). Except these values, the ratio cannot take any other values like 0.3 or 0.9 0.7 and so on. Therefore the ratio of wings to legs is a discrete random variable but not continuous.

1.2.7. Population

The totality of all statistical units in a specific region at a given time is known as population. Usually the term population is used by common man to represent people residing in a town / city / country. In statistics, the term population is used to represent the collection of all statistical units, having certain common character in a particular region at a particular time.

For example, total number of fish in a lake in a month forms a population, in statistics. Similarly, total blood in a patient body, total agricultural lands under a crop in a village / district in a year, total number children born in a hospital in a month / a year, total number of students studying different courses in a college, in an academic year, total number of sandal wood / rose wood / teak wood trees in a forest in a year, total number of AIDS patients in a city say Mumbai / Chennai/ Delhi in a year say 2008 – 09. All are examples for "Statistical Populations" in which the researcher or administrator or the concerned head of the institution is interested.

Population may contain finite or infinite units. If the population consists of finite number of units, such populations are known as finite populations.

For example, patients admitted in a hospital in a month, number of print mistakes/words in a book / news paper, number of students studying different courses in a college, are examples for finite populations. If we start counting, there will be an end for the process of counting such things are called "countable infinite". For example, number of leaves on a tree, hair on the head, threads in a piece of cloth / shirt, number of X-rays produced from a substance, are examples for countable infinite. If total units in the population are countable infinite, then the population is known is "countable infinite population".

In some situations, it is not possible to count even if we prepare to count. For example, number of stars, all numbers between 0 and 1, total water in the sea are examples of un-countable infinity. If the population consists of such un-countable infinite number of units is called "un-countable infinite population" or simply "un-countable population".

1.2.8. Census

Getting information or collecting the data from each and every individual belonging to a population is called 'Census'.

In general getting the information from every unit in the population is very difficult and time consuming. Still in some situations, we have to go for census. For example, preparation of voter list, where information is to be recorded from each and every eligible voter in a region. Another example is dialysis to a patient suffering from kidney failure or malfunctioning, then entire blood in the patient is to be cleaned externally through an instrument. Even though it is painful and time consuming, patient has to undergo the dialysis. Conducting census is tedious and takes long time to complete. Hence, in many practical problems, we collect the information on some units of the population which is known as a 'sample'.

1.2.9. Sample

A sample is defined as a portion of the population where the units in the sample are selected following a procedure.

1.2.10. Parameter

A function of population observations/data is called parameters.

1.2.11. Statistic

A function of sample observations is called statistic.

We generally estimate or predict the population characteristics or parameters using statistics, that is, sample observations/sample data. For example, doctor wants some blood characteristics of a patient, a sample blood is tested in the laboratory/diagnostic centre and based on the reports doctor tries to predict or estimate the total blood characteristics of the patient under study.

1.2.12. Statistics

Statistics is a science which deals with collection, organization, summarization, analysis of data and to interpret the results obtained, that is, to draw inferences.

1.2.13. Biostatistics

Application of statistical tools and techniques to infer biological / clinical data is known as 'Biostatistics'.

Statistical tools, methods and techniques can be applied to any type of data, in any discipline. For example, if the water is put in a glass will get glass shape and in a beaker will get a beaker shape and in test tube, will get a test tube shape. Similarly, if statistical tools are employed for business data it will become 'Business Statistics'. If they are employed for Legal data it will become 'Legal Statistics' and if they are employed for analyzing industrial data, it will become 'Industrial Statistics'. If they applied to improve quality of an Industrial output then it is called as 'Statistical Quality Control' and so on.

1.2.14. Statistical Inference

The procedure of concluding/predicting the characteristics of population using the sample information is known as "Statistical Inference".

1.3 SAMPLING TECHNIQUES

If some units in the population are selected following a Procedure, such selected group of units forms a sample selected from that population. The basic purpose of different sampling procedures is to see that the selected sample should reflect the characters of the population from which it is taken. That is the sample selected must be a good representative of the population from which it is selected. Procedures of selecting appropriate units of a population into the sample so that the selected sample reflects the characters of the population are known as "Sampling Techniques". Basically sampling techniques are classified into two categories, namely:

1. **Random sampling and (2) Non-Random sampling methods.**

1. **Random Sampling Methods are:**

   (*a*) Simple Random Sampling (SRS)
   (*b*) Stratified Random Sampling (StRS)
   (*c*) Systematic Random Sampling (SyRS)
   (*d*) Cluster Sampling (CS)
   (*e*) Double Sampling (DS)
   (*f*) Two Stage Sampling (TS)
   (*g*) Multi Stage Sampling (MS) and
   (*h*) Multi Phase Sampling (MF)

2. **Non-Random Sampling Methods are:**

   (*a*) Purposive Sampling (PS)
   (*b*) Quota Sampling (QS)
   (*c*) Snowball Sampling (SS)
   (*d*) Area Sampling (AS) and
   (*e*) Convenient Sampling (CS)

If the selected sample is a good representative of the population our predictions may be correct, otherwise our predictions may go wrong. If the selection procedure involves random selections, the estimations or predictions will become true in majority cases. Out of above listed procedures for selecting Random samples from a population, we will discuss most popularly used Random Sampling methods namely, SRS, StRS and SyRS in forth coming sections. Other sampling methods are having limited applications and are to be used under special circumstances not usually in biostatistics and hence are not discussed in this book.

1.4 SIMPLE RANDOM SAMPLING (SRS)

This method is to be used when all the units in the population are homogenous like blood in a patient's body or all products produced from the same machine, by same worker, using same raw material. Then, selecting 'n' units from the total 'N' units in the population, by giving equal chance (or) probability for every unit being selected into the sample, is known as Simple Random Sample (SRS) and the procedure adopted is known as "Simple Random Sampling" procedure.

1.4.1. The selection procedure of an SRS by lottery method is explained in the following steps as follows:

Step – I : Identify the units in the population by giving numbers from 1, 2, 3 ..., N.

Step – II : Write down these numbers on identical slips (or) chits such that one number on each chit.

Step – III : Select randomly a chit, after putting all 'N' chits in a bowel by folding properly and after shuffling well all chits.

Step – IV : The unit having the selected number forms a member/unit in the sample.

Above procedure is to be repeated until we obtain 'n' sample units.

This procedure of selecting sample is known as SRS by lottery method. Here again two methods are available. In step – III, after selecting a chit, (1) the selected chit will be replaced back into the bowel and (2) the selected chit is not replaced back into the bowel. First procedure is known as SRS with replacement and the latter one is known as SRS without replacement. What is the difference between these two methods and which is to be preferred is the basic question to be answered now. In the first procedure, since the already selected chit is replaced, there is a chance that the same chit may come in subsequent drawings and hence we have to select again already selected units. This is obviously a repetition of already selected unit and hence we may not get any extra information but number of units in the sample will be reduced because of repetitions. For example, if we want to select a SRS of size 30 and 5 units repeated, it means that we have the sample of size 25 only because 5 units got repeated. Thus effective sample size will be reduced. This is not a desirable situation because; reduction in sample size will result in increase in experimental/Standard Error of the Statistic. Hence we have to resort to without replacement.

If this is done, the chance / probability of selecting units into the sample, will vary from draw to draw (this concept is explained in chapter-5). This is because draws are not independent. Number of chits left in the bowel will be reduced by one for each draw and hence the probabilities for selecting units vary from draw to draw. By definition of SRS these probabilities should be same then only the selected sample is an SRS. To make probabilities equal, we have to resort to with replacement method, which increases the error. To avoid this criticism, we assume that the sample is drawn from large population. When population size is large, say 10,00,000 or 20,00,000 reduction by one may not affect much the corresponding probabilities. They can be considered as approximately same for all units. Thus when population is large enough, we prefer SRS without replacement. Even otherwise, we prefer to go for SRS without replacement than with replacement.

This method fails when '*N*' is large. Sometimes, we may not know the value of '*N*'. For example, number of persons suffering from AIDS in India / in Andhra Pradesh. In some situations, even if *N* value is known, adopting above explained procedure is cumbersome and consumes lot of time. It is not possible to identify each unit with numbers. For example, blood in the patient's body. In such situations, we use any one of the following methods.

1.4.2. Selection of SRS using Random Number Tables

When the population size '*N*' is large lottery method will fail because it is very cumbersome and time consuming procedure.

1. Instead we can use random number tables for selecting an SRS.
2. Random number tables are prepared in a special manner such that the digits from zero to 9 will repeat equal number of times, in a table. (Vide Random Numbers table in appendix).
3. Tippet's table is most popular one which gives random numbers.
4. Randomly select the page in the book consisting of random numbers and select randomly a column and a row.
5. Start reading the numbers from that randomly selected number in any direction.
6. Let '*r*' is the random number selected: if the r is less than or equal to *N* select the unit with number '*r*' into the sample and read next number.
7. If the selected random number *r* is greater than or equal to *N* ignore that number and read next number.
8. If any number is a repetition, if you consider the same unit, we obtain SRS with replacement and if you ignore the repeated random number and read the next random number, then we obtain SRS without replacement.
9. Repeat this procedure until we obtain '*n*' units.

1.4.3. Selecting SRS by using Calculator /Computer

1. One can select an SRS by selecting the random number '*r*' (or) by using calculator (or) computer. It is important to note that all the numbers selected through computer (or) calculator are in between 0 and 1.

i.e. $0 \le r \le 1$

Example: $r = 0.7352$.

2. If the number is as given above, select randomly any two digits say first and last digits (or) middle most two digits (or) first and third digits to select a random number of size two.
3. Similarly to select a random numbers of sizes 3 one can select randomly first 3 digits (or) last 3 digits (or) any 3 digits to get a three digit random number.
4. After selecting 'r' the rest of the procedure is same as explained above, from 7 to 10 in 1.4.2.

Example (1.4.1): In a university, there are 80 students studying M.Sc. Bio-technology in all four semesters. Their I.D. numbers are from 1001 to 1080. Select a simple random sample (SRS) of 8 students (1) with replacement and (2) without replacement.

Solution: Generate random numbers using random number tables or calculator.

For example, the generated random numbers are:

1028,1095,1062,1085,1002,1029,1105, 1034, 1298, 1028, 1082, 1142, 1010 , 1050, 1039, 1090, and 1012.

1. Selected 8 students with replacement are: 1028, 1062, 1002, 1029, 1034, 1028, 1010 and 1050.

   Here 1028 is repeated twice and hence effective sample size is only 7 but not 8.
2. Selected 8 students without replacement are: 1028, 1062, 1002, 1029, 1034, 1010, 1050 and 1039.

Thus if a population consists of N units, we obtain

$$\binom{N}{n} = n!/n!\,(N-n)! \text{ different samples.}$$

Here $n! = n \times (n-1) \times (n-2)\ldots 2 \times 1$. It is important to note that $n!$ is to be read as *n factorial* and 0! is always considered as 1. That is if $N = 4$ and $n = 2$ we have 6 different SRS without replacement samples.

1.5. STRATIFIED RANDOM SAMPLING (StRS)

1. When population is heterogeneous then SRS is not an appropriate sample which represents the population because the sample selected through SRS may not reflect the heterogeneity in the same manner as in population. Hence, the population is to be divided into small homogenous, sub-groups such that units within the groups are homogenous.
2. Such a homogenous sub-group is called "*Strata*". Let a population of size 'N' is divided into 'K' Strata such that 'N_1' units in 1st strata & N_2 in the 2nd strata .... N_k in the 'K^{th}' strata. $N_1 + N_2 + N_3 + \ldots + N_k = N$ i.e. $\Sigma N_i = N$.
3. From the above population we have to select a sample of 'n' such that 'n_1' units in 1st strata, 'n_2' units in 2nd strata, -,-,-, and 'n_k' units in k strata, such that: $\Sigma n_i = n$, where $n_i = (N_i \times n)/N$ where, $i = 1, 2, \ldots k$.

4. The selected sample of size n following above steps is called "Stratified Random Sample" and the procedure is known as "stratified random sampling" procedure.

Example (1.5.1): Consider a firm where 1000 employees are working of which, 600 are class IV employees and 300 are office clerks and 100 are officers. The company manager wants to select 100 employees as a random sample. If he selects these 100 employees, from one group, the sample is not a representative one. Here SRS is not an appropriate one. First, population of employees is to be divided into three strata of sizes N_1, N_2 and N_3 such that $N_1 = 600$, $N_2 = 300$ and $N_3 = 100$. Then respective sample sizes using above explained procedure, we have $n_1 = 60$, $n_2 = 30$, and $n_3 = 10$. Now for selecting 60 class IV employees from 600, one can apply SRS and selecting 30 clerks from 300 clerks, again apply SRS and finally to select 10 officers from 100, third time apply SRS independently. Thus SRS is three times independently if three strata are there. We can apply SRS because units in each stratum are homogeneous.

5. It is Important to note that (selecting 'n_i' units) since all the units in the strata are homogenous selecting 'n_i' units from "N_i" in same as applying an S.R.S. in each strata independently k times.
6. Hence, stratified RS can be considered as repeated application of SRS independently in each strata 'k' times.

1.6. SYSTEMATIC SAMPLING (SyS)

1. When units in a population are numbered and are arranged already in an order, like books in the library, houses in a colony (or) products produced in a continuous manner, from a machine then, selecting a sample by using a fixed interval, which is known as sampling interval, will become easy in identification of the units in the sample in a systematic manner.
2. One can select the sample units using an order hence, it is known as "systematic sampling".

Example (1.6.1): If the population consists of 20 units and a sample of size '4' is to be selected using systematic random sampling scheme. Then $K = 20/4 = 5$.

1 2 3 4 5 6 7 8 9 10 11 12 13 14 15 16 17 18 19 20

Select the first unit in the sample randomly from 1 to k, let the selected random number be denoted by 'r' then, remaining units in the sample are: r, $k + r$, $k + 2r$, $k + 3r$, ... If the selected random number from 1 to 5 is 3 then $r = 3$ and the sample units are: 3, 3 + 5 = 8, 3 + 10 = 13, 3 + 15 = 18. That is we have to select 3rd unit, 8th unit, 13th unit and 18th unit from the population.

3. In this procedure, only the first unit is selected at random. Based on this unit all other units are fixed. This procedure is known as "Linear Systematic Sampling".

Limitations of linear systematic sampling procedure:

1. In the above procedure, it is assumed that $N = nk$.

   Where, N = Population size

   n = Sample size

   k = Sampling interval

2. Sometimes the population 'N' may not be exactly equal to nk.

   When, $N \neq nk$ then, above procedure will result sometimes a sample of size 'n' and sometimes a sample of size $(n - 1)$. Hence we get samples of different sizes.

3. When sample size decreases error will increase (already discussed this point in SRS). In order to get a fixed sample size we adopt the following procedure.

4. Assume that the population units are arranged in a circle. Then, select any starting point from 1 to n. Then, the rest of the sample is r, $r + k$, $r + 2k$,... .

Example (1.6.1): Select a circular systematic sample of size 5 if the population consists of 23 units numbered from 1 to 23.

Solution: Assume that units from 1 to 23 are arranged in a circular form starting point is 12, and $K = 5$, then the selected sample units are: 12, 17, 22, 4 and 9.

Systematic sampling has special applications in industry. When produced products are coming on a conveyer belt and accumulate at a point, sample can be conveniently collected while coming on conveyer belt with half an hour or one hour interval gap one can select units or we can arrange an automatic machine to select one unit with an equal time interval. Similarly, raw materials supplied to a factory on a conveyer belt can be selected with random interval of time or fixed interval of time. Thus, systematic sample has operational convenience in industrial applications. Similarly this has special applications in forest research to estimate timber of a particular type like sandal wood, rose wood and teak wood. Similarly, in fisheries to estimate total number of fish in a tank/lake. Here also samples can be selected at equidistant in the forest or in the lake.

REVIEW QUESTIONS AND PROBLEMS

(A) Objective Type Questions

1. Totality of all units in a specified region at a specified time is known as ....

(*a*) sample (*b*) population
(*c*) parameter (*d*) statistic.

2. Statistic is a function of .... observations.

(*a*) sample (*b*) population
(*c*) infinite population (*d*) finite population.

3. Information collected from every unit in the population is known as ....
   (*a*) population (*b*) sample
   (*c*) statistic (*d*) census

4. Total number of SRS of size 2 without replacement from a population of size 6 are ....
   (*a*) 14 (*b*) 16
   (*c*) 15 (*d*) 30

5. Sub-population having homogeneous units is known as ....
   (*a*) strata (*b*) stratum
   (*c*) sample (*d*) statistic

6. When population consists of heterogeneity we use .... Sampling.
   (*a*) simple random (*b*) cluster random
   (*c*) systematic random (*d*) stratified random.

7. When population is homogeneous, we use .... sampling.
   (*a*) simple random (*b*) cluster random
   (*c*) systematic random (*d*) stratified random.

8. Sample size decreases .... will increase.
   (*a*) cost of the survey (*b*) duration of the survey
   (*c*) error (*d*) accuracy.

9. When population units are numbered and arranged in an order we use .... sampling.
   (*a*) simple random (*b*) cluster random
   (*c*) systematic random (*d*) stratified random.

10. In a systematic sampling, *K* is called ....
    (*a*) constant (*b*) sampling interval
    (*c*) sample size (*d*) population size.

B. Short Answers Questions

1. Explain the terms
   (*a*) population (*b*) sample
   (*c*) parameter and (*d*) statistic.

2. Define
   (*a*) Biostatistics and (*b*) statistical inference.

3. Distinguish between discrete and continuous random variables.

4. Explain the terms
   (*a*) Attributes and (*b*) Variables.

5. Give five examples of Attributes.
6. Give five examples of Discrete Random Variables.
7. Give five examples of Continuous Random Variables.
8. Select all possible samples of size two from a population consisting of four units 10, 15, 23 and 30.
9. Select a systematic sample of size 6 from units numbered from 101 to 130.
10. Select a SRS of size 5 from 50 items
    (*a*) with replacement and (*b*) without replacement.

C. Essay Type Questions

1. Explain the application of Statistics in Biological sciences, with suitable examples.
2. Explain the method of drawing an SRS of size n form a population of size N.
3. Distinguish between SRS with and without replacement. Which method you prefer? Why?
4. Explain the selection of systematic sampling and discuss its application in Industry.
5. Distinguish between linear and circular Systematic Sampling methods.
6. When do you use Stratified Random Sampling? Explain the method with a suitable example.
7. Discuss the role of statistical methods in clinical data analysis.
8. Explain the procedure of using random number tables.
9. List out various sampling methods and explain any two of them.
10. Explain the term biostatistics and discuss its applications.

References:

1. Gupta S.P. 1990 "Statistical Methods". Sultan Chand & Sons, New Delhi.
2. Wayne W. Daniel 2008 Biostatistics, 9th edition, John Wiley & Sons. Inc. Newyork.
3. P.N. Arora *et al*. 2007 "Comprehensive Statistical Methods" Sultan Chand and Company Ltd. First edn. New Delhi.
4. VK. Kapoor 1986 "Problems and solutions in Business statistics" Sultan Chand and Sons New Delhi.

Answers to Objective Questions

A: 1. – b, 2 – a, 3 – d, 4 – c, 5 – a, 6 – d, 7 – a, 8 – c, 9 – c, 10 – b.

2 COLLECTION, CLASSIFICATION AND TABULATION OF DATA

2.1. INTRODUCTION TO COLLECTION OF DATA

In the previous chapter, we have discussed the need for statistical tools and techniques are used in making statistically valid decisions by scientists, researchers, administrators, managers and business organizers and so on. Further, we also learnt that the basis for such decision making is the 'data' collected, or observed or recorded after conducting an experiment and so on. In all these cases, the data is obtained by the decision maker on his own or by investigators under the direction of the decision maker/the experimenter. Such type of collection of required data by the experimenter/by trained investigators is called 'Primary Data'. This type of enquiries requires large amounts of money and requires more time to collect the data and for the analysis. On the other hand sometimes getting the information from standard sources like Government Gazettes/publications or research publications or information published by standard organizations is more convenient. Such type of collecting the information/data from standard sources requires less time and money. Such type of data collected from other published sources is called 'Secondary Data'. It is important to note that lot of precautionary steps are to be taken to see the appropriateness and applicability of such data to the present context on which we want to infer/making the decisions. In many scientific enquiries, generally we conduct the experiment and results are recorded with proper care and at most accuracy. Hence, collection of data is usually through an experiment and hence other data collection methods are not concentrated much in this book. Thus the basic assumption is that the data is an experimental data, which is the Primary data for the experimenter and is recorded at most care without errors.

Sampling and non-sampling errors: Usually we conclude about the population characteristics based on the partial information that is the information available from a sample. This is called 'Inductive way of reasoning' and in this we may sometimes, commit errors. For example, consider that four blind persons want to explain 'How an elephant looks like' by touching an elephant. One person touching elephant's leg assumed that elephant is like a pillar. Second person touching the tail assumed that the elephant is like a snake like thing. Third person touching the ear, assumed that the elephant is like flat like thing. Fourth person touching the belly assumed that it is a drum like thing. Four persons got different pictures about the same elephant based on the information available. No one in these four can explain how the original elephant is? because, all the four persons, are blind people. Similarly, we also commit sometimes, if we conclude about a population based on the available sample information because the sample selected is not an appropriate sample representing the population.

This type of error is called 'Sampling Error'. That is, decisions taken based on the partial sample information sometimes may go wrong, if the sample selected is not a good representative of the population. This type error can be reduced by increasing the sample size '*n*' to the population size '*N*'. Thus sampling errors will decrease as the sample size '*n*' increases. Thus 'Census Data' that is, collecting the data from all the units in the population, does not contain 'Sampling errors'. But other type of errors like not getting information from the selected unit because of non availability of units at home, or not possible to record information because of natural calamities like floods, fire accidents or earth quakes, recording errors, some units are reluctant to give information on some sensitive issues like preference of the party he would like to vote in the coming elections, salary/income and so on. On such items we may not get correct information. Such errors are called "Non-sampling Errors'. Such errors can also present in sample surveys. Thus sample surveys contains both sampling and non-sampling errors where as census contains only non-sampling errors. It is found that errors in census are enormously large when compared to sample surveys. Hence we always prefer to go for sample surveys than census, unless otherwise, it is desirable or necessary like preparation of voter list or dialysis of blood in the kidney failure patients. Basic difference between sampling and non-sampling errors is that the former one decreases as sample size increases. Whereas, non-sampling errors increases to a large extent along with the sample size.

2.2. EDITING OF DATA

After collecting the data, first step in the analysis is editing.

Editing is nothing but scanning the data for any abnormalities or extreme values or uncommon things or recording errors and so on. Any such abnormalities are present in the collected data, those data items are to be removed from the collected data. Presence of such errors or extreme data will create problems in future analysis and reduces the efficiency of the estimates/statistics calculated. We recall this point at appropriate places while discussing the properties of the relevant estimates/statistics. Editing of data is explained with the following example.

Example (2.2.1): The following data represents marks of 20 students in bio-statistics paper belonging to a class. Edit the data and draw your conclusions.

82, 64, 169, 58, 75, –52, 64, 46, 89, 58, 64, 22, 59, 43, 91, 84, 64, 0.49, 83 and 68.

Solution: Using common sense one can easily suspect three data items in the above data. First one is 169, second one is –52 and the third one is 0.49 because usually marks in a subject cannot be of the forms. The reasons are (1) They cannot be more than 100 (unless otherwise stated) (2) marks cannot be negative in any subject and (3) marks cannot usually take decimals like 0.49 or 0.82. Thus these figures are errors and are to be rectified before taking the data for further analysis. After verification, with original documents found that it is 16 but not 169. Similarly, it is 52 but not –52 and it is 49 but not 0.49. Thus the corrected data after editing is as follows:

82, 64, 16, 58, 75, 52, 64, 46, 89, 58, 64, 22, 59, 43, 91, 84, 64, 49, 83 and 68.

On similar lines, using the past experience/common sense, one has to edit the data first, then only the data is eligible for further analysis. Editing is similar job of pre-operational conditions like cleaning the skin, giving enema and anesthesia to the patient and so on. Then only, the patient is eligible to undergo for an operation. Similar way, editing is similar type of job of preparing the patient/data, for operation/further analysis. Editing is compulsory irrespective of the method of data collection, that is, either the data is collected through census or sample surveys.

2.3 CLASSIFICATION OF DATA

Basically, any deviation from true value of the data item is called error. For example, to measure the weight of a person, we ask the person to stand on a weighing machine, and record the weight of that person as 52.5 kgs. This 52 kgs weight is not exactly the weight of the person, because, it includes the weight of the dress wore by the person, items in the pockets of dress and the weight of the food he has taken and so on. Therefore, his true weight may be around 49. 82 kgs, but we are recording it as 52.5 kgs. This difference is called "error" in the data of the weight of the person. Similarly, weighing machine, also will have Instrumental error. Thus recorded data items includes, all these errors. Hence, if we record a person's weight as 52.5 it means that true value may lie in the interval, say 50 – 55 or 45 – 55 or 50 – 60. Hence, we consider the interval 50 – 55 or 45 – 55 or 50 – 60 for the analysis instead of 52.5, because, this interval contains the true value and hence, decisions taken will have more statistical validity. This is called 'classification of data'. Thus classification is the technique of removing errors.

After editing, next step in the analysis is 'Classification of data'. Classification is a similar job of sorting letters in the post office, before delivery. For convenience, post men sorts out letters as per the route and houses in that route. All letters coming to one house are bunched so that delivery is easy. Similarly, data items are to be sorted out, for convenience of presentation. For classification, there should be one basis, like cities, areas in the city, street numbers, or door numbers useful for sorting, here also we choose one character/attribute/variable as basis for classification. There are basically four types of classifications. Namely: (1) Chronological classification, (2) Attribute classification, (3) Geographical classification and (4) Variable classification.

2.3.1. Chronological Classification

Here the basis of classification is time. As per the time, we classify the items in the population/sample. For example, books in the library can be classified as per the year of publication. Similarly, patients in a hospital can be classified according to date of joining or age of the patient or duration of onset of the disease. Similarly, students in a college can be classified according to the age of students or date of joining into the course, or date of birth. Research articles, can be classified according to date of publication in the journal. References in a research can be arranged as per date/year of publication. All these type of classifications are known as 'chronological classifications'.

2.3.2. Attribute Classification

In this type classifications, the basis of classification is an attribute like male or female patients, bounded or un-bounded books affected by a disease or not affected by a disease, Students belonging to Open Category (OC) or Backward Class (BC – A or B or C or D), schedule caste (SC), schedule tribe (ST) and so on. Here we classify the units as having the attribute / characteristic, units not having the attribute or the characteristic under consideration. Patients coming to a hospital can be classified according to the disease / complaint like, heart patients, neurology patients, ENT patients, eye patients, maternity patients, general ailment patients, dog bite patients, out patients, in patients, patients belonging to different blood groups. Similarly engineers as civil engineers, computer engineers, mechanical engineers and so on. These type of classifications are known as "Attribute Classifications'.

2.3.3. Geographical Classification

Here the basis of classification is geographical region. That is units belonging to a geographical region like visitors from abroad, and with the country, students of I.I.T 's in Delhi, Mumbai, Chennai, Kharagpur, Kanpur and so on, patients coming from rural and urban places, rural and urban voters, players of different countries like India, Sri Lanka, Australia, New Zealand, China, Pakistan and so on. These types of classifications are known as "Geographical Classifications".

2.3.4. Variable Classification

Here basis of classification is a variable like height, weight, temperature, marks, price, blood sugar, serum cholesterol, blood pressure, income, number births, number of visitors, traffic flow, prices of commodities and so on. These type of classifications are known as "Variables classification". Variable classification is further divided into two categories. Namely:

1. Inclusive method of classification.
2. Exclusive method of classification.

2.4. TABULATION

Presenting the classified data in the form of tables to have neat and compact way of presentation is called 'Tabulation'. The following are some general rules to be followed for tabulation.

Rule 1. Every table should be identified with a number representing chapter, section and individual table, for the purpose of identification.

Rule 2. Every table should have a title and sub-headings for columns.

Rule 3. Any table should not be over loaded with information unless it is necessary.

Rule 4. Every table should be clearly explained the measuring units in which data items are measured.

Rule 5. Every table should contain foot notes if they are necessary.

Above type classifications along with tabulation are explained in the following examples.

Example (2.4.1): The following data in table (2.4.1) represents year of publication of books added after 2000 to a public library. This can be considered as chronological classification:

Table (2.4.1): Table representing the books purchased after 2000 in the public library.

Year of publication	Number of books.
2001	2,562
2002	3,985
2003	5,648
2004	8,876
2005	10,578
2006	15,606
Total number of books added	42,255

Example (2.4.2): The following data in table (2.4.2) represents different backward class students studying in different groups in engineering colleges in Hyderabad. This is an example of attribute classification.

Table (2.4.2) : Table showing distribution of B.C. students gender wise.

Groups in Engineering course	Number of B.C. Students.		
	Male	Female	Total
Civil	25	02	27
Mechanical	30	05	35
Computer Science	45	35	80
Electronics and communications	42	28	70
Aeronautical Engineering	15	08	23
Total number of B.C. Students	157	78	235

Example (2.4.3): The following data in table (2.4.3) represents visitors to a museum from different states in the month of January 2009. This can be considered as an example of geographical classification.

Table (2.4.3): Visitors from different states to the museum in the month of January 09.

Name of the state	Children (less than 18 years)			Adults (greater than 18 years)		
	Male	Female	Total	Male	Female	Total
Andhra Pradesh	1,252	926	2,178	5,686	6,976	12,662
Karnataka	978	802	1,780	5,794	4,670	10,464
Kerala	3,586	2,238	5,824	4,708	4,658	9,366
Madhya Pradesh	2,148	2,876	5,024	3,498	4,185	7,683
Maharashtra	3,784	2,982	6,766	6,298	5,235	11,533
Tamil Nadu	4,129	5,356	9,485	7,508	7,437	14,945
Total Visitors	15,877	15,180	31,057	33,492	33,161	66,653

To prepare variable classification, we follow the following steps.

Step I: Note down the Largest and Smallest data item in the given data.

Step II: Adjust the range in a convenient form such that starting and ending points are '5' or multiples of '5's.

Step III: After determining the class interval write down various classes starting from the lower limit of adjusted range and each class interval equal to class interval decided. Then, go on classifying each observation by determining to which class it belongs to and put a tally mark against that class.

Step IV: It is important to note that when an observation (or) data item is equal to the upper limit of any class then the item is to be included in the next class. This method of classification is known as exclusive method of classification and is to be used when the variable under consideration is a continuous variable. Bunch 5 tally marks as one group by putting a cross, the fifth one as shown in the example (2.4.4).

Example (2.4.4): The following data represents weights of sample of 20 fish caught in a tank measured in grams classify the data and prepare the frequency distribution.

12, 15, 11, 13, 25, 42, 29, 52, 13, 08, 92, 42, 68, 47, 50, 40, 36, 95, 42 and 59

Solution: In the above example, largest value is 95 and smallest value is 08.

The range for the data is : Largest – Smallest = 95 – 08
= 83 grams.

Adjusted range is from 05 – 105.

It is important to note that adjusted range should contain the actual range calculated. Then class intervals are 5 – 15; 15 – 25; ..., 95 – 105. So the class interval is of length 10 grams. After determining the class intervals, read first data item. It is 12 hence, determine to which class it belongs to? It belongs to 5 – 15 class.

Therefore put one tally mark against that class. Next data item is 15, hence as explained in step – IV, in exclusive method of classification, the tally mark is to be put against the class 15 – 25 but not to the class 5 – 15. Similarly, five tally marks are to be bunched together, as shown in the table (2.4.4).

Table (2.4.4): Table showing tally marks and frequencies.

Class Interval	Tally Marks	Frequency
5–15	~~1111~~	5
15–25	1	1
25–35	11	2
35–45	~~1111~~	5
45–55	111	3
55–65	1	1
65–75	1	1
75–85	0	0
85–95	1	1
95–105	1	1
Total		20

Some more examples for exclusive method of classification are:

0 – 10	5 – 15
10 – 20	15 – 25
20 – 30	25 – 35
30 – 40	35 – 45
40 – 50	45 – 55

Step V : If upper limit is also included in the same class such a classification is called as inclusive method of classification and is to be used when the variable is discrete in nature.

Example of inclusive method classification contains class intervals as follows :

Class Intervals		
0 – 9		0 – 19
10 – 19		20 – 39
20 – 29	(or)	40 – 59
30 – 39		60 – 79
40 – 49		80 – 99

If all the classes are of equal size then it is called equal class intervals. Sometimes there is a necessity for classifying the data with unequal class intervals. For example, publication of results by examination branch requires the following type of class intervals.

Below	– 35
35	– 50
50	– 60
60	– 75
Above	– 75

In the above example, class intervals are unequal hence such classification is known as unequal class intervals. Further, we observe that there is no lower limit for the first class and upper limit for the last class. Hence, such classification is known as "Open – End classification".

2.5. FREQUENCY TABLES

After preparing tables with class intervals, tally marks and frequencies, the column of tally marks is not required. Removing the column of tally marks, if we write the remaining table that is with class intervals and the corresponding frequencies, we obtain, a 'Frequency table' or frequency distribution as follows:

For example, consider the table (2.4.4) and delete the column of tally marks, we obtain the frequency distribution of fish in the selected sample, according to their weights. The frequency distribution is shown as follows in the table (2.5.1). Frequencies are distributed to different class and hence the table is usually known as frequency table:

Table (2.5.1) Table showing frequency distribution of weights of fish.

Class Intervals in grams	Frequencies
5–15	5
15–25	1
25–35	2
35–45	5
45–55	3
55–65	1
65–75	1
75–85	0
85–95	1
95–105	1
Total	20

Relative frequency: Sometimes it is convenient to represent frequencies in terms of proportions rather than the actual number belonging to a particular class interval. For example, proportion of persons affected by a disease between 40 – 60 age group, or proportion of under nourished babies less than 2.5 lbs in a hospital in a year, or proportion of AIDS patients less than 18 years in a town and so on. In such cases one has to convert the frequencies of each class into proportions known as Relative Frequencies defined as the ratio of frequency of each class to its total frequencies. Calculation of relative frequencies is explained in the following example.

Example (2.5.1): The following table (2.5.2) represents the number of births in a hospital in the year 2008.

Table (2.5.2): Frequency distribution of number of births in a hospital during 2008.

Number of births per day	Number of days	Proportion days	Relative Frequency
0	12	12/366	0.03279
1	56	56/366	0.15301
2	135	135/366	0.36885
3	120	120/366	0.32787
4	19	19/366	0.05191
5	08	8/366	0.02186
6	05	5/366	0.01366
7	04	4/366	0.01093
8	04	4/366	0.01093
9	02	2/366	0.00546
10	01	1/366	0.00027
Total	366	1.0000	1.00000

Example (2.5.2): The following table (2.5.3) represents number of customers visited to a railway reservation counter in the month of December, 2008. This is an example to illustrate inclusive method of classification.

Table (2.5.3): Frequency distribution of customers at railway reservation counter in the month of December, 2008.

Number of customers	Frequency	Relative frequency
00–29	16	16/31 = 0.51613
30–59	12	12/31 = 0.38709
60–89	02	2/31 = 0.06452
90–119	01	1/31 = 0.03225
Total	31	1.00000

Thus data can be presented either in raw form or tabulated form explained earlier. If the data is presented in the raw form, then it is known as '***Raw Data***' and if it is presented in the tabular form or frequency distribution form then, it is known as 'Classified Data'.

REVIEW QUESTIONS AND PROBLEMS

A. Objective Type Questions

1. Data collected from experiment in the laboratory by Research Scholars is -------- data.

   (*a*) secondary (*b*) sample
   (*c*) census (*d*) primary.

2. Data collected about temperature and rainfall of different cities in India from news papers of 2008 is ---------- data.

   (*a*) secondary (*b*) sample
   (*c*) census (*d*) primary.

3. Sampling errors will decrease along with ---------- size increases.

   (*a*) population (*b*) sample
   (*c*) parameter (*d*) statistic.

4. Non-sampling errors will ------------- along with the sample size.

   (*a*) decrease (*b*) not change
   (*c*) increase (*d*) be negligible.

5. Patients belonging to different blood groups is -------- classification.

   (*a*) variable (*b*) geographical
   (*c*) attribute (*d*) chronological.

6. Records of a college classified the students according to marks obtained in mathematics subjects is ------------- classification.

   (*a*) variable (*b*) geographical
   (*b*) attribute (*d*) chronological.

7. List of doctors' country wise is ---------- classification.
   (*a*) variable (*b*) geographical
   (*c*) attribute (*d*) chronological.

8. Patients classified according to the duration of stay in the hospital is ---------- classification.
   (*a*) variable (*b*) geographical
   (*c*) attribute (*d*) chronological.

9. Length of the class interval for the class 10 – 19 in inclusive method of classification is -----------.
   (*a*) 9 (*b*) 10
   (*c*) 8 (*d*) 11.

10. If any data item is equal to the upper limit of any class then, it is to be included in the next class is known as ------------ classification.
    (*a*) inclusive (*b*) exclusive method
    (*c*) open – end (*d*) attribute.

11. When the data is discrete variable ----------- of classification is to be used.
    (*a*) inclusive method (*b*) exclusive method
    (*c*) open – end method (*d*) attribute method.

12. Example of open end classification is --------------.
    (*a*) 0 – 10, 10 – 20, 20 – 30, 30 – 40.
    (*b*) less than 50, 50 – 80, more than 80.
    (*c*) 0 – 9, 10 – 19, 20 – 29, 30 – 39,...
    (*d*) 15 – 30, 30 – 60, 60 – 75, 75 – 100.

B. Short Answers Questions

1. Distinguish between primary data and secondary data by giving suitable examples.
2. Distinguish between sampling and non-sampling errors with suitable examples.
3. Explain the concept of error in the data with a suitable example.
4. Explain the need for classification of raw data.
5. Explain necessity of editing the data.
6. Give two examples for attribute classification.
7. Explain the concept of geographical classification with two examples.
8. Explain the related rules for tabulation.
9. Explain the need for tabulation.
10. Distinguish the difference between raw data and classified data.
11. Explain the concept of frequency distribution with an example.
12. Explain the basic difference between inclusive and exclusive method of classification.

C. Essay Type Questions

1. Explain in detail, various types of classifications. Also give one example each for different classifications.
2. Explain secondary data and list out various sources of secondary data.
3. Write detailed notes on sampling and non-sampling errors.
4. Edit the data representing ages of 15 patients in a hospital taking treatment for heart problems. Also write your comments.

   55, 42, 156, 02, 25, - 51, 39, 88, 102, 74, 62, 00, 27, 92 and 100.
5. The following data represents number of babies born in 60 different government hospitals in the month of January, 2009.

Raw Data:	27	53	30	54	42	22	39	56	45	48	49	58
	52	56	53	32	59	49	26	40	40	29	69	53
	52	57	43	66	54	31	22	31	24	64	43	56
	32	55	52	34	54	42	32	59	35	46	62	57
	39	56	59	58	49	30	53	21	34	28	50	58.

   Prepare the frequency table by considering class intervals as 20 – 29; 30 – 39; 40 – 49 and 50 – 59, 60 – 69. Also calculate the class interval for the above classification.
6. In a study concerned with the presence of significant psychiatric illness in heterozygous carriers of the gene for the wolfram syndrome on 600 patients, resulted the following frequency distribution according to their ages in completed years.

Class Interval	Frequency
Less than 29	65
30–39	98
40–49	115
50–59	90
60–69	65
70–79	73
80–89	49
Greater than 90	45
	600

   Calculate the relative frequency and also answer what proportion of patients are:

   (*i*) Above 70 completed years
   (*ii*) below 30 completed years
   (*iii*) 50 to 60 completed years.
7. The following data represents number of patients admitted in a general ward on 60 different days. Prepare a frequency table by considering class interval as 5 patients.

27	21	53	54	32	42	56	38	28	30	61	46	53	21	18
15	25	12	22	46	49	23	23	35	45	16	64	21	23	46
45	23	45	24	61	55	32	38	49	62	55	62	27	53	28
29	22	36	46	34	17	20	27	52	49	26	16	47	56	24.

8. Explain relative frequency and calculate the same for the data given in question number 6 in this sections.
9. Explain the need of open-end classification. Give an example of open-end classification.
10. Distinguish between the frequencies and relative frequencies with an example.

References:

1. Gupta S.P. 1990 "Statistical Methods". Sultan Chand & Sons, New Delhi.
2. Wayne W. Daniel 2008 Biostatistics, 9th edition, John Wiley & Sons. Inc. Newyork.
3. P.N. Arora *et al*. 2007 "Comprehensive Statistical Methods" Sultan Chand and company Ltd. First edn. New Delhi.

Answers to Objective Questions

1 – d; 2 – a; 3 – b; 4 – c; 5 – c; 6 – a; 7 – b; 8 – a; 9 – b; 10 – b; 11 – a; 12 – b.

3 PRESENTATION OF DATA

3.1. INTRODUCTION

In the previous two chapters we have discussed various data collection techniques and presentation of the collected data in the form of frequency tables. We can also present the frequency tables or results in the form of diagrams or graphs to have a quick and neat presentation of data / results. It is often useful to present frequency tables in the form of diagrams /graphs. This type of presentation of data makes the unwieldy data intelligible and conveys the meaning in quick and permanent impressions in the human mind. Usually human mind is allergenic and having some aversion to numbers than figures. Figures or pictures delights the human mind and the impressions created by pictures are quick and long lost in human mind. Keeping this in view, we usually present the data / frequency tables in the form of diagrams / graphs. It is important to note that diagrams / graphs do not add any new meaning to the statistical facts, but they exhibit the hidden facts in the data and exhibit the data / results more clearly. An ordinary man can understand pictures / diagrams more clearly than figures. It is very opt to quote a famous saying that "a picture more worthy than 1000 words". Diagrams / graphs give a bird's eye-view of the whole mass of statistical data which is usually, large in size and volume.

3.2. DIAGRAMMATIC REPRESENTATION OF DATA

The representation of statistical data through charts and pictures is known as diagrammatic representation of data. A diagram is defined as the geometrical image or pictorial representation of a statistical data. A picture is said to be more effective than words or numbers for describing a particular phenomenon. Thus a diagrammatic representation of data proves quite effective, economic and quick device for the presentation, understanding and interpretation of statistical data.

> *"Cold figures are uninspiring to most people. Diagrams help us to see the pattern and shape of any complex situation. Just as a map gives us a bird's eye-view of the wide stretch of a country, so diagrams help us to visualize the whole meaning of a numerical complex at a single glance. Gives me an undigested heap of figures and I cannot see the wood for the trees. Give me a diagram and I am positively encouraged to forget until I have real grasp of the overall picture. Diagrams register a meaningful and long lasting impression almost before we think".*
>
> — *M.J. Moroney.*

3.2.1. Rules for construction of diagrams

R-1: Title: Each diagram should be given a suitable title, either at the top or at the bottom. It should clearly convey the main theme which the diagram intends to portray. The title should be brief, self-explanatory, clear and un-ambiguous.

R-2: Foot notes: Foot notes are to be given at the end/bottom of each diagram in order to get clarification about the designs or shades used in the diagram.

R-3: Source note: Source, from where the data is collected/taken, where ever it is possible is to be provided at the bottom of the diagram.

R-4: Neat and attractive: Diagram should be made very neat, clean and attractive by neat lettering, designs, dots, dashes, shades and colors to attract the attention of the reader.

R-5: Size of the diagram: The size of the diagram would depend on the size of the data and the purpose. For exhibitions, fairs, and public meetings one can go for wall poster sizes also. For advertisements in T.V.'s, news papers, magazines, research articles, one can go for suitable sizes. Size of the diagram is not the important criteria but the diagram can be understood clearly the meaning what it is intended to convey to the reader.

R-6: Selection of the scale: Scale of presentation should be consistent with the size of the paper and size of the data / observations to be displayed. For example, we want to represent production of a crop since 2000 onwards every year up to 2009. Then on X-axis we can start from 2000 year onwards. X-axis need not start with '0' i.e. the origin. Similarly on Y-axis also we can start from 1,000; 2,000; 3,000; ... 10,000. Not necessarily start from the point '0'. Scale on both axis should clearly explained on the bottom of the diagram.

R-7: Index: A brief index explaining various colors, shades, designs and lines used in the diagram are to be clearly explained under the diagram.

R-8: Simplicity: The diagram should be as simple as possible. Avoid dumping un-necessary and more information in a single diagram.

The basic purpose of a diagram is that even a layman can also understand what the diagram is conveying? A diagram should not be over-loaded with more information giving confusion in the mind of the reader.

R-9: Proportion between length and breadth: The length and breadth of the diagram should be consistent with the space available. Though there are not hard and fast rules to the ratio to the length to breadth, generally we follow a rule called 'Root Two Rule', that is $\sqrt{2:1}$ or 1.414 : 1 between larger side and the smaller side respectively.

R-10: Choice of a diagram: The choice of the diagram should be made with at most caution and care, based on the nature of the data and the purpose of the diagram. It should be consistent with the nature of the data, magnitude of observations and the type of the people for which the diagram is meant.

3.2.2. Type of Diagrams

A large variety of diagrams are available in literature, to represent statistical data. In this book we discuss only those diagrams which are commonly used in biological sciences.

They are :

1. Line Diagrams,
2. Bar diagrams,
3. Pie Diagrams,
4. Pictograms, and
5. Cartograms.

Now we proceed to explain above diagrams one by one with suitable examples.

3.2.3. Line Diagrams

Line diagrams are one-dimensional diagrams where length of the line is considered and varies according to the variable under consideration. These diagrams are simplest of all diagrams and are simple mathematical diagrams that are drawn on the plain paper by plotting the class types on X-axis and variable on Y-axis. With the help of such graphs, the effect of one variable over different classes under consideration is compared clearly. Thus line diagrams facilitate comparisons. Even time series data can be plotted through line diagrams. It is important to note that the distance between the lines is, generally kept uniform.

Example (3.2.1): The following data represents number of books published by a publisher from 2001 to 2006. Represent the data through a line diagram.

Year of publication	Number of books
2001	2,562
2002	3,985
2003	5,648
2004	8,876
2005	10,578
2006	15,606
Total number of books published	42,255

Solution: The data given in example (3.2.1) is represented through line diagram as shown in Fig. (3.2.1).

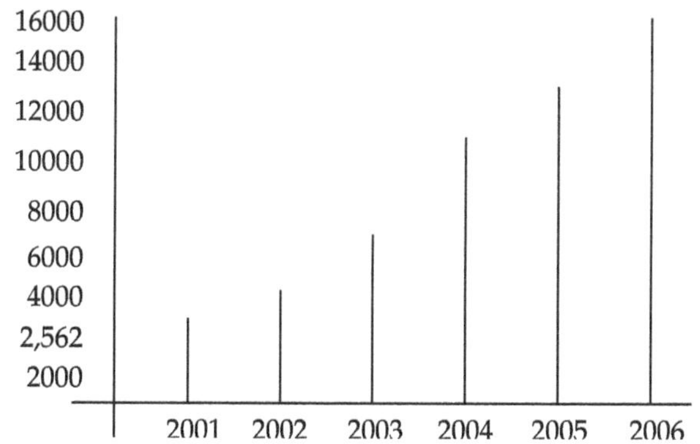

Fig. (3.2.1): *Line diagram representing number of books published.*

3.2.4. Bar Diagrams

Bar diagram is also a one dimensional diagram like a Line diagram. Instead of straight lines, we construct bars or rectangles, where length of the rectangle varies according to the variables and width of these bars or rectangles are not important, but rectangles of equal width are to be constructed. Widths of these bars or rectangles are merely to get attraction of the reader but do not convey any meaning. One can use different colors or designs or shades inside each bar. The meaning of these designs or colors and shades are to be explained in the Index. A Bar diagram is defined as a graph on which the data are represented in the form of bars or rectangles. It is important to note that the bars or rectangles are neither too short not too long. Numbers of bars or rectangles which are of uniform width with equal space between then on X-axis are to be drawn.

Bars may be drawn either vertically or horizontally. A good rule to use in determining the direction is that if the legend describing the bar can be written under the bars, when drawn vertically, vertical bars should be used, when it cannot be, horizontal ones must be used. This helps the reader to read the description of the legend easily without turning the graph. Usually the diagram will be more attractive, if the bars are wider than the space between them.

Bar diagrams are generally used for comparison of quantitative data. They are also used in presenting data involving time factor. For example, time series like prices of vegetables or share prices at different time points. Bar diagrams are different types namely:

1. Simple bar diagrams
2. Sub-divided or component bar diagrams
3. Multiple or grouped bar diagrams and
4. Percentage sub-divided bar diagrams

3.2.4a. Simple Bar Diagrams

These diagrams are to be used to compare two or more items related to a variable. For example, bullion rates in different months or cost of living of people living in different cities/countries, blood sugar of a patient in different months and so on. Thus the basic limitation of simple bar diagram is that, only one variable is to be presented on the diagram. To represent more variables, one has to use different simple bar diagrams. Basic difference between the line diagram and simple bar diagram is that "instead of lines we construct bars/rectangles". It is interesting to note that a line is a rectangle with no width.

Hence, line diagram is a bar diagram where we construct bars with no width. Except this, all other rules for the construction of simple bar diagram are same. That is widths of all bars should be uniform and space between each bar should be same and height of each bar represents the variable size. In order to distinguish the difference between bar diagram and line diagram same data in the example (3.2.1) is considered and constructed a simple bar diagram as follows.

Example (3.2.2): For the data in example (3.2.1) construct a simple bar diagram.

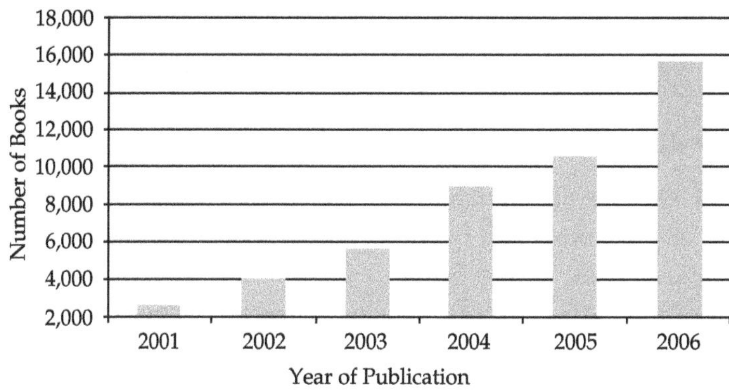

Fig. (3.2.2): *Simple bar diagram for number of books published.*

In simple bar diagram bars may be drawn either vertically or horizontally. A good rule is to use in determining the direction is that if the variable describing the bar can be written under the bars when drawn vertically, vertical bars should be used as shown in Fig. (3.2.2). When this is not possible, horizontal bars should be used. But it should be noted that the bars drawn are neither too short nor too long. The scale should clearly indicate the units considered on x–axis, for horizontal bars and y–axis for vertical bars. Widths of bars are not representing anything. It is an arbitrary factor just to attract the attention of the reader. Horizontal bars are written as follows as shown in Fig. (3.2.3):

Example (3.2.3): Draw horizontal bar diagram for the data representing number of male and female births in a hospital in a month.

Number of male births	Number of female births
52	68

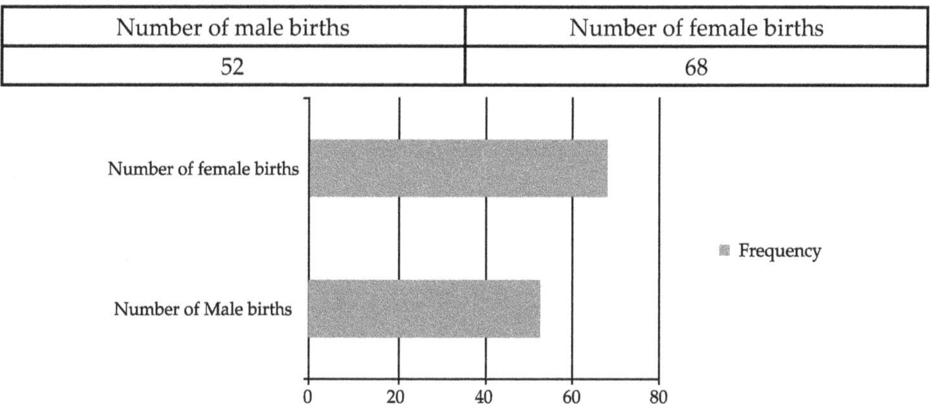

Fig. (3.2.3): *Horizontal bar diagram representing number of births.*

Uses of simple bar diagrams

Bar diagrams are generally used for comparison of quantitative data. They are also used to the data representing time series, where time factor is involved.

Limitations of simple bar diagrams

1. In simple bar diagram, width of bars only attracts the attention of the reader but does not represent anything. Because of this, simple bar diagrams are known as one dimensional diagrams.

2. In simple bar diagrams one can represent one variable only at a time. To represent more variables, different simple bar charts are to be drawn.
3. In simple bar diagrams one cannot represent totals.

3.2.4b. Sub-divided or Component Bar Diagrams

To overcome the second limitation of simple bar diagram, we prefer to draw sub-divided or component bar diagram. A component bar diagram is one which is formed by dividing single bar into several sub-parts or components. The total length of the bar represents totals or aggregate values. The design and the procedure of constructing it is similar to simple bar diagram except that in this form presentation each bar is sub-divided into different components. The method of construction of sub-divided or component bar diagram is explained in the following example.

Example (3.2.4): Construct component bar diagram for the following data representing different types of visitors to a government hospital from January to April 2007.

Months	Children	Adults	Old People	Total
January, 07	86	37	60	183
February, 07	58	86	75	219
March, 07	59	79	82	220
April, 07	88	62	85	235
Total	291	264	302	857

Solution: Here, we draw component bar diagram because, total visitors in different months are further divided into three categories, namely, children, adults and old people.

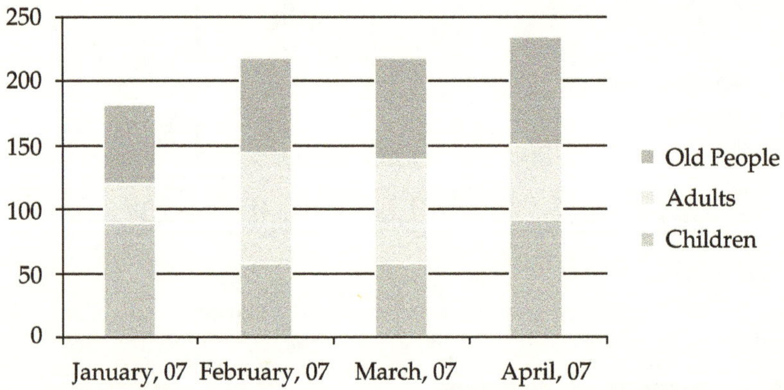

Fig. (3.2.4): *Vertical component diagram representing different type of visitors in different months.*

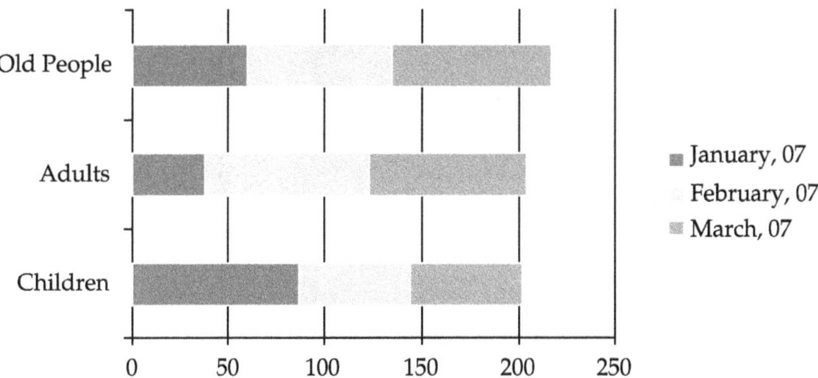

Fig. (3.2.5): *Horizontal component diagram representing different type of visitors in different months.*

3.2.4c. Multiple or grouped bar diagrams

A multiple or grouped bar diagram is used when number of items are to be compared in respect of two or three or more values. In this diagram individual bars are constructed for each sub-component and are grouped together. A multiple bar diagram is nothing but group of simple bars constructed adjacent to each bar. Construction of multiple bar diagram is similar to the construction of simple bar diagram except the difference that, multiple bars are to be constructed instead of single bar, each bar representing each sub-component. To distinguish multiple bar diagram with sub-divided bar diagram, the same data in the example (3.2.4) can be represented as follows:

Example (3.2.5): Represent the data in example (3.2.4) as multiple bar diagram.

Solution: Construct vertical or horizontal bars as shown in the figure such that each bar represents each sub-component. One can construct sub-divided bar diagram or multiple bar diagram as desired. Whichever is suitable, one can choose. It is important to note that width of each bar should be uniform. Gaps between each group of bars should be uniform.

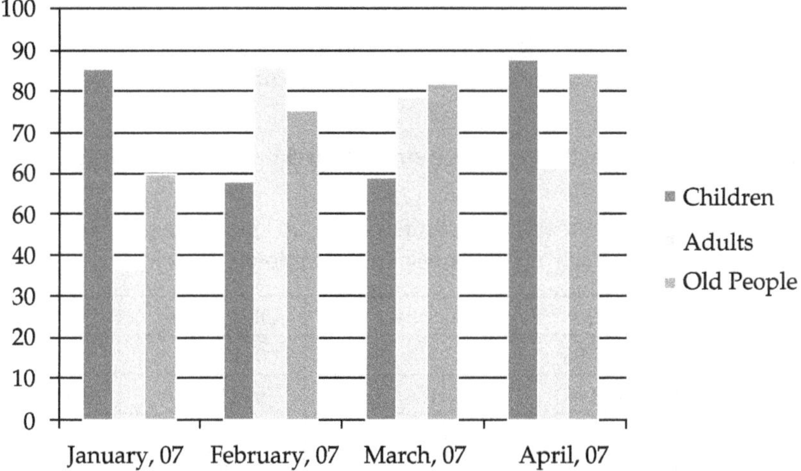

Fig. (3.2.6): *Vertical multiple bar diagram representing different type of visitors in different months.*

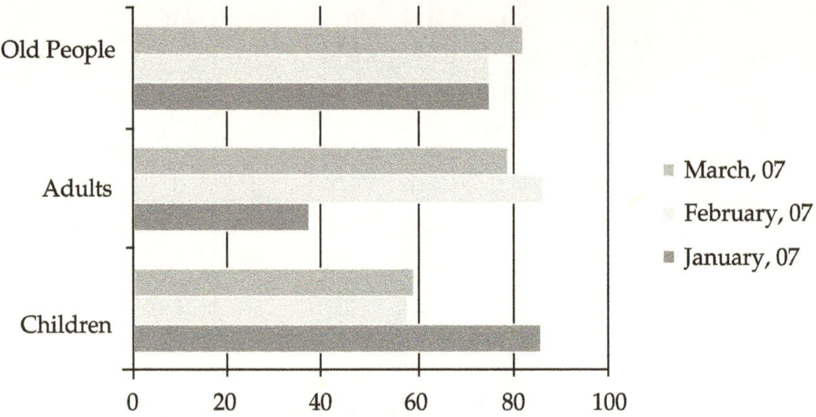

Fig. (3.2.7): *Horizontal multiple bar diagram representing different type of visitors in different months.*

3.2.4d. Percentage sub-divided bar diagrams

Percentage sub-divided bar diagram consists of one or more than one bars where each bar is of equal height equal to 100 %. It's construction is similar to the sub-divided bar diagram with only difference that in the sub-divided bar diagrams, segments example representing sub-components are considered where as in the percentage bar diagrams, the sub-components represent the percentages of sub-divisions. Construction of percentage sub-divided bar diagram is explained in the following steps.

Step – 1: Convert the quantities or sub-divisions into percentages of the whole.

Step – 2: Take the cumulative percentages.

Step – 3: Represent each category of items in different shades or colors or different designs.

Step – 4: Consider different periods on *X*-axis and variable on *Y*-axis.

Above steps are explained with an example. To distinguish the difference between sub-divided bar diagram and percentage sub-divided bar diagram, the data in example (3.2.4) is considered for the construction of percentage bar diagram.

Example (3.2.8): Construct percentage sub-divided bar diagram for the data in the example (3.2.4).

Solution: First convert each sub-division in to percentages. To get clarity percentages are written with parenthesis in the table given below.

Months	Children	Adults	Old people	Total
January, 07	86 (29.56)	37 (14.01)	60 (19.87)	183
February, 07	58 (19.93)	86 (32.58)	75 (24.83)	219
March, 07	59 (20.27)	79 (29.92)	82 (27.15)	220
April, 07	88 (30.24)	62 (23.49)	85 (28.15)	235
Total	291	264	302	857

In the next step calculate cumulative percentages as shown in the following table.

Months	Children cumulative %	Adults cumulative %	Old people cumulative %
January, 07	29.56	14.01	19.87
February, 07	49.49	46.59	44.70
March, 07	69.76	76.51	71.85
April, 07	100	100	100

After constructing cumulative percentage table, consider various visitors on x-axis and different months on y-axis, draw percentage bar diagram as shown in the figure.

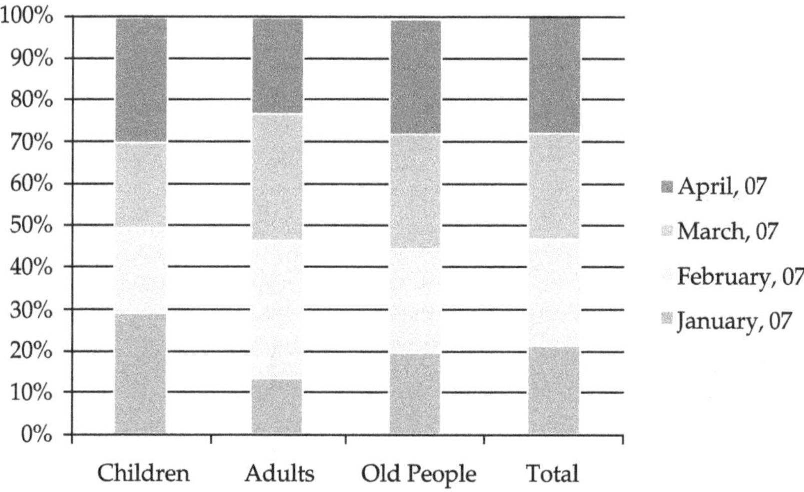

Fig. (3.2.8): *Percentage sub-divided bar diagram by considering months as components.*

If we want to consider different types of patients in different months, then calculate percentages over all visitors in different months. The procedure is explained as follows.

First construct percentages for different month's totals as follows:

Months	Children	Adults	Old people	Total
January, 07	86 (46.99)	37 (20.22)	60 (32.79)	183
February, 07	58 (26.48)	86 (39.27)	75 (34.25)	219
March, 07	59 (26.82)	79 (35.91)	82 (37.27)	220
April, 07	88 (37.45)	62 (26.38)	85 (36.17)	235
Total	291	264	302	857

Now we proceed to construct cumulative percentage table as follows.

Month	Children	Adults	Old people
Jan. cum. %	46.99	67.21	100
Feb. cum. %	26.48	65.75	100
March cum. %	26.82	62.73	100
Apr. cum. %	37.45	63.83	100

After constructing the cumulative percentage table, consider months on x-axis and various visitors on y-axis, draw percent bar diagram as shown in the figure.

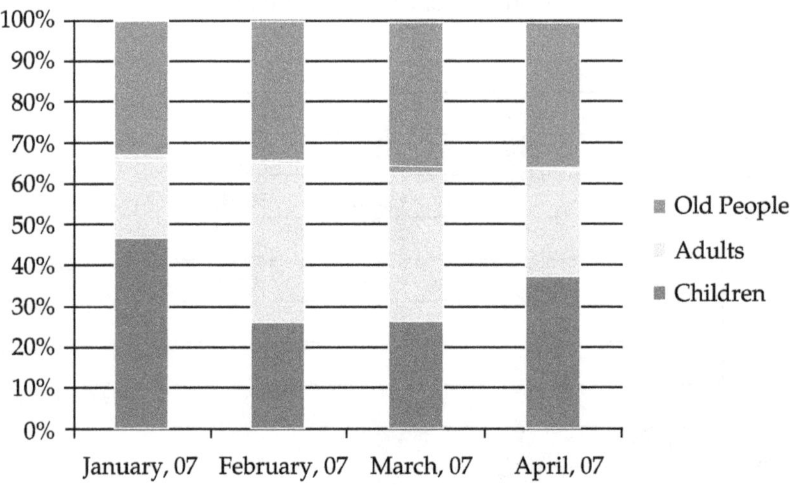

Fig. (3.2.9): *Percentage sub-divided bar diagram by considering various type of visitors as components.*

3.2.5. Pie Diagrams

Pie diagrams are also known as rupee diagrams or circle diagrams. A pie diagram is a circular graph, which represents the total value of the variable and different sectors of the graph represent various sub-components of the variable under study. Pie diagram is a special type of percentage sub-divided bar diagram and basic differences between pie diagram and percentage sub-divided bar diagrams are listed as follows:

S.No.	Percentage sub-divided bar diagram	Pie diagram
1.	We use rectangles	We use circles
2.	Total equated to 100	Total equated to 360 degrees
3.	We calculate percentages to represent sub-components	We convert sub-components into sectors with different degrees
4.	We calculate cumulative percentages	We calculate cumulative degrees
5.	Total is equated to rectange height 100.	Total is equated to circle degrees that is 360 degrees.

Because of reason 5 pie diagrams are also known as angular diagram. The name pie diagram is given to a circle diagram because in determining the circumference of a circle, we use the quantity known as "Pie" which is written as π, where $\pi = 180°$.

Method of construction of a Pie diagram

The total area of the circle or the pie chart is equal to $2\pi = 360$ degrees. The data to be represented through a circle such that total is equal to 360 degrees and parts or sub-divisions represented by sectors in the circle of pie diagram. Angles of these sectors represent the volume of the sub-division of the variable. Thus one has to convert sub-divisions into respective degrees of the sector. For example, total of a variable is 500 and the value of the sub-division is 200 then the corresponding sector should contain the angle as $200 \times (360/500) = 144°$. After determining angles of each sector, represent each sector such that each sector contains angle equal to the respective calculated angle. The procedure is explained with an example as follows.

Example (3.2.10): Construct pie charts for (1) visitors in different months and (2) various types of visitors for the data in example (3.2.4) which is as follows:

Months	Children (1)	Adults	Old people	Total
January, 07	86	37	60	183
February, 07	58	86	75	219
March, 07	59	79	82	220
April, 07	88	62	85	235
Total	291	264	302	857

Solution: In the first step we have to convert various sub-classes into degrees (1) by considering each month's totals equal to 360° and (2) by considering various categories of visitor's totals. These degrees are given in the following two tables respectively.

Table (3.2.1): Calculation of degree for month's totals

Months	Children (1)	Adults	Old people	Total
January, 07	86 × (360/183) = 169.18°	37 × (360/183) = 72.79°	60 × (360/183) = 118.03°	183 = 360°
February, 07	58 = 95.34°	86 = 141.36°	75 = 123.29°	219 = 360°
March, 07	59 = 96.55°	79 = 129.27°	82 = 134.18°	220 = 360°
April, 07	88 = 134.81°	62 = 94.98°	85 = 130.21°	235 = 360°
Total	291	264	302	857

Using table (3.2.1) we have to prepare cumulative degrees table as follows.

Months	Children (1)	Adults	Old people	Total
January, 07	169.18°	241.97°	360°	183 = 360°
February, 07	58 = 95.34°	236.7°	360°	219 = 360°
March, 07	59 = 96.55°	225.82°	360°	220 = 360°
April, 07	88 = 134.81°	229.79°	360°	235 = 360°
Total	291	264	302	857

Then start constructing various segments by starting from any point as shown in the figures:

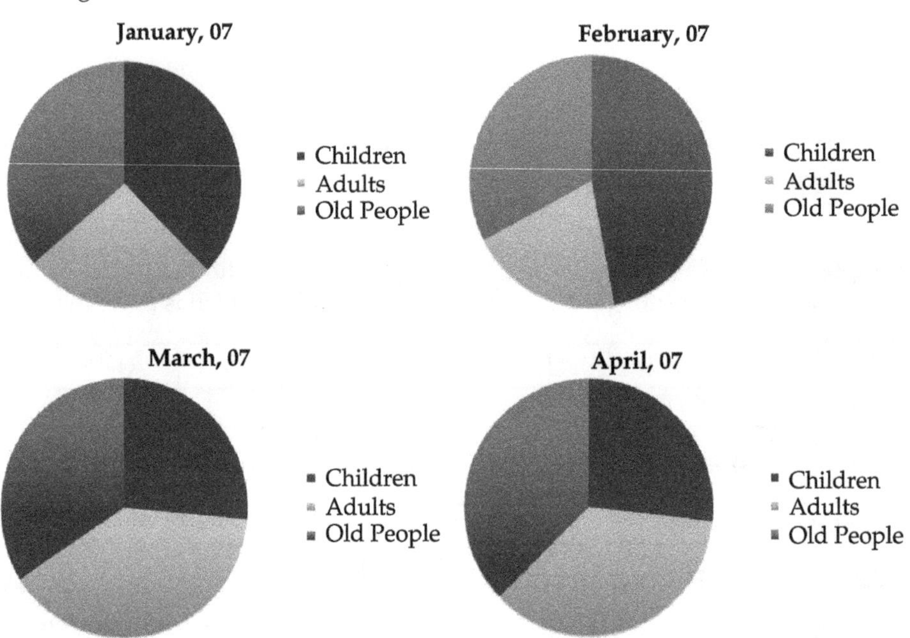

Fig. (3.2.10): *Pie charts for different month.*

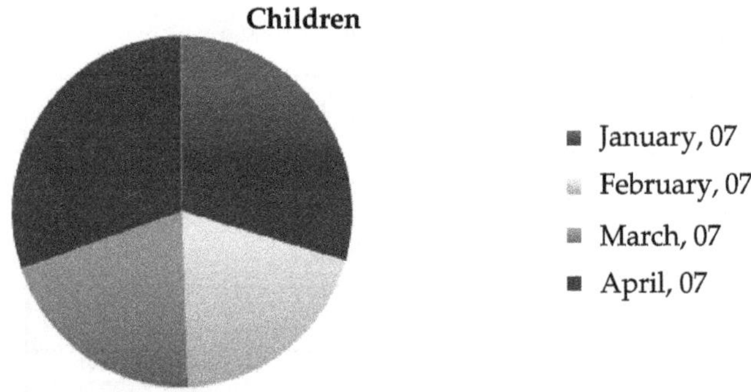

7. Dotted lines or straight lines can be used to join two points on the graph.
8. Every graph must have a title.
9. Scales considered on both axis should be explained.
10. If two or more variables are considered on the same graph distinguish the variables using thick lines or dotted lines or different colored lines for different variables considered.

3.3.3. Types of Graphs

Graphs basically are of two types, namely:

1. Graphs for frequency distributions and
2. Graphs for time series.

3.4. GRAPHS FOR FREQUENCY DISTRIBUTIONS

A frequency distribution can be represented in any form of the following graphs, namely:

1. Histogram
2. Frequency polygon
3. Frequency curve and
4. Ogives.

3.4.1. Histogram

A histogram is a graph containing rectangles each being constructed such that width of the rectangle represents the class interval and the length of the rectangle represents the frequency of that class. Thus both length and width of each rectangle represents class interval and the frequency respectively. Because of this, histograms are known as two dimensional graphs. Even though histograms looks like bar diagrams, former are two dimensional where as latter are one dimensional. In bar diagrams length of the bar correspond the value the variable but width of the bar does not convey anything. It is only to attract the attention of the reader. In histogram, the area of the rectangle (that is length x-breadth of the rectangle) is proportional to the frequency and the corresponding class interval of the class for which it represents. Thus if we have, equal class intervals, we obtain equal widths of rectangles in histogram otherwise, we obtain unequal widths of rectangles. A histogram is always used to depict a frequency distribution. Histograms are of two types, namely:

(*i*) Histograms with equal class intervals and

(*ii*) Histograms with unequal class intervals.

Construction of a histogram (with equal class intervals): Histogram is a bar diagram for a frequency distribution and the following points are to be kept in mind in construction of a histogram.

1. Convert the frequency distribution into exclusive method if it is given in inclusive method.
2. Always consider class intervals on x-axis and the frequencies on y-axis.
3. It is customary to take two extra intervals (or classes) one below and one above the given frequency distribution.
4. Select and suitable scale for class intervals on x-axis and another for frequencies on y–axis.
5. Each class interval with its specific frequency construct rectangle, such that class interval as width and frequency as length or height of the rectangle.
6. Since class intervals are of equal widths, we obtain a histogram with equal width of rectangles.

Construction of a histogram (with unequal class intervals):

1. If class intervals are un-equal, first select smallest class interval among the given intervals and convert all intervals equal to this smallest interval selected. Thus class intervals are to be adjusted and are to be converted to equal class intervals.
2. After adjusting the class intervals, frequencies of the classes are to be adjusted. The adjustment of frequencies is explained as follows:

   "if the class interval is twice larger than the smallest class interval, the frequency of the class is to be divided with two".

   "if the class interval is thrice larger than the smallest class interval, the frequency of the class is to be divided with three", and so on.

After adjusting the class intervals and frequencies, construction of histogram with unequal class intervals is same as that of histogram with equal class interval.

Example (3.4.1): Construct a histogram for the following frequency distribution representing the distribution of students according to marks in an examination.

Class intervals	Frequencies
0 – 10	25
10 – 20	33
20 – 30	72
30 – 40	55
40 – 50	45
50 – 60	52
60 – 70	48

Solution: We represent class intervals on x-axis and frequencies on y-axis. Taking class intervals as width of each rectangle construct the rectangles of length / height of each rectangle equal to the corresponding frequency as shown in the figure.

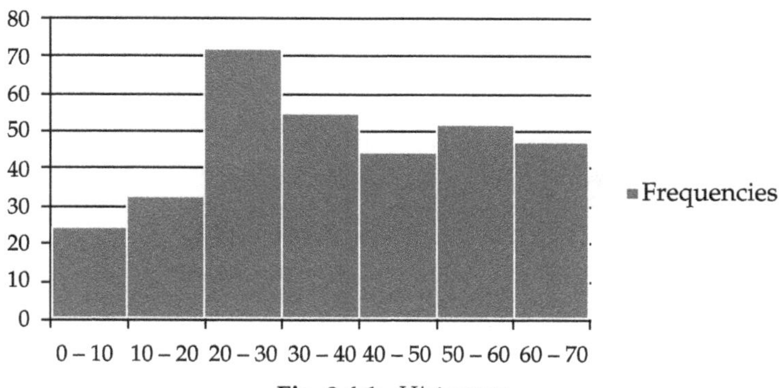

Fig. 3.4.1: *Histogram*

Example (3.4.2): Construct a histogram for the following data.

Class interval	Frequency
0 – 30	36
30 – 50	32
50 – 60	20
60 – 80	50
80 – 100	20

Solution: Given class intervals are unequal class intervals. In this case, first identify the smallest class interval. That is 50 – 60. Class interval = 10. First convert all class intervals equal to this class. That is 0 – 10, 10 – 20, .,.,., 90 – 100. After adjusting the class intervals now frequencies are to be adjusted as follows: First class intervals thrice larger than the smallest class interval. Hence, the frequency 36 is to be divided by 3. That is 36/3 = 12. Thus 0 – 10, 10 – 20 and 20 – 30 classes should contain frequencies equal to 12. Similarly, second class 30 – 50 is twice larger than the smallest interval. Therefore, the frequency 32 is to be divided by 2. That is 16 is to be considered for classes 30 – 40 and 40 – 50. Like that we have to construct adjusted frequency table as follows:

Adjusted class intervals	Adjusted frequencies
0 – 10	12
10 –20	12
20 – 30	12
30 – 40	16
40 – 50	16
50 – 60	20
60 – 70	25
70 – 80	25
80 – 90	10
90 – 100	10

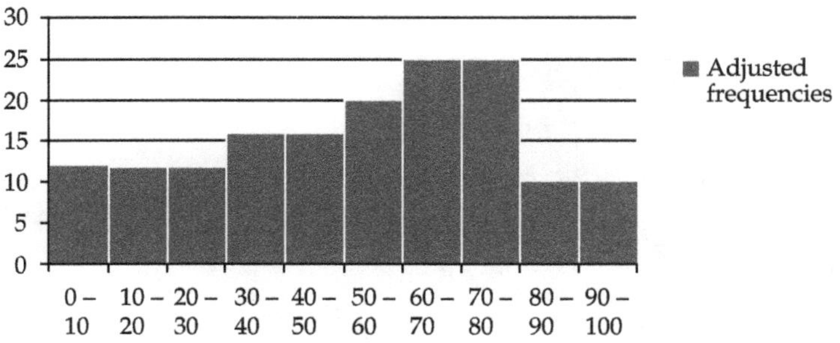

Fig. (3.4.2): *Histogram for unequal class intervals.*

3.4.2. Frequency polygon

In histogram, we cannot two or more frequency distributions which are to be compared. To do this, we require drawing frequency polygon. A frequency polygon is a line graph for the graphical representation of the frequency distribution. Two or more frequency curves can be drawn on the same graph so that comparison can be made easily.

Construction of frequency polygon:

Method – I:

1. Draw the histogram for the given frequency distribution.
2. Identify mid-points of upper horizontal side of each rectangle.
3. Join each mid-point to its adjacent point by straight lines.

Method – II:

1. Calculate mid-values for each class.
2. Consider mid-values on x-axis and frequencies on y-axis.
3. By choosing suitable scale plot the mid-points and the corresponding frequency on the graph.
4. Join these points with the adjacent ones with straight lines.

The figure so formed is called a frequency polygon.

Example: (3.3.3): The following data represents the expenditure incurred by different patients to cure a viral fever in two summers of 2008 and 2009. Represent the data through frequency polygons.

Expenditure in rupees on viral fever	2008 summer	2009 summer
100 – 150	52	79
150 – 200	70	92
200 – 250	68	102
250 – 300	58	63
300 – 350	60	89
350 – 400	32	56
400 – 450	28	38
450 – 500	12	16

Solution: Since, we have two series, one for 2008 and the other for 2009. We apply Method–II, this is because of the fact that writing histogram and identifying mid-points of upper horizontal side of each rectangle is cumbersome here. Hence, calculation of mid-values and plotting mid-values and the frequencies is easy method (usually we follow this procedure only). Thus we obtain the following table.

Mid-values	2008 summer	2009 summer
125	52	79
175	70	92
225	68	102
275	58	63
325	60	89
375	32	56
425	28	38
475	12	16

Consider mid values of x-axis and frequencies on y-axis, draw frequency polygons.

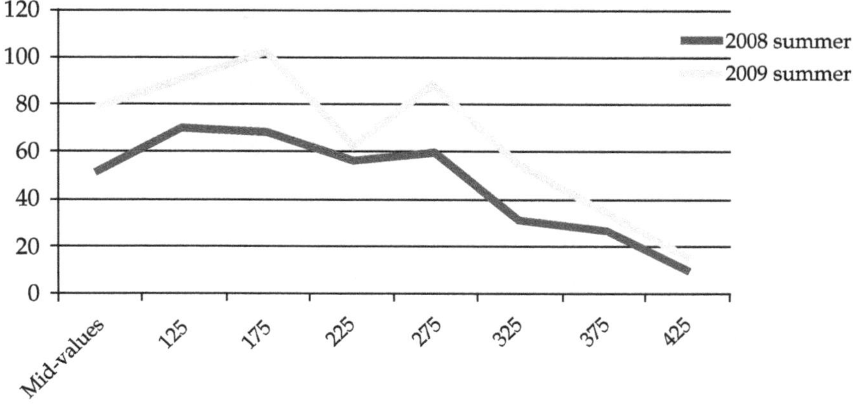

Fig. (3.4.3): *Frequency polygons for two summers 2008 and 2009.*

3.4.3. Frequency Curves

In a frequency polygon, instead of straight lines, if we join the points on the graph with smooth freehand curve, we obtain a frequency curve. Thus, a frequency curve is a nothing but smoothing of frequency polygon. Because of this, frequency curves are also known as smooth frequency curves. The purpose of smoothing is to avoid sharp turns which represent random effects or effects due to random causes. Thus a frequency polygon, if smoothed further, so as to minimize sudden changes, results into a frequency curve or smooth frequency curve. The curve should begin and end at the base line. To draw the frequency curve, firstly draw a histogram, then draw a frequency polygon and lastly, smooth it to get frequency curve. The basic object of drawing a frequency curve is to present graphically, the area covered by histogram in a more symmetrical manner.

Example (3.4.4): Draw the frequency curve for the following data representing number of days of stay in the nursing home for the post operational care, of a heart disease.

Number of days	0–15	15–30	30–45	45–60	60–75	75–90	90–105	105–120	120–135
Frequency	6	10	22	28	24	14	8	6	2

Solution: Consider mid-values of classes intervals on x-axis and frequencies on y-axis with suitable scale and plot points on the chart like frequency polygon. Instead of straight lines, join these points to adjacent points with a smooth freehand curve. The resultant figure is a frequency curve. Now we proceed to calculate mid-values for the given data in the following table.

Mid values	7.5	22.5	37.5	52.5	67.5	82.5	97.5	112.5	127.5
Frequency	6	10	22	28	24	14	8	6	2

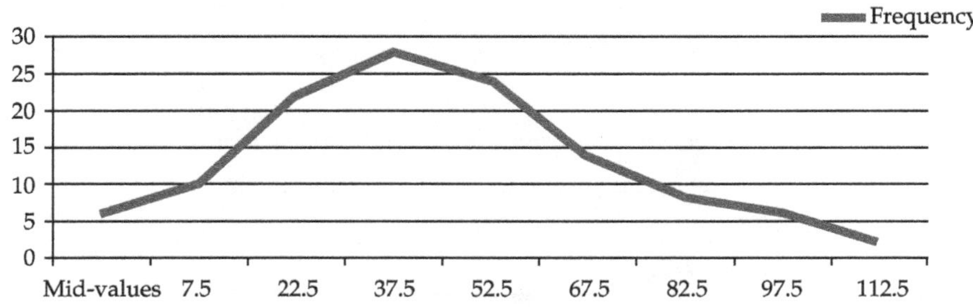

Fig. 3.4.4: *Frequency curve*

3.4.4. Ogives

Cumulative frequency curves are known as ogives. Now we proceed to explain how to calculate cumulative frequencies of (*i*) Less than the upper limit and (*ii*) Greater than the lower limit for a frequency distribution. Representing these cumulative frequency through frequency curve is known as an ogive. Ogives can be used to find median, mode, quartiles, deciles and percentiles graphically (these concepts are discussed in chapter-4). Ogives are of two types. Namely:

(*a*) Less than ogive and
(*b*) Greater than ogive.

Construction of ogives

To draw less than ogive, consider upper bounds of each class on x-axis and the corresponding less than cumulative frequencies on y-axis. Plot the points and a frequency curve, then we obtain a raising curve, which is known as "less than cumulative frequency curve" or "less than ogive". Similarly, if we consider lower bounds of each class on x-axis and greater than cumulative frequencies on y-axis and plot the points on the graph. If we join these points with the adjacent ones, we obtain a declining curve which is known as "greater than cumulative frequency curve" or "greater than ogive". Construction of ogives is explained with an example.

Example (3.3.5): Construct both ogives for the following data representing the frequency distribution of students with respect to their intelligent quotient (I.Q.).

I.Q.	60–70	70–80	80–90	90–100	100–110	110–120	120–130
Frequency	5	8	16	38	45	12	6

Solution: To draw both ogives, we require calculating both cumulative frequencies.

Table (3.3.5): Table of cumulative frequencies.

Class interval	Frequency	Less than cumulative frequencies	Greater than cumulative frequencies
60–70	5	5	130
70–80	8	13	125
80–90	16	29	117
90–100	38	67	101
100–110	45	112	63
110–120	12	124	18
120–130	6	130	6

Consider upper bounds of each class and the corresponding less than cumulative frequencies as shown below to draw less than ogive.

Upper limit	70	80	90	100	110	120	130
Less than cum. frequency	5	13	29	67	112	124	130

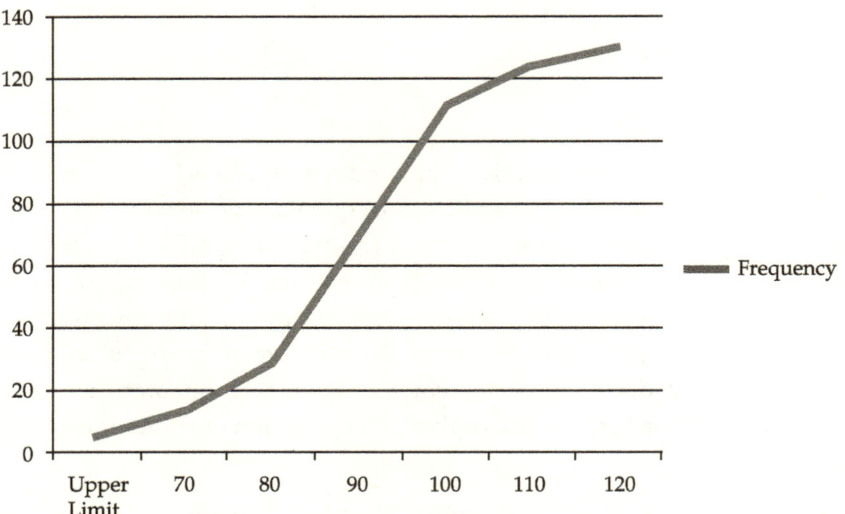

Fig. 3.3.5: *Less than ogive*

To draw greater than ogive, consider lower limits of each class on x–axis and greater than cumulative frequencies on y-axis and join the points to the adjacent ones through a smooth freehand curve.

The resultant figure is called "greater than cumulative curve" or "greater than ogive".

Lower limit	60	70	80	90	100	110	120
Greater than cumulative frequency	130	125	117	101	63	18	6

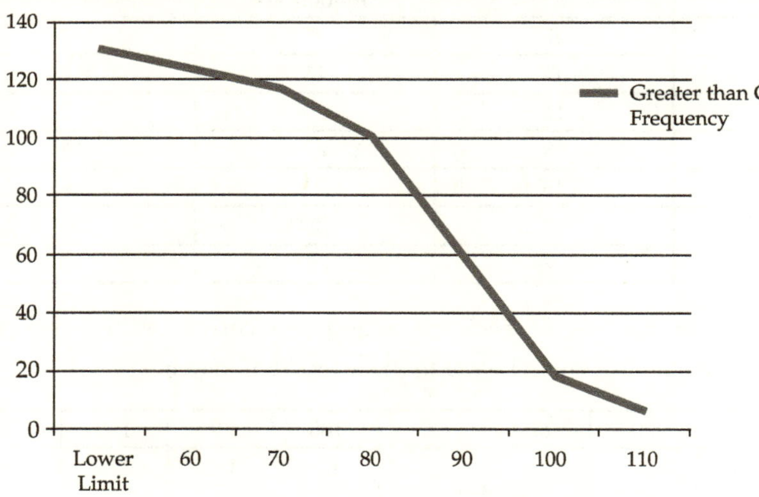

Fig. 3.3.6: *Greater than ogive*

3.5. GRAPHS FOR TIME SERIES

The data collected on a variable, like prices of different commodities, production of industrial output, population of a town, over a period of time is known as "time series". Consider time on x-axis and the variable(s) on y-axis if we draw a graph, then it is known as "graph of time series" or "line graph", which is used to determine trend, and seasonal effects present in the time series data. This is the simplest, easiest and no technical skills are required to construct this graph. Basically, these graphs are of two types, namely:

1. graph of one variable and
2. graph of many variables.

3.5.1. Graph of One Variable

When only one variable is to be represented, the desired graph is obtained on plotting the time on x-axis and the variable on y-axis by choosing a suitable scale on both the axis. Here, we generally use two techniques, namely:

(*a*) False base line technique and

(*b*) Clinked or broken line technique.

These principles can also be used in other graphs also discussed earlier.

3.5.2. False Base Line

The fundamental principle of drawing a graph is that, horizontal / vertical scale must start with zero. If the lowest value to be plotted on the x-axis or y-axis is relatively high, then for an effective depicture of these fluctuations, the vertical axis scale, that is, the scale on the x-axis or y-axis is to be stretched by using "false base line". In such situation, The x-scale or y-scale is broken and the space between the origin and the first unit of x-scale or y-scale is denoted by drawing two zigzag horizontal or vertical lines. This technique is known as false base line. Using this technique, the space between zero and lowest value of the variable is omitted. This technique is explained as follows with an example.

Example. (3.5.1): Draw the graph for the following time series data by using false base line for both x-axis and y-axis.

Year	2000	2001	2002	2003	2004	2005	2006	2007	2008	2009
Number of heart patients	335	348	308	302	332	348	358	369	372	380

Solution: Since the year starts fron 2000, x-axis should start from 2000 but not from zero. Thus the space on the graph between zero to 2000 is to be eliminated. This can be done by using false base line for x-axis.

Similarly, smallest value on y-axis is 302 and hence should start from the value 300, but not from zero on y-axis. Thus the space from zero to 300 on y-axis is to be eliminated. This is done again by using false base line on y-axis. Using this technique, for both x-axis and y-axis, figure (3.5.1) is drawn.

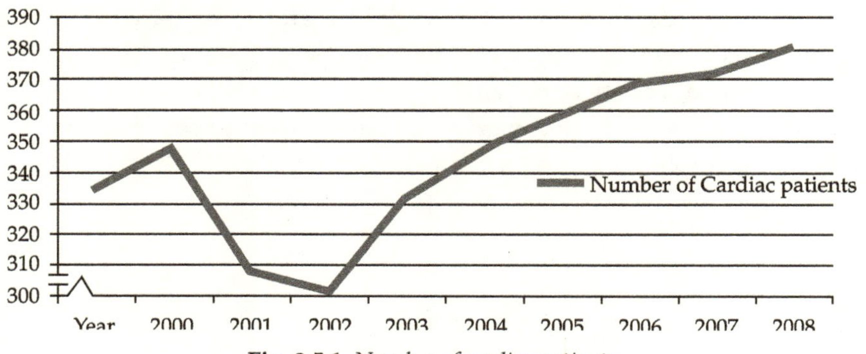

Fig. 3.5.1. *Number of cardiac patients*

3.5.3. Broken Scale

Instead of using a false base, we can also use broken vertical scale. The scales should normally, begin with zero and proceed uniformly. But when the variations in x-axis or y-axis figures are small as compared with their general level, they cannot be shown properly if this rule is strictly followed. In such cases, it is permissible to have a broken horizontal/vertical scale as shown in the figure (3.5.1) both on x–axis and y-axis respectively.

Example (3.5.2): Represent the following data graphically using broken scale on both the axis.

X	0.2	0.3	0.4	0.5	0.7	0.8	0.9
Y	1.73	1.38	1.52	1.98	1.45	1.69	1.25

Solution: Consider X on x-axis and Y on y-axis. Since the values on x-axis is in between 0 and 1 the scale on x-axis using broken line is given as shown in Fig. (3.5.2). Similarly, values on y-axis are in between 1 and 2 we have to use broken line technique for y-axis also. Using broken line technique for both the axis we obtain the Fig. (3.5.2).

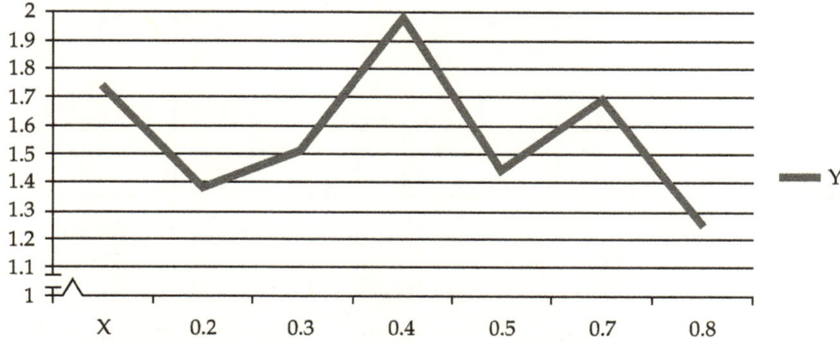

Fig. 3.5.2. *Use of broken lines.*

3.5.4. Graphs of Several Variables

One can consider more than one variables on y-axis simultaneously which facilitates the comparison between different variables or different places of time series data. Such graphs are known as "graphs of several variables", which is explained as follows.

Example (3.5.3): The following data represents patients suffered for diarrhea in different cities in three cities A, B and C. Represent the data through graph of time series of several variables.

Year	City-A	City-B	City-C
2001	120	130	110
2002	130	149	100
2003	145	123	112
2004	132	112	142
2005	105	125	128
2006	140	130	145

Solution: Using false base line on x-axis and y-axis and considering number of affected persons in different cities on y-axis we obtain the Fig. (3.5.3) as follows. Since the smallest value on x-axis is 2001 and on y-axis the smallest value is 100 we have used the technique of false base line on both axes.

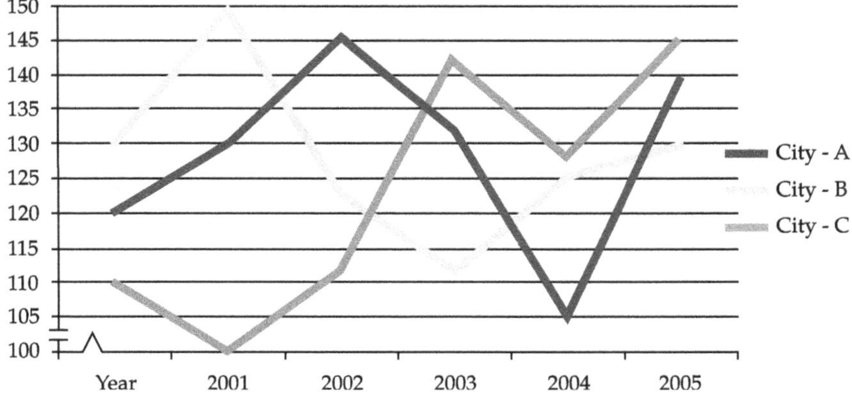

Fig. 3.5.3. *Graph of time series data of several variables*

3.6. RANGE GRAPHS

In many real life situations, particularly in medical field, we come across variables, which have both maximum and minimum values. For example, blood-pressure (B.P.), serum cholesterol, blood glucose and so on should always be in between a minimum and a maximum values. Similarly, temperatures of different places have minimum and maximum values. The difference between maximum minus minimum value is called "The Range". Both maximum and minimum values can be represented on y-axis. Such charts are known as "Range Charts". The following points are to be remembered while constructing the range graph.

1. Take time on x-axis and variables on y-axis.
2. Draw two curves representing maximum and minimum values of the variable.
3. The gap between these curves represent the range of variation.
4. The range of variation can be represented with different colors or shades or designs.

Example (3.6.1): Represent the following data through the range chart. The data is measured in degrees Celsius.

Month	1	2	3	4	5	6
Max. temp	42	40	41	39	38	35
Min. temp	29	27	27	28	25	22

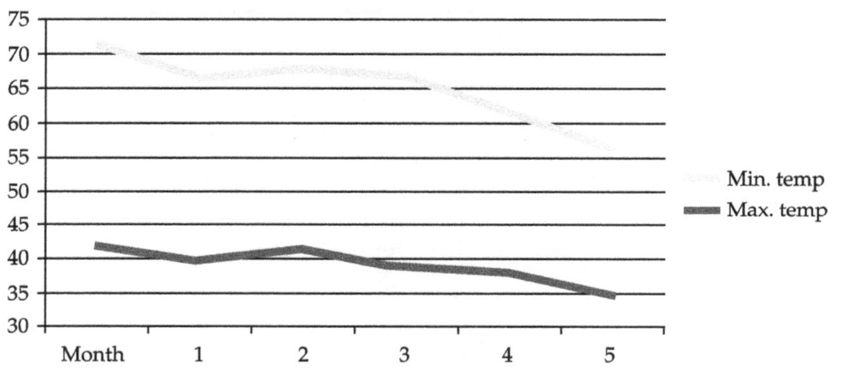

REVIEW QUESTIONS AND PROBLEMS

A. Objective Type

1. Bar charts are ------------------ dimensional diagrams.
   (*a*) two (*b*) three
   (*c*) one (*d*) multi
2. Histograms are ----------------- dimensional graphs.
   (*a*) two (*b*) three
   (*c*) one (*d*) multi
3. If midpoints of upper horizontal side of a histogram are joined with straight lines to the adjacent points, the resultant figure is known as ------------------.
   (*a*) ogives (*b*) frequency polygon
   (*c*) frequency curve (*d*) sub-divided bar diagrams.
4. Cumulative frequency curves are known as ------------------.
   (*a*) ogives (*b*) frequency polygon
   (*c*) frequency curve (*d*) sub-divided bar diagrams.

5. Smoothing the frequency polygon is known as --------------.
   (*a*) ogives (*b*) frequency polygon
   (*c*) frequency curve (*d*) sub-divided bar diagrams.
6. Pie diagrams are also known as ----------------- diagrams.
   (*a*) ogives (*b*) rupee
   (*c*) cumulative (*d*) range.
7. Multiple bar diagrams are alternative to ----------- diagrams.
   (*a*) ogives (*b*) frequency polygon
   (*c*) frequency curve (*d*) sub-divided bar diagrams.
8. Basic disadvantage of diagrammatic or graphical representation is -------------.
   (*a*) they are difficult to draw
   (*b*) we require much skills
   (*c*) difficult to understand
   (*d*) we cannot represent more than two variables at a time.
9. For drawing graphs of time series we should always consider ----------- on x-axis.
   (*a*) variables (*b*) time
   (*c*) cumulative sums (*d*) ranges.
10. Reducing the space between zero and smallest value of the variable is known as ------------------------.
   (*a*) false base line (*b*) scaling the axis
   (*c*) reduction technique (*d*) broken line.

B. Short Answer Questions

1. Distinguish the difference between diagrams and graphs.
2. Explain various advantages and disadvantages of diagrammatic representation of data.
3. Explain the method of construction of sub-divided bar diagrams.
4. Explain the method of construction of pie diagrams.
5. What is a histogram? Explain with an example.
6. Explain any one method of construction of frequency polygon.
7. Distinguish between frequency polygon and frequency curve.
8. Explain the method of construction of ogives.
9. Explain the use of false base line.
10. Explain range charts.

C. Essay Type Questions

1. Explain various rules for construction of diagrams.
2. Explain various types diagrams along with their construction.
3. Explain various rules for construction of graphs.

4. Explain various types of graphs along with their construction.
5. Explain the method of construction of graphs for time series.
6. The following data represents different type patients having variety of intake of food habits.

Different places	Rice eaters (in '000)	Wheat eaters (in '000)	Ragi eaters (in '000)
City A	53	42	33
City B	47	50	28
City C	59	65	34
City D	26	47	43
City E	38	34	51
City F	29	38	22

(*a*) Represent the above through sub-divided bar diagram.
(*b*) Draw multiple bar diagram for the above data.
(*c*) Draw pie charts for different cities.
(*d*) Draw line diagrams for different cities.
(*e*) Draw percentage sub-divided bar diagrams for different cities.
(*f*) Draw percentage sub-divided bar diagrams for different variety of food habits.

7. The following data represent distribution of different heart patients according to their weights.

Weight in Kgs.	Male	Female	Total
45 – 50	12	7	19
50 – 55	18	19	37
55 – 60	27	22	49
60 – 65	24	40	64
65 – 70	12	33	45
70 – 75	8	12	20
75 – 80	4	6	10
80 – 85	2	4	06

(*a*) Draw suitable graph for the above data.
(*b*) Draw histogram for the total patients.
(*c*) Draw pie charts for different weighted patients, both for male and female patients separately.
(*d*) Draw frequency polygon and frequency curves for the above data.
(*e*) Draw ogives for total number of patients with different weights.

8. "Diagrams and graphs are more effective in attracting attention of reader than any other method of presentation of statistical data" – comment.
9. Following data represents the distribution of different students with respect to marks in bio-statistics.

Class interval	Frequency
0 – 10	12
10 – 20	14
20 – 40	16
40 – 50	14
60 – 70	8
80 – 90	16
90 – 100	5

(*a*) Draw the histogram and frequency polygon for the above data.
(*b*) Draw both ogives.
(*c*) Draw frequency curve.
(*d*) Draw pie diagram.

10. The data represents sugar levels in diabetic mellitus patient measured (*i*) fasting and (*ii*) post prandial in mg/dl in different months.

Patient I.D/Month	Fasting blood sugar	Post parandial
5009 / January	90	224
5018 / February	87	118
5126 / March	103	168
3104 / April	96	154
4132 / May	120	210
2764 / June	132	210
1734 / July	123	221
5492 / August	149	236
2448 / September	143	192
1228 / October	181	275

(*a*) Draw range graph for the above data.
(*b*) Draw graphs separately for fasting blood sugar and post prandial blood sugar.
(*c*) Determine the trend in the patient with respect to blood sugar.

References:

1. Gupta S.P. 1990 "Statistical Methods". Sultan Chand & Sons, New Delhi.
2. Wayne W. Daniel 2008 Biostatistics, 9th edition, John Wiley & Sons. Inc. Newyork.
3. P.N. Arora *et al.* 2007 "Comprehensive Statistical Methods" Sultan Chand and company Ltd. First edn. New Delhi.
4. VK. Kapoor 1986 "Problems and solutions in Business statistics" Sultan Chand and sons New Delhi.

Answers for Objective Questions

1 – c; 2 – a; 3 – b; 4 – a; 5 – c; 6 – b; 7 – d; 8 – d; 9 – b; 10 – a.

4 DIFFERENT STATISTICAL MEASURES

4.1 INTRODUCTION

In the previous three chapters, we have discussed various methods of data collection and it's presentation through diagrams and graphs. Presentation of the data, in diagrams and graphs helps the reader to take more appropriate decisions quickly. These methods help to take decisions by comparison. Basic disadvantage of diagrammatic and graphical representation of statistical data is that they represent approximate values but not accurate values for the variables. Hence, these approximate values, sometimes lead to wrong conclusions. For example, height if a person A is 5.23 feet and height of another person B is 4.93 feet. If we approximate, both values should be equal to 5 feet (using common principle of rounding off a figure) and based on this information if we conclude that A and B are of equal height, then our decision is wrong. We are in scientific world and decisions are to be taken based on accurate values but not on approximate values. To do this we require statistical measures which give more accurate values, so that our decisions are more reasonable and reliable.

In the present chapter, we introduce various statistical measures which can give more accurate and precise results so that the decisions taken using such results have more statistical validity.

They are

(*i*) Measures of central tendencies
(*ii*) Measures of variation
(*iii*) Coefficient of variation
(*iv*) Skewness and
(*v*) Kurtosis

These statistical measures along with related measures are discussed in the rest of this chapter.

4.2. MEASURES OF CENTRAL TENDENCIES

Measures of central tendencies are also known as measures of location parameter or simply averages. Basic objective is to facilitate comparison among several variables. Thus basic purpose of averages is to select a single observation from a group of data, which is useful for comparison of two or more variables. Such a selected single number from a group of numbers is called "Central Value" or "Important Value" or an "average". Since, it is selected from a group of data; naturally it should represent the entire data. Thus an average is a representative number, selected through a procedure from a group of data.

The term average is used slightly with a different meaning in statistics than used by a common man in day to day life. For example, an average student in common terminology means that the student is neither too intelligent nor too dull but a mediocre type. But in statistics, the term average is used as a representative, representing the entire group of data. Since an average is a representative representing the group, it should satisfy certain properties which are known as "desirable properties of a good average". These desirable properties are listed as follows:

4.2.1. Desirable Properties of a Good Average

Professor G.U. Yule suggested that, following are the properties, which are to be satisfied by a good or an ideal measure of central tendency.

1. It should be easy to understand and easy to calculate.
2. It should be easy to interpret.
3. It should be rigidly defined so that different people may not interpret it differently.
4. It should be based on every item of data.
5. It should be have sampling stability. It means that if the average is computed from similar samples, the result also must be similar.
6. It should not be influenced by extreme values.
7. It should be useful for further statistical analysis.
8. It should be least affected by the fluctuations of the sampling.

4.2.2. Types of Averages

There are many types of averages available in literature. For example: (1) arithmetic mean (2) median (3) mode (4) geometric Mean (4) harmonic mean (5) weighted averages (6) moving averages and so on. But, we discuss in this book, only first three averages namely (1) Arithmetic mean (2) Median and (3) Mode, keeping in view of the syllabus of biostatistics. These three are most popularly used averages. Other averages are having limited applications in biological sciences.

4.2.3. Arithmetic Mean

Arithmetic mean is also known as simply "mean" which is defined as the ratio of sum of data items to the number of data items. If $x_1, x_2, \ldots, x_n$ are data items then arithmetic mean or mean is defined as :

$$\text{Mean} = \text{A.M.} = (x_1 + x_2 + \ldots + x_n)/n$$

or

$$\sum_{i=1}^{n} x_i/n \qquad \ldots(4.2.1)$$

This is the formula for raw data.

Usually, arithmetic mean is denoted by the symbol $\bar{X}$ to be read as X–bar. Mean satisfies seven desirable properties except one. That is it is much affected by extreme values. Extreme values are too large values or too small values.

4.2.4. Merits, Demerits and Uses of Mean

Merits :

1. It is easy to calculate.
2. It is easy to understand.
3. It is rigidly defined by a mathematical formula.
4. Its calculation is depending on all the observations.
5. It is having sampling stability.
6. It is un-affected by fluctuations of sampling
7. It is the best measure to compare two or more data sets.

Demerits:

1. It may not be represented in actual data and hence, it is a theoretical value only.
2. It is much affected by extreme values. That is mean is much affected by too large or too small values of the data.
3. It is not possible, if all the values in the data are not known.
4. It cannot be determined for the quantitative data.
5. Sometimes, it gives meaningless results.
6. It cannot be determined in open-end class or classes with unequal width of class intervals.
7. It cannot be determined graphically.

Uses:

1. It is more popularly used in many real life problems.
2. It is used in estimation of parameters of a population.
3. It is extensively used in many practical situations.
4. It is extensively used in market research.
5. It is popularly used in biological studies and medical research.

Apart from the above discussed, arithmetic mean satisfies some special mathematical properties. These properties are satisfied by mean alone and other averages do not possess these properties.

Special Mathematical Properties of Arithmetic Mean

1. Sum of the deviations of observations taken from its arithmetic mean is always zero '0'. That is $\sum_{i=1}^{n} (xi - \bar{X}) = 0$. This property is similar to the concept of "center of gravity". For any object, if we subtract mass to the left of centre of gravity of the object from the mass to the right of centre of gravity of the object, we naturally get zero. Thus mean provide the centre of gravity for the given data series. This property is explained with an example as follows:

Example (4.2.1): Consider the series 15, 25, 12, 18 and 30, then mean = 100/5 = 20. Now subtract 20 from each observation as follows:

15 – 20 = – 5; 25 – 20 = +5; 12 – 20 = –8; 18 – 20 = – 2; and 30 – 20 = +10.

Now add these differences, we get zero. That is, – 5 + 5 – 8 – 2 + 10 = 0.

2. The product of the average with number of items in the data will results the sum of the items. That is $n \times \bar{X} = \sum_{i=1}^{n} xi$

Using this property many bits are asked in competitive examinations. This is explained with the following examples:

Example (4.2.2): A and B on the average has Rs. 100 and A has Rs. 100. What is the amount with B?

Solution: We feel like selecting the answer zero, in fact, it is a wrong answer. A and B on the average has Rs. 100. Therefore 2 × 100 = 200. Since A has 100 rupees, B also has 200 – 100 = 100 rupees.

Example (4.2.3): The average mark of a class consisting of 12 students in biology is 68 marks. When a new student joined into the class, the average increased to 70 marks. Find the marks obtained by the newly joined student.

Solution: Average mark of 12 students is 68.

Therefore, total marks = 12 × 68 = 816.

When a new student joined, class strength will become 13

Therefore, 13 students total marks are = 13 × 70 = 910.

Hence marks obtained by the newly joined student = 910 – 816 = 94 marks.

Thus newly joined student got 94 marks in Biology.

3. If $\bar{X}_1$ is average of data items of size 'n_1' and $\bar{X}_2$ is average of another data of size 'n_2' then the combined mean for both the groups denoted by $\bar{X}_c$. Then $\bar{X}_c = (n_1\bar{X}_1 + n_2\bar{X}_2)/(n_1 + n_2)$.

This property is another important property where we can find combined mean for different groups if individual group mean and strength are known. We need not know the actual observations, still we can find combined mean.

Example: (4.2.4): A class consisting of 15 students got 65 as average mark and another class consisting of 20 students got the average as 70.

Calculate the combined average of both classes.

Solution: Total marks of first class = 15 × 65 = 975.

Similarly, total marks of second class = 20 × 70 = 1400

Therefore, total marks of both classes 975 + 1400 = 2375.

Total strength of both classes = 15 + 20 = 35.

Therefore, combined average = 2375/35 = 67.85714 marks.

4. $\sum_{i=1}^{n}(x_i - A)^2$ is minimum only when $A = \bar{X}$. This property is similar to the concept that distance between any two points is minimum only when the path is a straight line. Thus shortest distance between any two places is considered as aerial distance between them. This is because of the fact that in air we can travel in a straight line path.

That is sum of squared deviations of observations taken from arithmetic mean is always minimum. This property is similar to the property that distance between two points or places is minimum or smallest only when line joining them is a straight line. This property is explained with an example as follows:

Example (4.2.5): Consider the series 15,20,25,30,35 and its mean is 25. Subtract the mean from each observation and square the differences as follows: $15 - 25 = (-10)^2 = 100$; $20 - 25 = (-5)^2 = 25$, $25 - 25 = (0)^2 = 0$; $30 - 25 = (5)^2 = 25$; $35 - 25 = (10)^2 = 100$ Now add these squared differences = 100 + 25 + 0 + 25 + 100 = 250 units. The property says that other than the mean 25, if you consider any other number and do the squares of differences, the sum will be larger than 250. For instance, consider 30 and do the same operation as follows:

$15 - 30 = (-15)^2 = 225$; $20 - 30 = (-10)^2 = 100$; $25 - 30 = (-5)^2 = 25$; $30 - 30 = 0$ and $35 - 30 = (5)^2 = 25$. Therefore total of squared differences is 375 which is larger than 250. Reader is advised to try with any other number and verify that squared differences is larger than 250. This is true with any series of data.

5. If the mean of 'n' observations $x_1, x_2, \ldots, x_n$ is $\bar{X}$ then mean of $(x_1 + a)$, $(x_2 + a), \ldots, (x_n + a)$ is $(\bar{X} + a)$. That is if any constant is added to each observation, then the mean also should be added by the same constant to get the mean of new series.
6. If the mean of 'n' observations $x_1, x_2, \ldots, x_n$ is $\bar{X}$ then mean of $(x_1 - a)$, $(x_2 - a), \ldots, (x_n - a)$ is $(\bar{X} - a)$. That is if any constant is subtracted from each observation, then the mean also should be subtracted by the same constant to get the mean of new series.
7. If the mean of 'n' observations $x_1, x_2, \ldots, x_n$ is $\bar{X}$. If each observation is multiplied by a constant $c \neq 0$, then mean of new series is $c\bar{X}$.
8. If the mean of 'n' observations $x_1, x_2, \ldots, x_n$ is $\bar{X}$. If each observation is divided by a constant $c \neq 0$, then mean of new series is $\bar{X}/c$.

4.2.5. Calculation of Arithmetic Mean for Raw Data

Calculation of arithmetic mean for raw or un-classified data uses the formula given in (4.2.1).

Example (4.2.6): Following data represents marks of 12 students in Bio-statistics.

55, 47, 25, 17, 45, 62, 89, 10, 62, 72, 82 and 66.

Calculate arithmetic mean for the above data.

Solution: Calculate sum of the observations. That is 55 + 47 +.,.,., + 66 = 632.

Number of observations = n = 12

Using the formula (4.2.1) $\bar{X}$ = 632/12 = 52.66667 Marks.

Remarks:

1. It is interesting to note that the mean 52.6667 is not at all a member in the given data set. This is what it meant by demerit 5. Sometimes mean gives meaningless results.
2. It can be easily verified that other properties are true.

For example, if any data item is slightly changes, average or the mean will change automatically.

4.2.6. Calculation of Arithmetic Mean for a Frequency Distribution

Calculation of mean for classified data or frequency distribution is of two types, namely: (a) direct method (b) short-cut (or) step deviation method. Now we proceed to explain these two methods in the following paragraphs.

(a) Direct method:

Calculation of arithmetic mean for a frequency distribution through direct method is explained in the following steps:

Step–1 Calculate mid-values for each class denoted by 'm_i', where m_i = (Upper Limit + Lower Limit) /2 or $(U_i + L_i) / 2$ $i = 1, 2,.,., K$. Here K represents number of classes.

Step–2 Let f_i denote the frequency if ith class. $i = 1, 2 ,.,.,., K$.

Step–3 Calculate the product of f_i and m_i for each class.

Step–4 Calculate the total of the products $f_i\, m_i$. That is $\sum_{i=1}^{k} f_i\, m_i$

Step–5 Arithmetic mean $\bar{X} = \left(\sum_{i=1}^{k} f_i\, m_i\right)/N$, where

$$N = \sum_{i=1}^{k} f_i = \text{Total of the frequency.}$$

Using above explained steps now we proceed to calculate mean for some problems.

Example (4.2.7): Following data represents distribution of students according to marks in biology. Calculate the arithmetic mean for the data.

Class interval	0 – 20	20 – 40	40 – 60	60 – 80	80 – 100
Frequency	15	25	45	43	22

Solution:

Class interval	Mid-values (m_i)	Frequency (f_i)	Product of $f_i\, m_i$
0 – 20	10	15	150
20 – 40	30	25	750
40 – 60	50	45	2250
60 – 80	70	43	3010
80 – 100	90	22	1980
Total		150 = N	$8140 = \sum_{i=1}^{k} f_i\, m_i$

$$\text{Arithmetic mean} = \bar{X} = \left(\sum_{i=1}^{k} f_i\, m_i\right)/N = 8140/150 = 54.26667 \text{ marks.}$$

Above method will become cumbersome, if m are in decimals and f are large in size. In such situations, we use shortcut method which is explained as follows.

(b) Step deviation method or short cut method:

Various steps to calculate arithmetic mean in step deviation method is explained as follows.

Step –1 Calculate mid-values for each class denoted by 'm_i', where m_i = (Upper Limit + Lower Limit)/2 or $(U_i + L_i)/2$ $i = 1, 2,.,., K$. Here K represents number of classes.

Step – 2 Calculate deviations denoted by $d_i = (m - A)/c$, where c is the class interval and $i = 1, 2,.,.,., K$

Step – 3 Let f_i denote the frequency if ith class. $i = 1, 2,.,.,., K$.

Step – 4 Calculate the product of f_i and d_i for each class.

Step – 5 Calculate the total of the products $f_i\, d_i$. That is $\sum_{i=1}^{k} f_i\, d_i$

Step – 6 Arithmetic Mean $\bar{X} = A + \sum_{i=1}^{k} (f_i\, d_i)/NC$ (4.2.2)

where $N = \sum_{i=1}^{k} f_i$ = Total of the frequency.

Example (4.2.8): Following is the distribution of patients admitted in a year according to their completed years of age. Calculate the arithmetic mean using step deviation method.

Age	10 – 19	20 – 29	30 – 39	40 – 49	50 – 59	60 – 69	70 – 79
Frequency	113	158	295	562	397	113	82

Solution:

The data is given in inclusive method and hence, is to be converted into exclusive method of class intervals. To do this, calculate the difference between the lower limit of the second class and the upper limit of the first class, that is 20 – 19 = 1. Divide this difference by two. That is ½.

Hence add ½ to the upper limit and subtract ½ from the lower limit or add upper limit of previous class to the lower limit of the next class and divide this sum be two to get new upper and lower limits. This adjustment is to be made for all classes. Thus we have the following table with new class intervals.

Class interval	Mid-values (m_i)	$d_i = (m_i - A)/c$	Frequency (f_i)	$d_i \times f_i$
9.5 – 19.5	14.5	– 3	113	– 339
19.5 – 29.5	24.5	– 2	158	– 316
29.5 – 39.5	34.5	– 1	295	– 295
39.5 – 49.5	44.5 = A	0	562	0
49.5 – 59.5	54.5	1	397	397
59.5 – 69.5	64.5	2	113	226
69.5 – 79.5	74.5	3	82	156
Total			1720 = N	$171 = \sum_{i=1}^{k} f_i d_i$

Here A = Assumed mean

Therefore $$\bar{X} = A + \left(\frac{\sum_{i=1}^{k} f_i d_i}{N} \right) C = 44.5 + (-171/1720) \times 10$$

$$= 44.5 - 0.99419 = 43.50581 \text{ years}$$

or 43.5 years (approximately).

4.2.7. Median

Arithmetic mean satisfies all the desirable properties of a good average, except that, it is much affected by extreme values. To overcome this difficulty of arithmetic mean, another method of selecting the average is introduced known as Median. By definition median is a middle most value. Basic property of median is that it divides the data into two equal halves such that number of data items on its left side is equal to the number of data items on its right side. To calculate the median, the following procedure is used.

Median is defined as the middle most or the central value of the variable in a set of observations, when the observations are arranged either in an ascending or descending order of their magnitude.

4.2.8. Calculation of the Median

(a) For raw data

Step I : Arrange the given data in an increasing order (ascending) (or) decreasing order (descending)

Step II : Median: The item occupying $((n + 1)/2)^{th}$ place (if n = odd number) (4.2.3)

Median: (item occupying $(n/2)^{th}$ place + item in $((n/2) + 1)^{th}$ place)/2. (4.2.4)

if n is an even number. That is in this case median is the average of the middle most two numbers.

Example: (4.2.9): Calculate the median for the following data.

Marks: 55, 47, 25, 17, 45, 62, 89, 10, 62, 72 and 82.

Solution: Arrange the given data in an ascending order of magnitude.

Ascending order: 10, 17, 25, 45, 47, **55**, 62, 62, 72, 82, 89.

Number of observations n = 11 (odd number). Therefore, using the formula (4.2.3) we have the item occupying $(11 + 1)/2 = 6^{th}$ place in the arrangement. That is 55 marks. This means that 5 students in the series are below or equal to 55 marks and 5 students in the series are above or equal to 55 marks. Thus median divides the data into two equal halves.

Remark: It is interesting to note that instead of 89, if we have 189 or 1089, the median value does not change. Similarly, instead of 10, if we have 5 or 2 the median value does not change. Thus median is not affected by extreme values.

Example (4.2.10): Calculate the median for the following series.

Marks: 55, 47, 25, 17, 45, 62, 89, 10, 62, 72, 82 and 66.

Solution: Arrange the data in ascending order of magnitude.

Ascending Order: 10, 17, 25, 45, 47, 55, 62, 62, 66, 72, 82, 89.

Number of observations n = 12 (even number). Therefore we have to use the formula (4.2.4). $[n/2 = 12/2\ 6^{th}$ item + $(n/2) +1 = 7^{th}$ item]/2. That is median = (55 + 62)/2 = 58.5 marks. This means that 6 students got less than or equal to 58.5 marks and 6 students got greater than or equal to 58.5 marks.

Remark: It is interesting to note that instead of 89, if we have 189 or 1089, the median value does not change. Similarly, instead of 10, if we have 5 or 2 the median value does not change. Thus median is not affected by extreme values.

(b) Calculation of median for classified data:

In order to calculate median for classified data or for a frequency distribution following steps are to be followed.

Step – 1: First calculate less than cumulative frequencies for the given data.

Step – 2: Determine the values of N and $N/2$.

Step – 3: Determine to which class the value $N/2$ belongs using cumulative frequencies calculated in step – 1. This class is called Median Class (M.C.)

Step – 4: Mode = $L + \dfrac{\left(\dfrac{N}{2} - c.f\right)}{f} \times C.$ ...(4.2.5)

Where L = Lower limit of the M.C.

N = Total of the frequencies.

$c.f.$ = Cumulative frequency up to the M.C.

f = Frequency of the M.C.

C = Class interval of the M.C.

Example (4.2.11): Calculate median for the following frequency distribution.

Class interval	0 – 20	20 – 35	35 – 50	50 – 60	60 – 75	Above 75
Frequency	125	142	385	462	120	82

Solution: First calculate cumulative frequencies and determine the median class (M.C.). Then determine other values, namely, L, c.f., *f* and *c* values and substitute these values in the formula (4.2.5).

Class interval	Frequency	Less than cumulative frequency
0 – 20	125	125
20 – 35	142	12 + 142 = 267
35 – 50	385	267 + 385 = 652
50 – 60 = M.C.	462	652 + 462 = 1114
60 – 75	120	1114 + 120 = 1234
Above 75	82	1234 + 82 = 1316 = N

Therefore $N/2$ 1316/2 = 658. To determine median class, we can observe that cumulative frequencies are 652 up to the class 35 – 50. Therefore 658 must lie in the class 50 – 60. Hence, 50 – 60 is the median class (M.C.). For this problem $L = 50$, $c.f. = 652$, $f = 462$, $C = 10$. Substitution these values in the formula (4.2.5) we have:

Median = 50 + [(1316/2 – 652)/ 462] × 10 = 50 + [(658 – 652)/462] × 10

= 50 + (6/462) × 10 = 50 + 0.12987 = 50.12987 marks

= 50 marks (approximately).

This implies that 658 students got marks less than or equal to 50 marks and another 658 students got marks greater than or equal to 50 marks. Thus median divides the data into two equal halves.

4.2.9. Merits, Demerits and Uses of Median

Merits:

1. It is easy to understand
2. It is not affected by extreme values.
3. It can be located graphically.
4. It is the best measure for qualitative data like, beauty, honesty, intelligence, pain and so on.

5. It can be easily located frequency distributions with unequal class intervals.
6. It can be determined even by inspection.
7. It can be determined in open-end classification.

Demerits:

1. It is not useful for further statistical analysis.
2. It is not depending on all items in the data.
3. It is not having sampling stability.
4. It is not rigidly defined.
5. It is not suitable in those situations where due importance is given to extreme values.

Uses:

1. Median is the middle most value in the frequency distribution of given series and hence used in open – end classes.
2. Median is called positional average and hence has operational convenience.
3. Median can be determined graphically, by plotting upper limits and less than cumulative frequencies, draw less than ogive. Determine $N/2$ on y-axis and draw parallel line to x-axis to cut the curve. From that intersection point draw vertical line, parallel to y-axis to cut x-axis. The point at which the vertical line cuts x-axis is the median point.
4. Median is used in many practical problems, where arithmetic mean gives meaningless results.
5. Median is particularly useful in qualitative nature data.

4.2.10. Quartiles, Deciles and Percentiles

In order to divide the data into two equal halves, we use the concept of median. Similarly, if we want to divide the data into four equal parts, we use the concept of "*Quartiles*". There are three quartiles denoted by Q_1, Q_2 and Q_3, Q_1 is called first quartile. 1/4th observations will be on the left of Q_1 and 3/4th observations will be on the right of $Q_1 \cdot Q_2$ = Median and Q_3 = Third quartile. 3/4th observations will be on the left side of Q_3 and 1/4th observations will be on the right side of Q_3. Quartiles are calculated on similar lines of median by using the same formula except that N is to be divided by 4, instead of 2. Thus, formula for Q_i are:

$$Q_i = L + \frac{\left(i\frac{N}{4} - c.f\right)}{f} \times C. \; i = 1, 2, 3. \qquad (4.2.6)$$

Where L = Lower limit of the Q_i class.

N = Total of the frequencies.

$c.f.$ = Cumulative frequency up to the Q_i class.

f = Frequency of the Q_i class.

C = Class Interval of the Q_i class.

On similar lines, we can divide the series into 10 equal parts, by using "*Deciles*". Thus deciles are nine in number denoted by D, i = 1, 2, .,.,., 9. While calculating deciles, N is to be divided by 10. Thus formulae for deciles are:

$$D_i = L + \frac{\left(i\frac{N}{10} - c.f\right)}{f} \times C. \quad i = 1, 2, .,.,.,9. \qquad (4.2.7)$$

If we divide the data into 100 equal parts, then they are called "Percentiles", denoted by P_i, i = 1, 2, .,.,., 99. While calculating percentiles, N is to be divided by 100. Formula for percentiles is given by:

$$P_i = L + \frac{\left(i\frac{N}{100} - c.f\right)}{f} \times C. \quad i = 1, 2, .,.,.,99. \qquad (4.2.8)$$

Example: (4.2.12): Following data represent the frequency distribution of 5000 students according to their marks in a competitive examination. 500 students are to be called for an interview. Determine the passing mark to be announced. Also determine Q_1, Q_3, D_4, D_7, P_{52}, P_{86} and P_{95} values.

C.I.	< 50	50 – 70	70 – 90	90 – 100	100 – 110	110 – 130	130 – 145	145 – 150
Freq.	40	480	592	678	684	1120	1254	152

Solution: Calculate less than cumulative frequencies.

Class interval	Frequencies	Less than cumulative frequencies
Less than 50	40	40
50 – 70	480	40 + 480 = 520
70 – 90	592	520 + 592 = 1112
90 – 100	678	1112 + 684 = 1790
100 – 110	684	1790 + 678 = 2474
110 – 130	1120	2474 + 1120 = 3594
130 – 145	1254	3594 + 1254 = 4848
145 – 150	152	4848 + 152 = 5000

To determine qualifying mark to call 500 students, we proceed as follows.

500 candidates out of 5000 is 10 per cent. Therefore we have to find the percentile such that 90 % should be on the left side and 10 % should be on the right side. Thus we have to find P_{90} or D_9 = 90 (5000/100) or 9(5000/10) = 4500.

P_{90} or D_9 = 130 + [(4500 – 3594)/1254] × 15 = 130 + 10.837 = 140.837.

= 141 marks.(approx.)

In order to call 500 students, qualifying mark should be considered as 141.

For calculation of Q_1 consider 5000/4 = 1250.

Therefore $Q_1 = 90 + [(1250 - 1112)/678] \times 10 = 90 + 2.0354 = 92.0354$
$= 92$ marks (approx.)

Similarly $Q_3 = 130 + [(3 \times 1250 - 3594)/1254] \times 15 = 130 + 1.86603$
$= 131.86603 = 132$ marks (approx.)

$D_4 = 100 + [(4(5000/10) - 1790)/684] \times 10 = 100 + 3.07018$
$= 103.07018 = 103$ marks (approx.)

$D_7 = 110 + [(7(5000/10) - 2474)/1120] \times 20 = 110 + 18.32143$
$= 128.32143 = 128$ marks (approx.)

$P_{52} = 110 + [(52(5000/100) - 2474)/1120] \times 20 = 110 + 2.25$
$= 112.25 = 12$ marks (approx.).

$P_{86} = 130 + [(86 \times 50 - 3594)/1254] \times 15 = 130 + 8.44498$
$= 138.44498 = 138$ marks (approx.)

$P_{95} = 130 + [(95 \times 50 - 3594)/1254] \times 15 = 130 + 13.82775$
$= 143.82775 = 144$ marks (approx.).

Example (4.2.13): The following data represents the frequency distribution of 200 students according to their heights measured in c.ms. Determine Q_1, median (Q_2) and Q_3 graphically.

Height (in cms)	135–140	140–145	145–150	150–155	155–160	160–165	165–170	170–175
Frequency	14	19	28	44	42	24	17	12

Solution: First we have to calculate Less Than Cumulative Frequencies (L.T.C.F.) in the following table.

Height (in cms)	Frequency	Less than cumulative frequency
135 – 140	14	14
140 – 145	19	14 + 19 = 33
145 – 150	28	33 + 28 = 61
150 – 155	44	61 + 44 = 105
155 – 160	42	105 + 42 = 147
160 – 165	24	147 + 24 = 171
165 – 170	17	171 + 17 = 188
170 – 175	12	188 + 12 = 200

Now consider upper limits of each class and less than cumulative frequencies in a separate table and draw less than ogive.

U.L	140	145	150	155	160	165	170	175
L.T.C.F.	14	33	61	105	147	171	188	200

Since $N/4 = 200/4 = 50$, $2(N/4) = 100$ and $3(N/4) = 150$ draw parallel lines to x-axis at 50, 100 and 150 on y-axis. These lines cut the curve at three distinct places. From those points draw three lines parallel to y-axis to cut x-axis. These points on

x-axis represents Q_1, Q_2 = median and Q_3 respectively. This procedure of finding median or quartiles is explained in the following figure. Therefore on similar lines, we can determine

$$Q_1 = 144 \text{ cms (approx.)}$$

$$Q_2 = \text{Median} = 150 \text{ (approx.)}$$

and $$Q_3 = 155 \text{ (approx.)}.$$

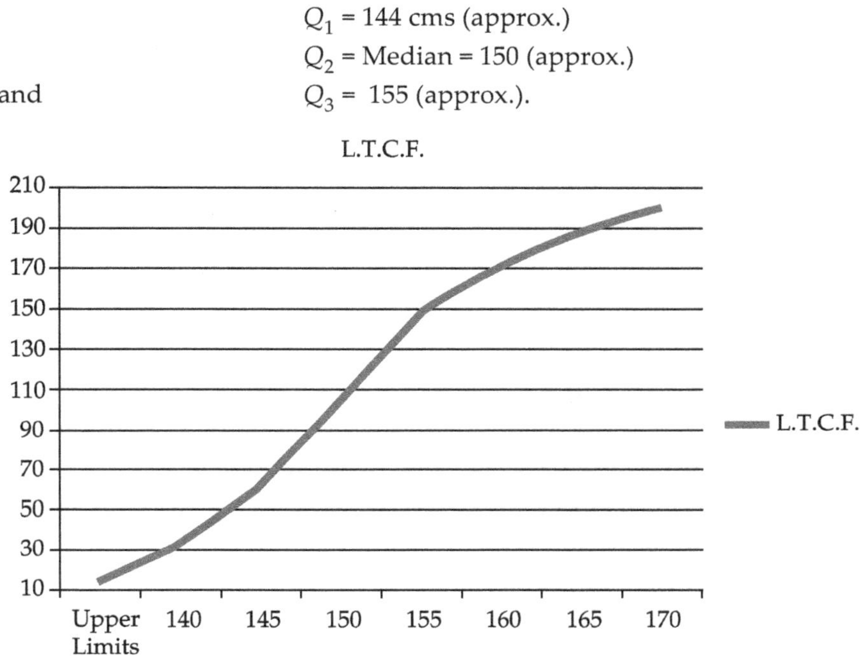

Fig. 4.2.1: *Determination of median and quartiles graphically*

First vertical line cutting the curve at 144 determines, the first quartile Q_1, and the second vertical line (middle line) cutting the curve at 150 determines, the second quartile = median = Q_2, and the third vertical line at 155 determines third quartile Q_3.

On similar lines, one can determine any deciles or percentiles drawing appropriate lines from y-axis to x-axis via the frequency curve.

Remark: It is advised the reader to calculate the exact values of first, second and third quartiles using the respective formula and verify answers obtained through the graph. We can observe that graphical method provides approximate solutions to the questions but not accurate values. To have accurate solutions, one has to calculate the answers using the formula. Calculating the answer through the formula is known as mathematical solutions. Thus solutions obtained through a graph are called graphical solutions. One can easily observe that mathematical solutions more accurate than graphical solutions.

4.2.11. Mode

By definition, Mode is the most typical/popular value in a series of data items. Thus, the mode value repeats more number of times in a given data. For example, in the series 23, 45, 27, 45, 67, 45, 36, 34, 45, 36, 27, 52, 45, 34 and 45, the number 45 repeated 6 times. Therefore 45 is the mode for the given series, because 45 repeated more number of times than other numbers. Mode is popularly used in garment making and shoe manufacturing to determine model size. Mode popularly used in market research, to determine model T.V.'s, model services, model transport, model dress, model family size and so on. Mode can also be determined graphically, by drawing frequency curve. The peak point at which the curve reaches maximum height is called mode point.

4.2.12. Calculation of Mode for a Frequency Distribution

Calculation of mode for raw data is nothing but obtaining frequency for each observation representing number of repetitions by each observation and the observation which has highest frequency is called Mode. In a frequency distribution, the class which has maximum frequency called Modal Class (Mo.C.) To calculate mode for a frequency distribution, we use the following formula:

$$\text{Mode} = \text{Mo} = L + \left[\frac{f_1 - f_0}{2f_1 - f_2 - f_0}\right] \times C \tag{4.2.9}$$

Where f_0 = Frequency of the class prior to the model class
f_1 = Frequency of the model class
f_2 = Frequency of the class after the model class
L = Lower limit of the model class
C = Class interval of the model class.

Using the above formula, finding out of mode is also known as method of interpolation.

Example: (4.2.14): Determine the mode mathematically and graphically for the following frequency distribution representing sale a medicine number of boxes per day in three months.

C.I.	21–22	23–24	25–26	27–28	29–30	31–32	33–34	35–36
Days	3	14	22	18	16	8	6	3

Solution: Since the given class is an inclusive classification, first we have to convert the given class into exclusive method. Following the procedure explained earlier, we have:

Class interval (number of boxes sold)	Frequency
20.5–22.5	3
22.5–24.5	14
24.5–26.5 (modal class)	22
26.5–28.5	18
28.5–30.5	16
30.5–32.5	8
32.5–34.5	6
34.5–36.5	3

For the given problem the class 24.5 – 26.5 is the model class because, the corresponding class frequency is highest. That is 22.

Hence we have $f_0 = 14$, $f_1 = 22$, $f_2 = 18$, $L = 24.5$ and $c = 2$. Substituting these values in the formula (4.2.9), we have:

$$\text{Mode} = 24.5 + [(22 - 14)/(2 \times 22 - 14 - 18] \times 2 = 24.5 + [8/(44 - 32)] \times 2$$
$$= 24.5 + 1.33333 = 24.83333 = 25 \text{ boxes per day (approx.)}.$$

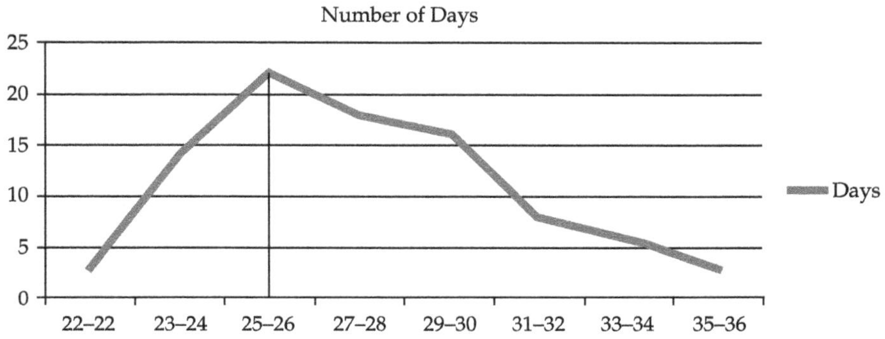

Fig. 4.2.2: *Determination of mode graphically.*
Number of boxes of medicine sold per day.

4.2.13. Merits, Demerits and Uses of Mode

Merits:

1. It is very easy to understand.
2. It is not affected by extreme values in the data.
3. It is the most suitable for qualitative data.
4. It can be located graphically.
5. It can be determined in open-end classification.
6. It can be determined even if class intervals are unequal.
7. It can be determined by inspection in many real life situations

Demerits:

1. It is not useful for further algebraic treatment.
2. It is not depending on every item of the data.
3. It is not rigidly defined. For example, if two or three observations repeated equally, then all those observations should be considered as modes.
4. It is a positional average.
5. It does not have sampling stability.
6. It is not suitable in those situations, where, due importance is to be given for extreme data items.

Uses:

1. It is popularly used where, data cannot be measured numerically, in surveys.
2. It is best suited to deal qualitative data.
3. It is popularly used in medical and biological research.
4. It is popularly used in market research.

Among mean, median and mode, mean satisfies majority of the pre-requisites of a good average and hence mean is most popularly used in many fields of research. Among the averages, mean is the most commonly and frequently used average. Only difficulty with the mean is that it is much affected by extreme values. To overcome this difficulty, after collecting the data, editing is to be done compulsorily, where, we eliminate extreme values, if they are present in the data. Thus mean can be used safely for such edited data. Mean is also known as measures if central tendencies because mean lies somewhere in between the largest and smallest data item. Similarly, mean is also known as measures of location parameter, because it identifies the location or address of the on x-axis. This is explained with an example that if a road accident occurred on a high way and you want to give information to the ambulance for help. We generally identify the accident spot as **between 50th and 60th kilometer on N.H. 3., at 40th kilometer after New Delhi, towards Agra, and so on.**

Similar way, average identifies the address of the data or location of data on x-axis. Hence, mean is also known as "Location Parameter". Other averages like geometric mean or harmonic mean, moving averages are having special uses and having limited applications in time series data analysis. Hence, these averages are not included in this book. Now we proceed to discuss "Measures of Variation" in the following section.

4.3. MEASURES OF VARIATION OR DISPERSION

Averages alone cannot give entire information about a data series. For example, consider the following series:

Series–I	Series–II	Series–III	Series–IV
15	10	12	6
15	12	18	14
15	18	0	18
15	20	30	22
Total : 60	60	60	60
Mean : 15	15	15	15

In all the four series, mean is 15 and hence, if concluded that all the four series are same, our decision goes wrong. Hence, there is a need to have an idea about the variability or dispersion among the observations under consideration. How individual data items spread around the mean is called variation or dispersion. In the series – I all items are equal to the mean hence variability is zero. In series – III variation is very large because, minimum value is zero and maximum value is 30, next series – IV lesser variability than series-III. Series–II has still smaller variance than series–III and series–IV. Generally, we prefer that data where variation is small. **Lesser variation, represents greater the efficiency.** Thus efficiency of an estimate is measured through its variability. Therefore, there is a need to calculate and study the variation or dispersion present in the data, along with **averages**.

Since, measure of variation is also a representative, representing variation present in the data, pre-requisites discussed for a good average discussed in (4.2.1) should also must hold good for a **good measure of variation or dispersion.**

There are four methods of measuring variation or dispersion, namely:

1. The range.
2. Quartile deviation or inter quartile range.
3. Mean deviation and
4. Standard deviation.

4..3.1. The Range

The range is the simplest and easiest measure of variation or dispersion which is defined as the difference between the largest and the smallest data item in the given series. For example, the range for the series 23, 59, 72, 45, 24, 12, 39, 45 and 60 is 72 – 12 = 70 units.

Thus the formula for the range = $L - S$, where L = Largest data item and S = Smallest data item in the given series.

Example (4.3.1): Calculate the range for the following data:

Height (in cms)	135–140	140–145	145–150	150–155	155–160	160–165	165–170	170–175
Frequency	14	19	28	44	42	24	7	12

Solution: In the given problem,

$$L = 175 \text{ and } S = 135.$$

$$\text{Hence range} = L - S = 175 - 135 = 40 \text{ cms.}$$

4.3.2. Merits, Demerits and Uses of the Range

Merits:

1. It is simple to calculate and easiest to understand.
2. It is an absolute measure of dispersion.
3. It is popularly used in industry and biological sciences.
4. It does not require intricate mathematical knowledge.

Demerits:

1. It is not useful for further algebraic treatment.
2. It depends on extreme values.
3. It is not based on all data items in the series.
4. It does not have sampling stability.

Uses:

1. It is frequently used in statistical quality control.
2. It is used in forest research in estimating timber and in fisheries department to estimate weight of the fish.
3. It is popularly used in meteorology department.
4. It is used in market research.

4.3.3. Inter Quartile Range

Inter quartile range is a measure of dispersion based on upper or third quartile (Q_3) and the lower or first quartile (Q_1) of a series. Inter quartile range is also known as *Quartile Deviation* (*Q.D.*) and is defined as:

$$\text{Quartile Deviation (Q.D.)} = (Q_3 - Q_1)/2. \qquad ...(4.3.1)$$

Example (4.3.2): Calculate Q.D. for the series:

25, 12, 43, 62, 17, 82, 65, 59, 78, 49, 89, 15, 76, 90, 48 and 36.

Solution: First arrange the data in ascending order or magnitude.

Ascending order: 12, 15, 17, 25, 36, 43, 48, 49, 59, 62, 65, 76, 78, 82, 89, 90.

Here $N = 16$. $Q_1 = 16/4 = 4$th item in the arranged series = 25

$Q_3 = 3(16/4) = 12$th item in the arranged series = 76

Quartile deviation : Q.D. = $(Q_3 - Q_1)/2 = (76 - 25)/2 = 51/2 = 25.5$ is the inter quartile range.

Calculation of Q.D. for a Frequency Distribution

For a given frequency distribution, first we have to calculate first and third quartiles and use the formula given in (4.3.1) to find quartile deviation. This is explained with the following example:

Example: (4.3.3): Calculate quartile deviation for the following frequency distribution given in the example (4.2.13).

Solution: In the example we have already calculated that Q_1 = 144 cms and Q_3 = 155 cms. Therefore Q.D. = (155 – 144)/2 = 5.5 cms.

4.3.4. Merits, Demerits and Uses of Q.D.

Merits:

1. It is easy to understand and simple to calculate.
2. It is not affected by extreme values.
3. It is specially used in open end classification.
4. It is much better than the range.

Demerits:

1. It is not based on all data items.
2. It is not capable of further algebraic treatment.
3. It is not having sampling stability.
4. It is not a good representative to measure scatter of data items around the mean value.

Use:

1. It is mainly used in descriptive statistics, where data cannot be measured in numbers or in numeric form.
2. It is used in social sciences and market research.

4.3.5. Mean Deviation or Average Deviation

Above discussed methods namely, the range and quartile deviations are not based on all data items in the series. To do so, we have to calculate deviation of each observation from the mean in a data set and calculate the average of these deviations. Such a measure is known as Mean Deviation (M.D.). Mean deviation for a given set of data items is defined as the arithmetic mean of all absolute deviations. That is after ignoring the sign of deviations, obtaining the mean.

Example (4.3.4): Consider the following data representing marks of 10 students in biostatistics: Marks: 62, 52, 79, 81, 45, 89, 23, 68, 72 and 29.

Calculate the M.D., range and Q.D.

Solution: We have mean is 600/10 = 60. Now we have to subtract the mean 60 from each observation. Thus we have:

Deviations	Absolute	Deviations
62 – 60 = 2	2	
52 – 60 = – 8	8	Therefore M.D. = 182/10 = 18.2 marks.
79 – 60 = 19	19	We can observe that for the same data
81 – 60 = 21	21	The range is 89 – 23 = 66 marks.
45 – 60 = – 15	15	To calculate Q.D. arrange the data in
89 – 60 = 29	29	ascending order as follows:
23 – 60 = – 37	37	23, 29, 45, 52, 62, 68, 72, 79, 81 and 89
68 – 60 = 8	8	Thus Q_1 = (29 + 45)/2 = 37 marks.
72 – 60 = 12	12	Similarly, Q_3 = (79 + 81)/2 = 80 marks
29 – 60 = – 31	31	Hence Q.D. = (80 – 37)/2 = 21.5 marks
Total 0	182	

Calculation of Mean Deviation for a Frequency Distribution

To calculate M.D. for a frequency distribution, we use the formula

$$\text{M.D.} = \left(\left[\sum_{i=1}^{n} |d_i \ f_i| \right] / N \right) \times C \qquad (4.3.2)$$

Where $d_i = (m_i - A)/C$

f_i = frequency if ith class.

m_i = mid-value of ith class.

N = Total frequency.

A = Assumed mean

C = Class interval.

Example (4.3.5): Calculate mean deviation for the following frequency distribution.

Height (in cms)	135–140	140–145	145–150	150–155	155–160	160–165	165–170	170–175
Frequency	14	19	28	44	42	24	17	12

Solution:

Heights (in cms)	Frequency f_i	Mid-values m_i	Deviations $d_i = (m_i - A)/C$	$\lvert f_i \times d_i \rvert$
135 –140	14	137.5	– 4	56
140 – 145	19	142.5	– 3	57
145 – 150	28	147.5	– 2	56
150 – 155	44	152.5	– 1	44
155 – 160	42	157.5 = A	0	0
160 – 165	24	162.5	1	24
165 – 170	17	167.5	2	34
170 – 175	12	172.5	3	36
Total	200			256

Using (4.3.2) M.D. = (256/200) × 5 = 6.4 marks.

4.3.5. Merits, Demerits and Uses of Mean Deviation

Merits:

1. It is easy to understand and simple to calculate.
2. It is better than quartile deviation and range.
3. It depends on every item of the data.
4. It is less affected by extreme values.
5. It is least when deviations are taken from median.

Demerits:

1. Ignoring the direction of deviations is the basic criticism. While taking absolute deviations, we ignore the direction of the deviation.
2. It is rarely used in social sciences.
3. It is rarely used in statistical inference.
4. It is less efficient than the standard deviation.

Uses:

1. It is mainly used in economics to study the distribution of income and wealth in a society.
2. It is used in garments making, shoe making and market research.

4.3.6. Standard Deviation

Basically, the criticism on mean deviation is that it ignores the direction of deviations. That is in the calculations, we equate –500 to +500, which is mathematically wrong. We cannot consider loss of Rs. 10,000/- with a gain of Rs. 10,000/-. Hence to avoid this criticism, Karl Pearson suggested to squire each deviation and to nullify the effect of squiring, finally, we take square root to the mean of squared deviations.

This new measure is called Standard Deviation (S.D.) denoted by the symbol σ (Sigma). Standard Deviation is also known as **Root Mean Square Deviation** and is defined as:

$$\text{S.D.} = \sigma = \sqrt{\Sigma(x_i\ \bar{x})^2/n} \quad \text{(for raw data)} \qquad (4.3.3)$$

where

$\bar{X}$ = Arithmetic mean

n = number of observations.

Alternatively,

$$\text{S.D.} = \sigma = \sqrt{\{[\Sigma x^2/n] - [(\Sigma x/n)]^2\}} \quad \text{(for raw data).} \qquad (4.3.4)$$

Square of standard deviation is known as Variance and is denoted by σ^2.

Variance explains the spread or deviation of observations or data items around the mean in the given data.

Example (4.3.6): Calculate standard deviation and variance for the following data.

3, 4, 8, 9, 6, 2, 7, 5 and 1.

Solution: Mean = $\bar{X}$ = 45/9 = 5.

$3 - 5 = (-2)^2 = 4$	$2 - 5 = (-3)^2 = 9$	Sum of squares of deviations
$4 - 5 = (-1)^2 = 1$	$7 - 5 = (2)^2 = 4$	$= 4 + 1 + 9 + 16 + 1$ $+ 9 + 4 + 0 + 16$
$8 - 5 = (3)^2 = 9$	$5 - 5 = (0)^2 = 0$	= 60.
$9 - 5 = (4)^2 = 16$	$1 - 5 = (4)^2 = 16$	S.D.= $\sigma = \sqrt{60/9}$
$6 - 5 = (1)^2 = 1$		**= 2.58199 marks.**

Alternatively: $(3)^2 + (4)^2$.,.,. $(1)^2 = 9 + 16 + 64 + 81 + 36 + 4 + 49 + 25 + 1 = 285$.

$$\text{S.D.} = \sigma = \sqrt{[(285/9) - (45/9)^2]} = \sqrt{[31.6667 - 25]} = \textbf{2.58199 marks.}$$

Variance = $(2.58199)^2$ = 6.66667 units.

4.3.7. Merits, Demerits and Uses of Standard Deviation

Merits:

1. It is based on all items of the data.
2. It takes into account the direction of the deviations from the mean.
3. It is rigidly defined.

4. It is useful for further algebraic treatment.
5. It is having sampling stability.
6. It is a good representative of measure of deviation when extreme values not present.

Demerits:

1. It is difficult to compute, when compared to other measure.
2. It gives more importance to extreme values in the data.
3. It is not simple to understand.
4. It requires much time and labor to compute.

Uses:

1. It is widely used in biological and medical fields.
2. It is used in fitting a normal curve to a frequency distribution.
3. It is most widely used measure of dispersion in many fields of research.
4. It is used in statistical inference.

Remark: In measures of averages; the arithmetic mean, and in variation, standard deviations are most popular measures in any field of Research. Arithmetic mean explains the location and standard deviation explain the amount of spread present in any data series. These two measures are very useful to compare two or more series and to take decision. This concept is similar to explain a skin disease to doctor. First we should give information, where it is affected like on the hand or leg or stomach and how much area is affected around the circle of 1 cm or 2cms and so on. Similar way, mean explains location and S.D. explains variation present in the data.

4.3.8. Calculation of Standard Deviation for a Frequency Distribution

Calculation of standard deviation for a frequency distribution involves following steps:

Step – 1: Calculate mid-values m_i's for each class.

Step – 2: Take any m_i as assumed mean A and calculate d_i's, where, $d_i = (m_i - A)/C$. Here C = Class interval (equal class intervals in the frequency distribution is a must for this method).

Step – 3: Multiply the frequency f_i with d_i and calculate $\Sigma f_i d_i$.

Step – 4: Multiply once again $f_i d_i$ column with d_i to get $f_i d_i^2$ and calculate $\Sigma f_i d_i^2$.

Step – 5: Substitute the corresponding values in the formula for S.D.

$$\text{S.D.} = \sigma = \sqrt{\{[\Sigma f_i d_i^2/N] - [(\Sigma f_i d_i/N)]^2\}} \times C \quad \text{where } N = \Sigma f_i.$$

Example (4.3.7): Following data represents tail lengths of Albino rats measured in centi meters (cms). Calculate S.D. and variance.

Length in cms	2.5–3.0	3.0–3.5	3.5–4.0	4.0–4.5	4.5–5.0	5.0–5.5	5.5–6.0	6.0–6.5
Frequency	25	43	68	72	56	49	35	22

Solution:

C.I	Freq. f_i	m_i	d_i	$f_i d_i$	$f_i d_i^2$
2.5–3.0	25	2.75	–3	–75	225
3.0–3.5	43	3.25	–2	–86	172
3.5–4.0	68	3.75	–1	–68	68
4.0–4.5	72	4.25 = A	0	0	0
4.5–5.0	56	4.75	1	56	58
5.0–5.5	49	5.25	2	98	196
5.5–6.0	35	5.75	3	105	315
6.0–6.5	22	6.25	4	88	352
Total	370 = N			118	1386

$$\text{S.D.} = \sigma = \sqrt{\{[1386/370] - (118/370)^2} \times 0.5 = \sqrt{3.74595} - 0.10171 \times 0.5$$

$$= 0.9545 \text{ cms.}$$

$$\text{Variance} = \sigma^2 = 0.91106 \text{ cms.}$$

Important Note: All the measures of central tendencies and measures of variances discussed so far, in this chapter are measured depending on measuring units. That is, if the data is measured in kgs, these measures also should be in kgs. If the data is measured in cms, these measures also must be in cms. If the data is in marks, these measures also in marks and so on. If we want to compare two or three sets of data which are in measuring units, they should be converted into a common measuring unit. For example, if we want to compare two or three family expenditure on clothing, oil, wheat, and fruits, each item is in different measuring unit. That is cloth is measured in meters, oil is measured in liters, wheat in kilograms and fruits in numbers or dozens. Then comparison will become difficult. An alternative procedure is to consider the cost of these items measured in rupees or dollars or pounds and compare the expenditure of each family on these items. Sometimes, this conversion is also not possible. Consider the following example:

Example (4.3.8): A is a cricket player whose average is 154 runs with 81 runs as variance. Similarly, B is a hockey player, whose average is 8 goals with 4 goals as variance. We want to select one player among A and B for a prize. Which player we have to select for the prize?

In the above situation, conversion to common units is not possible. We cannot equate a cricket run with a hockey goal. To compare these two players, we require a measure free from measuring units. This can be done by using **"Coefficient of Variation"** which is explained as follows:

4.4. COEFFICIENT OF VARIATION

Coefficient of Variation (C.V) is a Statistical measure useful to compare two sets of data which are in two different measuring units and is defined as:

$$\text{C.V.} = (\sigma/\bar{x}) \times 100 \text{ or } (\text{S.D./Mean}) \times 100. \qquad (4.4.1)$$

In the example (4.3.8), if we find C.V of (A) = (9 runs / 154 runs)100 = 5.8442.

Similarly, C.V. of (B) = (2 goals/8 goals) 100 = 25.

Whose, C.V. is smaller, variance in that player is smaller. Hence, smaller C.V. player, as more consistent player. Therefore, player A is more consistent player and hence to be selected for the prize.

Important Note: This measure of C.V. become, free from measuring unit because, units get cancelled in the calculation of C.V. For C.V., we should not write measuring units like, kgs, Rs, cms, runs or goals.

4.5 SKEWNESS

In order to understand the concept of Skewness, first one has to understand the concept of **"Symmetry"**. Symmetry implies similarity on both left hand right hands from the middle. Left hand side shape should be mirror replica of right hand side. For example, our human body is symmetrical in the sense that : length of the left hand should be equal to the length of right hand, left and right eyes from nose should be at equidistant, left and right legs should be equal length and so on. Vertically divide the human body, left side portion is a mirror replica of right side portion. Thus Human body is symmetric. This concept of symmetry is explained another example that vehicle key is symmetric where door lock key is not symmetrical. The following figures are symmetrical

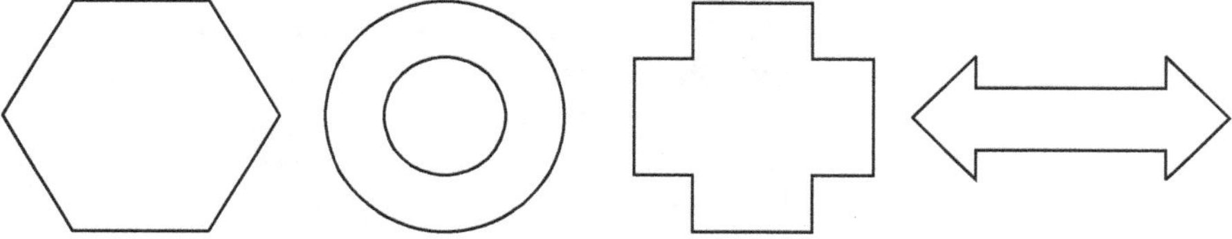

where as following pictures are asymmetrical or non-symmetric.

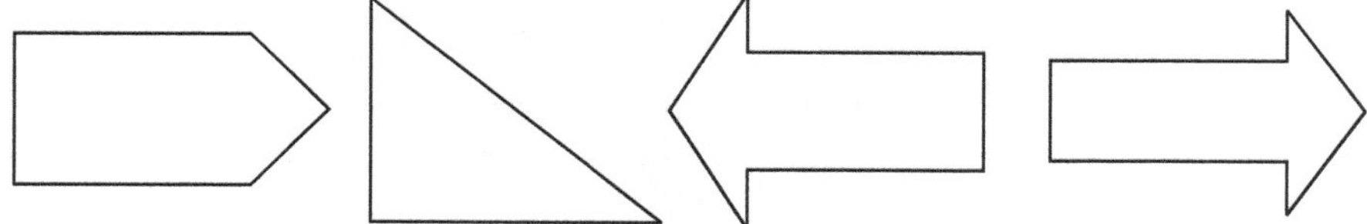

Lack of symmetry is measured through *skewness*. In a symmetrical distribution, Mean = Median = Mode. Thus this concept is used to measure asymmetry present in the data. In any distribution, If Mean ≠ Median ≠ Mode, such a distribution is known as **"Lack if symmetry"** or **"Skew symmetrical"** or **"Assymetrical"** distribution. In a skew symmetrical distribution, an empirical relation holds good between Mean, Median and Mode, which is given as follows.

$$(\text{Mean} - \text{Mode}) = 3\,(\text{Mean} - \text{Median}) \qquad (4.5.1)$$

Or

$$\text{Mode} = 3\,\text{Median} - 2\,\text{Mean} \qquad (4.5.2)$$

When two class frequencies are equal, we can use the relation (4.5.2) to determine the value of Mode. A symmetric curve is a bell shaped curve as shown in the figure. Calculating Mean, Median and Mode, we can determine the lack of symmetry or skewness present in the frequency distribution. A symmetrical curve looks like a bell shaped curve as shown in the following figure.

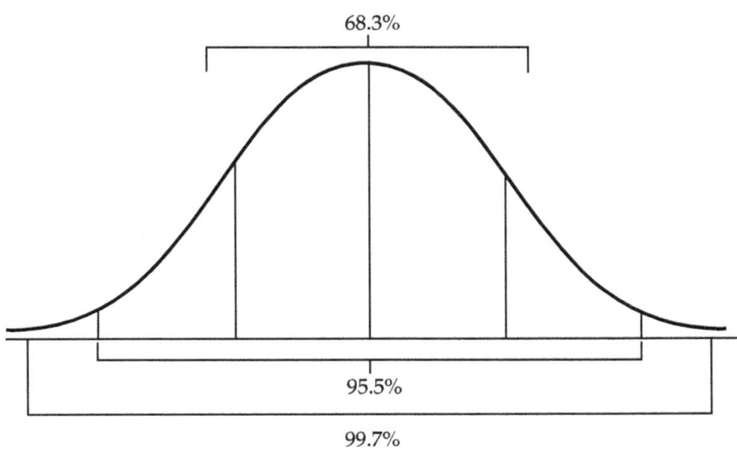

Fig. 4.5.1: *A symmetrical frequency distribution*

Skewness is of two types, namely (a) Negatively skewed distribution and (b) Positively skewed distribution. In a negatively skewed distribution, Mode will be larger than Mean and Median lies in between them. Whereas, in a positively skewed distribution, Mean will be larger than Mode and Median lies in between them. Thus if (Mean – Mode) is negative, we determine that the frequency curve is negatively skewed curve. If it is positive, we consider it as a positively skewed curve. Karl Pearson suggested the measure **(Mean – Mode)/ S.D.** or **3 (Mean – Median)/S.D.,** as coefficient of skewness. A negatively skewed curve is given in Fig. (4.5.2) and a positively skewed curve is given in Fig. (4.5.3).

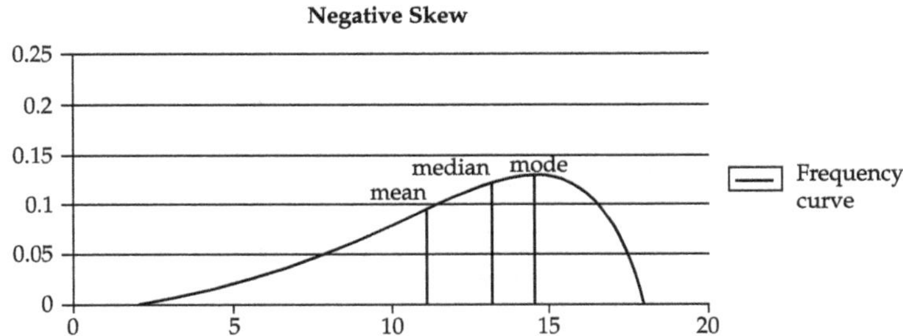

Fig. 4.5.2: *A negatively skewed curve.*

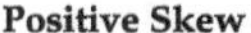

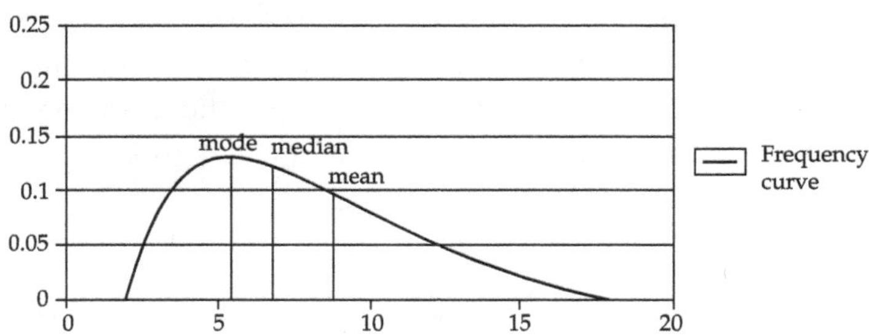

Fig. 4.5.3: *A Positively skewed curve.*

There is a slight difference between the dispersion or variation and skewness which is explained as follows:

Dispersion or vairation	Skewness
1. It measures the extent of variation in a series.	1. It measures the direction of variation or dispersion.
2. It tells about the spread of individual values about the central value i.e., mean.	2. It explains the departure or deviation from symmetry or it measures lack of symmetry.
3. It shows the degree of variability.	3. It shows whether the concentration is on higher side or lower side.
4. It judges the truthfulness of the central tendency.	4. It judges the difference between different central tendencies.
5. It measures the average deviation.	5. It is not an average, but measures differences among averages.

Example (4.5.1): Calculate Karl Pearson's coefficient of skewness for the following frequency distribution of 700 students in Bio-statistics paper.

C.I.	0–20	20–40	40–60	60–80	80–100
Frequency	125	135	155	145	140

Solution: First calculate mid-values and deviations, Mean, and Standard Deviation and then Median and Mode.

C.I.	f_i	M_i	d_i	$f_i \cdot d_i$	$f_i \cdot d_i^2$
0 – 20	125	10	–2	–250	500
20 – 40	135	30	–1	–135	135
40 – 60	155	50 = A	0	0	0
60 – 80	145	70	1	145	145
80 – 100	140	90	2	280	560
Total	700 = N			40	1340

Calculation of Mean and S.D.

$$\text{Mean} = [(\Sigma f_i \cdot d_i)/N] \times C = 50 + (40/700) \times 20$$

$$= 50 + 1.14286 \text{ marks} = 51.14286 \text{ marks.}$$

$$\text{S.D.} = \sigma = \sqrt{\{[\Sigma f_i d_i^2/N] - [(\Sigma f_i d_i /N)]^2\}} \times C$$

$$= \sqrt{\{(1340/700) - (40/700)^2\}} \times 20 = \sqrt{(1.91429 - 0.00327)} \times 20$$

$$= 1.38239 \times 20 = 27.64793 \text{ marks.}$$

Calculation of Median

C.I.	Frequency	Less than cumulative frequency (LTCF)	
0 – 20	125	125	N/2 = 700/2
20 – 40	135	260	= 350
40 – 60	155	415	Therefore 40–60 is
60 – 80	145	560	the Median class
80 – 100	140	700	
	700		

$$\text{Median} = L + (((N/2) - \text{C.F})/f)\, C$$
$$= 40 + ((350 - 260)/155) \times 20 = 40 + (90/155) \times 20$$
$$= 40 + 11.6129 = 51.6129 \text{ marks.}$$

Calculation of Mode:

C.I.	Frequency
0 – 20	125
20 – 40	135 = f_0
40 – 60	155 = f_1
60 – 80	145 = f_2
80 – 100	140

$$\text{Mode} = L + ((f_1 - f_0)/(2f_1 - f_0 - f_2)) \times C$$
$$= 40 + ((155 - 135)/(2 \times 155 - 135 - 145)) \times 20$$
$$= 40 + (20/30) \times 20 = 40 + 13.3333 = 53.3333 \text{ marks.}$$

Mean = 51.14286 marks.
Median = 51.6129 marks.
Mode = 53.3333 marks and
S.D. = 27.64793 marks.

Karl Pearson's Coefficient of Skewness = (Mean – Mode)/ S.D.
= (51.14286 – 53.3333)/27.64793 = – 0.07923.

Or 3(51.14286 – 51.6129)/27.64793 = – 0.05038.

Given frequency distribution is a negatively skewed distribution. It is slightly skewed towards left side than Symmetrical Curve.

4.6. KURTOSIS

Kurtosis is another statistical measure, useful to compare two or more sets of data and take decisions. Sometimes, the three measures, averages, variation and skewness are same for some data or frequency distributions (rarely), in those situations, kurtosis will help us to compare them and take appropriate decisions. Kurtosis measures the convexity or degree of peakedness of the frequency curve. Kurtosis the degree or the extent of peakedness or flatness of a curve of a frequency distribution. The measure of kurtosis indicates the shape of the top of a Frequency Curve. Kurtosis is defined by some statisticians as:

'A measure of kurtosis indicates the degree to which the curve of a frequency distribution is peaked or flat topped'

— Crosexton and Cowden.

'The degree of kurtosis of a distribution is a measure relative to the peakedness of a normal curve'

— Simpson and Katkes.

'Kutosis refers to the degree of peakedness of the hemp of the frequency distribution'

— C.M. Mayess.

4.6.1. Types of Kurtosis

Kurtosis is of three types, namely (a) platy kurtic (b) meso kurtic or normal and (c) lepto kurtic. If the curve is flatter than meso kurtic curve, then it is called platy kurtic curve and if the curve is relatively high peaked than the meso kurtic curve, then it is known as lepto kurtic curve. These curves are explained with the following figure.

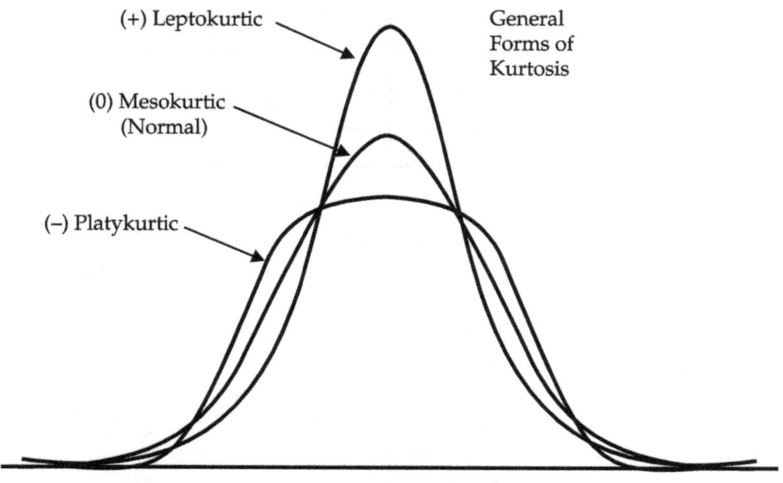

Fig. 4.6.1: *Different types of kurtosis.*

Usually, kurtosis is measured through moments. These concepts of moments are out of the scope of the book of bio-statistics. Hence measure of kurtosis is not discussed. The purpose of this section is just to introduce the concept, types and utility of the concept of kurtosis.

Note: More details of normal distribution and normal curve will be discussed in fifth chapter.

REVIEW QUESTIONS AND PROBLEMS

A. Objective Type Questions

1. Average is a measure of -------------- tendency.

(*a*) initial (*b*) central
(*c*) ending (*d*) linear.

2. The Mean of 22, 18, ---, 10, 15 is 20. Find the missing value.

(*a*) 32 (*b*) 30
(*c*) 31 (*d*) 35.

3. The median of 42, 15, 25, 32, 10, 40 and 35.

(*a*) 32 (*b*) 35
(*c*) 25 (*d*) 40.

4. The Mode in the series 25, 22, 25, 21, 25, 25, 26, 25, 20, 25, 21 is -----------.

(*a*) 21 (*b*) 22
(*c*) 25 (*d*) 26.

5. If Mean = Median = Mode is known as --------- curve.

(*a*) uniform (*b*) platy Kurtic
(*c*) symmetic (*d*) lepto Kurtic.

6. Mean is greater than mode in a --------- skewed distribution

(*a*) uniformly (*b*) positively
(*c*) negatively (*d*) absolutely.

7. Mean is less than mode in a -------- skewed distribution.

(*a*) uniformly (*b*) positively
(*c*) negatively (*d*) absolutely.

8. Standard deviation is also known as ----------- deviation.

(*a*) root mean square (*b*) mean square
(*c*) square (*d*) variance.

9. Absolute deviations are considered in ------------ deviation.

(*a*) standard (*b*) median
(*c*) mean (*d*) mode.

10. Measure of lack of symmetry is called ---------.

(*a*) skewness (*b*) kurtosis
(*c*) dispersion (*d*) average.

11. Skewness in a symmetrical distribution is -----------.
    (*a*) – 1 (*b*) 1
    (*c*) 0 (*d*) 0.5.
12. Kurtosis measures ---------- of the frequency distribution.
    (*a*) peakedness (*b*) dispersion
    (*c*) assymetry (*d*) variation.
13. Relation between Mean, Median and Mode in a symmetrical distribution is -------------------.
    (*a*) Mean > Median > Mode
    (*b*) Mean < Median < Mode.
    (*c*) Mean = Median = Mode
    (*d*) Mean ≠ Median ≠ Mode.
14. Sum of squares of deviations of the mean taken from each observation is always -----------------.
    (*a*) zero (*b*) minimum
    (*c*) maximum (*d*) negative.
15. Sum of the deviations of the arithmetic mean taken from each observation is always -------------------.
    (*a*) zero (*b*) minimum
    (*c*) maximum (*d*) negative.

B. Short Answer Questions

1. Write a short note on various measures of central tendencies.
2. List out various properties of a good average.
3. Write a short note of various measures of variation.
4. List out various properties of a good measure of dispersion.
5. Compute average deviation from median for the following data.
   12, 6, 7, 8, 8, 9, 10, 11, 13, 13, 11, 9, 8, 10.
6. Write short note on coefficient of variation.
7. Write short note on skewness.
8. Distinguish between measure of variation and skewness.
9. Calculate standard deviation and variance for the data:
   12, 10, 18, 16, 23 and 11
10. Calculate C.V. for the following data: 8, 5, 15, 12 and 20.
11. Calculate Karl Pearson's coefficient of skweness for the following Data representing runs in 11 test series.
    95, 125, 102, 125, 128, 125, 176, 125, 76, 125 and 151 runs.
12. Write short note on kurtosis.

C. Essay Type Questions

1. The following data represents weights of fish measured in Kgs. Calculate Mean, Median, Mode for the following data.

C.I.	Frequency
0 – 10	4
10 – 20	6
20 – 30	18
30 – 40	10
40 – 50	12

2. Compute Mean, Median and Mode for the following frequency distribution which represents the weights of 533 swines measured in Lb's.

Class mid point	Frequency	C.I.
85	1	75–95
105	7	95–115
125	39	115–135
145	66	135–155
165	143	155–175
185	1120	175–195
205	80	195–215
225	53	215–235
245	16	235–255
265	9	255–275
285	7	275–295

[**Hint:** first calculate class intervals as given in column three]

3. Calculate the Mean, Median, Mode, Standard Deviation and Karl Pearson skewness for the following data.

Class Interval	Frequency
110 – 120	22
120 – 130	42
130 – 140	60
140 – 150	20
150 – 160	6

4. The following data represents number of gamma rays produced from a machine in the laboratory. Calculate Mean, Standard Deviation.

X	f
0	40
1	30
2	20
3	10
4	0

5. Calculate: Range, Mean deviation, standard deviation and variance for the following data.

Class Interval	0 – 20	20 – 40	40 – 60	60 – 80	80 – 100
Frequency	32	49	52	36	31

6. Calculate Mean deviation and Std. deviation and C.V. for the following data.

Class Interval	0 – 10	10 – 20	20 – 30	30 – 40	40 – 50
Frequency	14	16	34	24	12

7. A is a cricket player with average of 150 runs and standard deviation as 25 runs. B is another hockey player with average 6 goals and standard deviation 2 goals. Select one player, among these two players, for a prize.
8. Write detailed notes, explaining various advantages, disadvantages and uses of various measures of averages.
9. Write detailed notes, explaining various advantages, disadvantages and uses of various measures of variation.
10. Discuss various types of skewness and kurtosis with suitable examples.

References

1. Gupta S.P. 1990 "Statistical Methods". Sultan Chand & Sons, New Delhi.
2. Wayne W. Daniel 2008 Biostatistics, 9th edition, John Wiley & Sons. Inc. Newyork.
3. P.N. Arora *et al.* 2007 "Comprehensive Statistical Methods" Sultan Chand and Company Ltd. First edn. New Delhi.
4. VK. Kapoor 1986 "Problems and solutions in Business statistics" Sultan Chand and Sons New Delhi.

Answers:

1 – b; 2 – d; 3 – a; 4 – c; 5 – c; 6 – b; 7 – c; 8 – a; 9 – c; 10 – a; 11 – c; 12 – a; 13 – c; 14 – b; 15 – a.

5 PROBABILITY

5.1. INTRODUCTION

In this world, many events are occurring with certain amount of uncertainty. For example, today it may rain or may not rain; or we may plan for a picnic or may not; if an operation is to undergo, it may be successful or a failure; if we write an examination, we may get though it or not and so on. We have to take decisions, under such changing or uncertainties. **"How to measure this Uncertainty?"** is the basic question. Probability is the method of measuring the chance or uncertainty in the occurrence of an event. In real life many factors influencing such events and hence, are happening with some uncertainty. For example, if a student write an examination, chance of passing depends upon his hard work, regularity in attending the classes, type of question paper, his health condition and so on. Similarly chance of getting rain on a day depends on climatic conditions, wind speed, temperature, cloud formation, wind direction and so on. Chance of a seed to germinate successfully and to grow as a tree, again depend on soil fertility rate, quality of the seed, temperature of the soil, type of water, type of soil and so on. Probability is a way of measuring uncertainty present in happening of an event keeping in view of all these factors influencing the event. Probability of happening an event A is denoted by $P(A)$ and is defined as the ratio of favorable number of cases to the event A to the total number of cases under consideration. Thus Probability in a simplest way is defined as the way of measuring or expressing the chance of occurrence of a certain event quantitatively. Before going for further details of probability, now we concentrate on some basic definitions.

5.2. BASIC CONCEPTS AND NOTATIONS

5.2.1. Random (or) Statistical Experiment and the Trial

An experiment is defined by the property, that is observations under a given set of circumstances and do not always lead to the same observed outcome but rather different outcomes. Basically an experiment is done to know the behavior of certain un-known result or outcome. If an experiment is conducted once, then it is called a **"trial"**. It is important to note that, all experiments are not random (or) statistical experiments.

Definition (5.2.1) : Random (or) Statistical Experiment:

A *Random* (or) *Statistical Experiment* is one in which the following three conditions are satisfied, namely:

1. All possible outcomes of an experiment must be known before conducting the experiment. — *totality condition.*
2. Result of any given trial is not known, unless the experiment is completed. —*randomness condition*
3. Experiment must be repeatable under similar conditions, as many times as possible, as desired by the experimenter. —*repeatability condition.*

Example (5.2.1): Consider a coin tossing experiment. This is a random (or) statistical experiment because:

1. All possible outcomes are known i.e., result of any trial will be a **head** or a **tail**. No other possibilities will arise. Like coin standing on its edge or after the toss, the tossed coin may not come back and so on.
2. If I go on tossing the coin, the result I will get at 15th time, is not known now. I know that it will be a head or a tail. But exactly what I will get at 15th trial will be known only after conducting the 15th trial.
3. I can repeat the experiment as many times as desired by me under similar conditions. This implies that, the force that I can apply in the first trial need not be exactly same at 100th time or 200th time, but it is approximately same in each trial. In this sense, the experiment must repeatable under similar conditions. (But not identical conditions).

Since coin tossing experiment satisfies all the three conditions, it is a random (or) statistical experiment. Similarly, die throwing experiment is a random experiment where total possible outcomes are 1 or 2 or 3 or 4 or 5 or 6. For simplicity, random experiments are known as experiments in further discussions.

5.2.2. Outcome

The result of a random experiment if it conducted will become a trial and the result of that trial is known as "*Outcome*" of that trial.

5.2.3. Sample Space

List of all possible outcomes of a random experiment is called the "*Sample Space*" of that experiment and is denoted by the symbol S or Ω.

For example for coin tossing experiment, Ω = **{Head, Tail}.** Similarly, for die throwing experiment $\Omega = \{1, 2, 3, 4, 5, 6\}$. Number of elements in the sample space is denoted by N. If N is finite, then it is called finite sample space and if it consists of infinite elements then it is known as infinite sample space.

5.2.4. Event

A sub-set of the sample space or a set of outcomes is called an "*Event*".

For example, when a die thrown, player A wins the game if an even number turns up then, winning of A is an event is given by $A = \{2, 4, 6\}$ which is a sub-set of the sample space of throwing a die. It is important to note that the event is different from outcome. (These terms are used as synonyms by many people in general. In fact, it is not so). If an event consists of only one outcome, then it is called "*Simple Event*" and if it consists of more than one outcome, then it is called "*Compound Event*".

5.2.5. Mutually Exclusive Events or Outcomes

If in an experiment, occurrence of event or an outcome prevents or rules out the occurrence of other events or outcomes, in the same trial, then such events are called "*mutually exclusive events or outcomes*".

For example, in a die throwing experiment, if 4 turns up in any trial (say) in the same trial other numbers like 1 or 2 or 3 or 5 or 6 will not occur. Similarly, if 5 turns up, 1 or 2 or 3 or 4 or 6 will not appear in the same trial. Such events or outcomes are called mutually exclusive events or outcomes.

Similarly if an event of even number results in any trial, then event of odd number in the same trial is not possible. Therefore, events getting even number or odd number are mutually exclusive events. Similarly, in new born babies, the baby is a male or female but not both. Thus getting a male or a female baby are mutually exclusive events. Similarly, a day can be a rainy day or a non-rainy day, but not both. Hence, a rainy day or a non-rainy day, are mutually exclusive events. An operation is done, it may be successful or a failure one but not both and hence, they are mutually exclusive events.

5.3. DEFINITIONS OF PROBABILITY

Probability is defined in many ways, of which classical and statistical definitions are relevant to biological studies. Hence, we are confining to these two definitions only in this book.

5.3.1. Classical Definition of Probability

Probability of an event A is denoted by $P(A)$ and is defined as:

$$P(A) = m/N \qquad (5.3.1)$$

Where N = Total number of outcomes

m = number of favorable outcomes to the event A.

Example (5.3.1): If a die is thrown, find the probability of getting an even number.

Solution: In a die throwing experiment $\Omega = \{1, 2, 3, 4, 5, 6\}$. $N = 6$

Let our event of interest getting an even number is denoted by A.

Thus $A = \{2, 4, 6\}$ that is $m = 3$.

Hence, $P(A) = m/N = 3/6 = ½ = 0.5$.

Example (5.3.2): A bag consists of 5 red balls, 3 green balls and 2 yellow balls. Then a ball is drawn randomly, calculate the probability of getting (1) a red ball (2) an yellow ball and (3) a green ball.

Solution: Since total number of balls in the bag = $N = 10$.

1. Event A = Getting a red ball.
   Number of favorable to A = Number of red balls = $m = 5$.
   Therefore $P(A) = 5/10$ (or) 0.5
2. Let A = getting an yellow ball. Hence $m = 2$
   $P(A) = 2/10 = 1/5 = 0.2$.
3. Let A = getting a red ball. Hence $m = 3$.
   Therefore $P(A) = 3/10 = 0.3$.

Example (5.3.3): If a card is drawn from a well shuffled deck of cards, find the probability that (1) It is a queen (2) It is a red card (3) It is a diamond (4) It is a spade 8.

Solution: A deck of cards contains 52 cards (Joker is not considered for these problems). Hence $N = 52$.

1. There are 4 queens. Hence $m = 4$.
   P(getting queen) = 4/52 = 1/13 = 0.07692.
2. There are 26 red cards. Therefore m 26.
   P (a red card) = 26/52 = 1/2 = 0.5.
3. There are 13 diamond cards. Hence $m = 13$
   P (a diamond) = 13/52 = 1/4 = 0.25.
4. There is only one spade 8. Therefore $m = 1$
   P (a spade 8) = 1/52 = 0.01923.

Example (5.3.4): What is the probability that a leap year, selected at random has 53 saturdays.

Solution: A leap year consists of 366 days and 52 complete weeks and two days extra. These extra two days can occur following possible ways.

(1) Sunday, monday; (2) monday, tuesday; (3) tuesday, wednesday; (4) wednesday, thursday; (5) thursday, friday; (6) friday, saturday; and (7) saturday, sunday. Hence $N = 7$.

Among the above seven possibilities, to get 53 saturdays, events (6) and (7) are favorable. Hence $m = 2$.

Therefore P(getting 53 saturdays in a leap year) = 2/7 = 0.28571.

Example (5.3.5): In a hospital there are 15 doctors, 35 nurses and 10 class iv employees. If we randomly select one person, find the probability the person is (1) a doctor (2) a nurse and (3) a class iv employee.

Solution: Total number of persons in the hospital are $N = 15 + 35 + 10 = 60$

(1) Here $m = 15$. P (a doctor) = 15/60 = ¼ = 0.25.

(2) Here $m = 35$ P (a nurse) = 35/60 = 7/12 = 0.58333.

(3) Here $m = 10$ P (a class iv employee) 10/60 = 1/6 = 0.16667.

5.3.2. Sure Event

If the probability of any event is equal to 1 then such an event is called *"sure event"* or *"definite event"* or *"certain event"*

5.3.3. Void Event

If the probability of any event is equal to 0, then such an event is called *"void event"* or *"impossible event"* or *"null event"* and is denoted by the symbol Φ (To be read as Phi) thus $P(\Phi) = 0$.

Thus probability always lies in between 0 and 1. Thus $0 \leq P(A) \leq 1$.

In the above problems, we have used classical definition of probability. Basic drawback of this definition is that N should be finite. Thus we can use this definition for finite sample spaces. If N is infinite this definition fails. Hence we require another definition to probability known as "statistical definition" or "empirical definition" proposed by Von Mises, which is explained as follows:

5.3.4. Statistical or Empirical Definition of Probability

"If the experiment is repeated a large number of times under essentially similar conditions, the limiting value of the ratio of the number of times the event A happens to the total number of trials increases infinitely, is called the probability of the event A".

That is
$$P(A) = \lim_{n \to \infty} (m/n) = L \quad (5.3.2)$$

Provided the limit L exists and is finite and unique.

This approach is also known as relative frequency approach because the ratio m/n is called as relative frequency. This approach to define the concept of probability is explained with an example as follows:

Consider tossing of a coin and toss a fair coin 10 times and let our event of interest is to get head. Count how many times head came in 10 tosses. Let number of heads be 6 (say) then calculate the ratio m/n = 6/10. Now increase number of trials be 20, 40, 50, 100, 150, 200, 250.,.,., and calculate the ratio every time by counting number of heads. This ratio converges to ½ . Thus ½ is considered as the probability of getting head. This concept is explained graphically as follows: Let number of trials and heads are tabulated as follows.

Number of trials = n	Number of heads = m or frequency	Relative frequency or ratio (m/n)
100	65	65/100 = 0.65
200	98	98/200 = 0.49
500	258	258/500 = 0.516
1000	489	489/1000 = 0.489
1200	625	625/1200 = 0.521
1500	732	732/1500 = 0.488
1800	915	915/1800 = 0.556
2000	1012	1012/2000 = 0.506
2500	1252	1252/2500 = 0.501
3000	1503	1503/3000 = 0.501

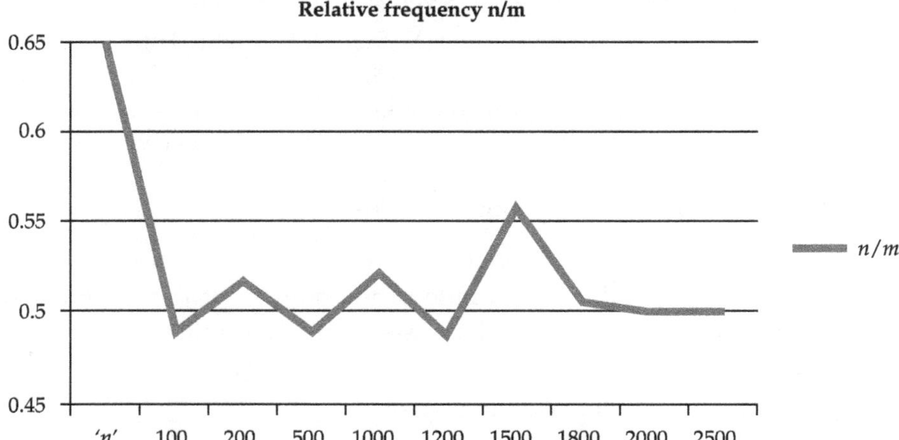

Fig. 5.3.1: *Relative frequency curve converging to ½ or 0.5 for* ***P(A)***

On similar lines, we can find probabilities for any event by collecting the data on the event and obtaining the class intervals, frequency and relative frequency.

Example (5.3.6): Following data represents different categories of babies with respect to their first day weights measured in lbs. There are 7000 births in a city in a year. Calculate probabilities for different events.

Weight (lbs)	Less than 2.5	2.5 to 3.0	3.0 to 4.5	Above 4.5
Frequency	2012	1062	2866	1060

Solution: Probabilities for different categories of babies are calculated by using statistical approach is done through relative frequencies as follows:

Weight of babies (lbs)	Frequency = m	Relative frequency m/n
Less than 2.5	2012	2012/7000 = 0.287
2.5 to 3.0	1062	1062/7000 = 0.152
3.0 to 4.5	2866	2866/7000 = 0.409
Above 4.5	1060	1060/7000 = 0.152
Total	7000 = n	7000/7000 = 1.000

Probabilities for various events are given in column 3. For example, to get a baby with weight between 3.0 to 4.5 lbs is 0.409. Similarly to get a ill-healthy baby (less than 2.5 lbs) is 0.287 and to get a healthy baby above 4.5 lbs is 0.152 and so on.

5.4. THEOREMS ON PROBABILITY

Basically there are two important theorems on probability, namely:

1. addition theorem or theorem on total probability and
2. multiplication theorem or theorem on compound probability.

Statements and applications of these theorems are discussed now. Proofs of the theorems are out of scope of the syllabus.

5.4.1. Addition Theorem of Probability

If A and B are two events then:

$$P(A \text{ or } B) = P(A) + P(B) - P(A \text{ and } B). \quad (5.4.1)$$

If A and B are disjoint,

$$P(A \text{ or } B) = P(A) + P(B) \text{ i.e. } P(A \text{ and } B) = 0. \quad (5.4.2)$$

Example (5.4.1): An urn contains 5 red balls, 3 green balls and 2 yellow balls. If a ball is drawn at random, find the probability that it is a red or a green ball.

Solution: Let us denote A = getting a red ball and B = getting a green ball.

The selected ball will be a red one or green one but not both.

Hence $P(A \text{ and } B) = 0$

$$P(A \text{ or } B) = P(A + B) = P(A) + P(B)$$
$$= 0.5 + 0.3 = 0.8.$$

Aliter:

Total number of balls = N = 10. Our event of interest is A or B means that getting a red or a green balls = 5 red + 3 green balls are favorable to our event. Hence m = 8.

Then P(getting a red ball or a green ball) = 8/10 = 0.8.

Example (5.4.2): If a dye is thrown, Calculate the probability of getting an even number.

Solution: Here N= 6 and P(getting 1) = 1/6, P(getting 2) = 1/6

P(getting 3) = 1/6, P(getting 4) = 1/6, P(getting 5) = 1/6 and

P(getting 6) = 1/6. Our event of interest is to get an even number i.e. 2 or 4 or 6.

Hence P(getting 2 or 4 or 6) = P(getting 2) + P(getting 4) + P(getting 6)

$= 1/6 + 1/6 + 1/6 = 3/6 = 0.5.$

Aliter: [see example (5.3.1)].

Example (5.4.3): In a die throwing experiment, Player A wins the game if 1 or 5 turns up; Player B wins the game if 2 or 3 turns up and Player C wins the game, if 8 turns up. Calculate probabilities for player A, Player B and Player C.

Solution:

Here $N = 6$ and Player A wins the game if 1 or 5 turns up.

Hence $m = 2$. Therefore $P(A) = 2/6 = 1/3 = 0.33333$. Using Addition theorem, we have P(getting 1 or 5) = $P(1) + P(5)$

$= 1/6 + 1/6 = 2/6 = 1/3 = 0.33333.$

Similarly, for player B P(getting 2 or 3) = $2/6 = 1/3 = 0.33333$.

And for player C P(getting 8) = $0/6 = 0$.

5.5. CONDITIONAL PROBABILITY AND MULTIPLICATION THEOREM

For the introduction of multiplication theorem, we require the concept of conditional probability. The concept of conditional probability reduces the searching area in the sample space for calculation of probabilities for events, if some information is known to you already. Conditional probability of an event B given that A has already occurred, is denoted by $P(B|A)$ or $P(B$ given $A)$ which is defined as follows:

5.5.1. Definition of Conditional Probability

If A and B are two events,

$$P(B|A) = P(A \text{ and } B)/P(A) \text{ if } P(A) > 0 \quad (5.5.1)$$

$$P(A|B) = P(A \text{ and } B)/P(B) \text{ if } P(B) > 0 \quad (5.5.2)$$

$P(B|A)$ is called the conditional probability of B given that A has already occurred. Similarly $P(A|B)$ is called the conditional probability of A given that B has already occurred. If the events A and B are independent, then

$P(A|B)$ will become $P(A)$ and $P(B|A)$ will become $P(B)$ itself.

5.5.2. Multiplication Theorem of Probability

If A and B are two events,

$$P(A \text{ and } B) = P(A)\,P(B|A) \text{ Or } P(B)\,P(A|B). \quad (5.5.3)$$

In particular if A and B are independent,

$$P(A \text{ and } B) = P(A)\,P(B). \quad (5.5.4)$$

Or if $P(A$ and $B) = P(A)\,P(B)$ then we say that A and B are independent. $P(A$ and $B) = P(A)\,P(B)$.

Note: It is important to note that the concept of disjoint is different from the concept of Independence. For example, group of male patients and group of female patients are disjoint. Here there is no possibility of having both the genders by the same element. Hence common portion is zero. Further, being a diabetic patient and the gender are two independent characteristics. Diabetic patients may be in both the genders.

Example (5.5.1): A bag contains 5 white, 8 red and 2 yellow balls. Four balls are drawn at random find the probability that selected balls contains all the three color balls.

Solution: To select 4 balls from 15 balls, we can select in $\binom{n}{k}$ ways. Here $\binom{n}{k} = n!/k!$ $(n-k)!$. Here $n! = n\,.\,(n-1)\,.\,(n-2).\,,.,.,\,2.1$. That is $4! = 4.3.2.1 = 24$.

Similarly $8! = 8.7.6.5.4.3.2.1 = 40{,}320$. $\binom{n}{k}$ the expression is to be read as $n\ c\ k$. This concept is more clearly explained in the next section. Further we should consider always 0! as 1. Thus selecting 4 balls from 15 balls in $\binom{15}{4}$ 15!/4!11! = (15.14.13.12)/1.2.3.4

= 32760/24 = 1365 ways.

Therefore $N = 1365$.

Selected four balls can occur in the following three ways.

Case – 1: 2 white and 1 red and 1 yellow or

Case – 2: 1 white and 2 red and 1 yellow or

Case - 3: 1 white and 1 red and 2 yellow.

$P(\text{case} - 1) = \binom{5}{2} \cdot \binom{8}{1} \cdot \binom{2}{1} / \binom{15}{4}$ = 10.8.2/1365 = 160/1365 = 0.11722.

$P(\text{case} - 2) = \binom{5}{1} \cdot \binom{8}{2} \cdot \binom{2}{1} / \binom{15}{4}$ = 5.28.2/1365 =280/1365 = 0.20528.

$P(\text{case} - 3) = \binom{5}{1} \cdot \binom{8}{1} \cdot \binom{2}{2} / \binom{15}{4}$ = 5.8.1/1365 = 40/1365 = 0.029304.

$P(\text{getting all the three colors}) = P(\text{case} - 1 + \text{case} - 2 + \text{case} - 3)$
$= P(\text{case} - 1) + P(\text{case} - 2) + P(\text{case} - 3)$ = 480/1365 = 0.35165.

Note: In solving the example (5.5.1), note that we have used both addition and multiplication theorems. For biological students, generally questions are asked in a simple manner as discussed above. Complicated problems are usually avoided because, we generally expect biological student with less mathematical background.

5.6. PROPERTIES AND UTILITIES OF PROBABILITY

The concept of probability is popularly used in many fields of research to take decisions involving uncertainty. Probability has the following properties:

1. Probability is non-negative i.e. $P(A) \leq 0$.
2. Probability of null event is zero i.e. $P(\Phi) = 0$.
3. Probability of the sample space is 1 i.e. $P(\Omega) = 1$.
4. Probability always lies in between 0 and 1 i.e. $0 \leq P(A) \leq 1$.

5. $P(A^c) = 1 - P(A)$, where A^c represents other than A to be read as A compliment.
6. $P(A \text{ or } B) = P(A + B) = P(A) + P(B)$ if A and B are disjoint.
7. $P(A \text{ and } B) = P(A \cdot B) = P(A) \cdot P(B)$ if A and B are independent.

Probability is mainly used in Life Insurance Corporation of India to calculate premiums to be paid by different age group customers, by calculating risk factors in different ages. Similarly, it is used in industry, medical research, biology, meteorology, market research, determination of share prices and so on, where lot of un-certainty is prevailed in these fields. Where ever un-certainty is present, one has to use the concept of probability to measure the amount un-certainty present.

REVIEW QUESTIONS AND PROBLEMS

A. Objective Type Questions

1. Probability of a sure event is ----------.

(*a*) 0 (*b*) 0.5
(*c*) 1 (*d*) 0.25.

2. Probability of a null event is -----------.

(*a*) 0 (*b*) 0.5
(*c*) 1 (*d*) 0.25.

3. Probability of the sample space is -------.

(*a*) 0 (*b*) 1
(*c*) 0.5 (*b*) 0.25.

4. If probability of any event is zero then it is known as ------ event.

(*a*) sure (*b*) void
(*c*) certain (*d*) disjoint.

5. If A and B are independent, then $P(A/B)$ is -----------.

(*a*) $P(A)$ (*b*) $P(B)$
(*c*) 0 (*d*) 1.

6. If A and B are disjoint the $P(A \text{ or } B)$ -----------.

(*a*) $P(A) + P(B)$ (*b*) $P(A)/P(B)$
(*c*) $P(A) \cdot P(B)$ (4) $P(A) - P(B)$.

7. If $P(A \text{ and } B) = P(A) \cdot P(B)$ then A and B are --------- events.

(*a*) sure (*b*) null
(*c*) independent (*d*) disjoint.

8. Conditional probability $P(A \mid B)$ in independent trials is --------.

(*a*) $P(A)$ (*b*) $P(B)$
(*c*) 0 (*d*) 1.

9. Range for the probability is ----------.

(*a*) –1 to +1 (*b*) 0 to 1
(*b*) greater than 1 (*d*) less than zero.

10. Probability measures ------------ in happening of an event.
    (*a*) un-certainty (*b*) certainty
    (*c*) un-reality (*d*) reality

B. Short Answer Questions

1. Define
   (*a*) sample space (*b*) event and
   (*c*) random experiment.
2. Distinguish between an event and outcome. When will an event become an outcome?
3. Explain random experiment by giving two examples.
4. If A and B are independent and $P(A \text{ or } B) = 0.8$ and $P(A) = 0.5$, then calculate $P(B)$.

   [**Hint:** $P(A \text{ or } B) = 0.8$ and A and B are independent.

   That is $P(A \text{ and } B) = P(A) \cdot P(B)$ and $P(A) = 0.5$. Substitute these values in (5.4.1) we have $0.8 = 0.5 + P(B) - 0.5\ P(B)$ i.e. $0.3 = P(B)[1 - 0.5]$

   Hence $P(B) = 0.3/0.5 = 0.6$]

   Note it is wrong to calculate as $P(B) = 0.8 - 0.5 = 0.3$.
5. State the addition and multiplication theorems on probability.
6. Explain the concept of conditional probability with an example.
7. List out various properties of probability.
8. Explain various applications of probability.
9. Explain the classical and Von Mises approach to probability.
10. Calculate the probability that a non-leap year consists of 53 fridays.

C. Essay Type Questions

1. Write detailed notes on probability and its applications.
2. Explain the statistical approach to the probability with suitable examples.
3. Write down the sample space of throwing two dies simultaneously

   And calculate the probabilities for (*a*) getting same numbers on both dies (*b*) if we add numbers on the dies total must be 8 or 10 or 12 (*c*) getting a total 2 or 4.
4. An urn contains 6 red balls, 4 green balls, 3 yellow balls and 2 white balls. If 5 balls are drawn at random, calculate the probability that the selected balls contains all the four colors.
5. Following data represents the attack of different diseases in a city in a year. Calculate probabilities for various diseases under consideration.

Disease	Heart	Kidney	Cancer	Fever	Skin
Frequency	3084	4690	8972	2468	4696

6. A coin is tossed 6 times. What is the probability of getting (*a*) exactly 2 heads (*b*) at least 5 heads (*c*) at most 2 heads.
7. Out of 10 outstanding students in an University there are 4 male and 6 female students. Four students are selected randomly from these 10 students. Find the probability that there are (*a*) 2 male and 2 female students (*b*) all are male students and (*c*) all are female students.
8. There are 50 animals in the laboratory, numbered from 1 to 50 serially. If an animal is selected at random find the probability that the selected animal has (*a*) an even number (*b*) a prime number (*c*) a number divisible by 5.
9. An urn contains 8 red, 4 white and 3 yellow balls. If 4 balls are drawn at random, find probability that (*a*) all are red balls (*b*) 2 white and 2 yellow balls and (*c*) all color balls.
10. *A* card is drawn from a well shuffled pack of 52 cards. The events *A* and *B* are, *A*: getting a card of spade and *B*: getting an ace. Show that *A* and *B* are independent events.

References

1. Gupta S.P. 1990 "Statistical Methods". Sultan Chand & Sons, New Delhi.
2. Wayne W. Daniel 2008 Biostatistics, 9th edition, John Wiley & Sons. Inc. Newyork.
3. P.N. Arora *et al*. 2007 "Comprehensive Statistical Methods" Sultan Chand and company Ltd. First edn. New Delhi.
4. VK. Kapoor 1986 "Problems and solutions in Business statistics" Sultan Chand and sons New Delhi.

Answers:

1 – c; 2 – a; 3 – b; 4 – b; 5 – a; 6 – a; 7 – c; 8 – a; 9 – b; 10 – a.

6 PROBABILITY DISTRIBUTIONS

6.1. INTRODUCTION

In the last chapter, we have observed that the maximum value that the probability can take is one and hence if we add all the probabilities for different events in a sample space, we get the total equal to one. In other words, in any problem, if we add all the probabilities of all possible events, it should be equal to one. It implies that the total probability one is distributed to various events in different, different manner. This distribution of total probability one to various events is known as probability distribution. For example, consider the coin tossing experiment, where there are two possible outcomes, namely a head or a tail. Further we know that $P(\text{Head}) = ½$ and $P(\text{Tail}) = ½$ and if we add, $½ + ½ = 1$.

Similarly, in a die throwing experiment there are six possibilities i.e. 1, 2, 3, 4, 5 and 6 each with probability 1/6. This means that $P(k) = 1/6$ for $k = 1, 2, 3, 4, 5, 6$. In the above two cases, total probability is distributed equally, to all the outcomes. Hence they are called equally likely outcomes. In reality, outcomes of a random experiment need not have equal probabilities to all outcomes or events. For example, weight of a new born baby, does not have equal probabilities, for different events. [vide example (5.3.6)]. Similarly, if we board the bus, probability for safe journey or probability of meeting with an accident are not equal. Similarly, if we operate a heart patient, success and failure of the operation are not equally likely. Thus many events in the real life, are not equally likely. Some events have more probability and some events have less probability. But, if we add all the probabilities, we get a total 1. In other words, total probability 1 is distributed to different events, in various different ways. These distributions are known as *"Probability distributions"*. The distribution sometimes may be equal like coin tossing experiment or die throwing experiment. In such situations, the distribution is called uniform distribution of total probability 1 to different events and the graph of such distribution is a straight line as shown in the following table and corresponding figure.

Table (6.1.1): Probabilities for various outcomes in a die throwing experiment.

Outcomes	1	2	3	4	5	6
Probability	1/6 = 0.167	1/6 = 0.167	1/6 = 0.167	1/6 = 0.167	1/6 = 0.167	1/6 = 0.167

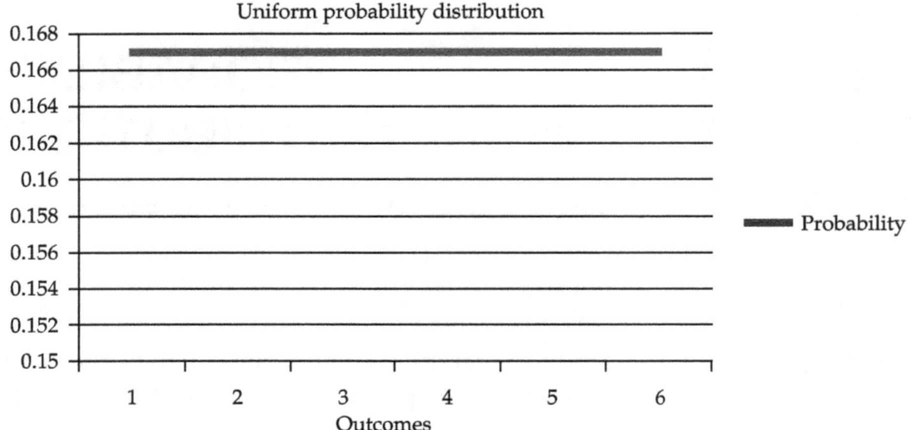

Fig. 6.1.1: *Graph of probability distribution in die throwing experiment.*

Sometimes, the distribution of the probabilities may not be equal but unequal. This is similar to the concept that a parent may distribute his property equally to both of his sons. If he has both sons and daughters, the distribution may not be equal to all his children. Depending on the nature of the distribution, there are many probability distributions. Among them, the following four are most popularly used distributions. Namely:

1. Binomial distribution,
2. Poisson distribution,
3. Normal distribution, and
4. Exponential distribution.

Before going to discuss about these distributions, there is a need to introduce the concept of "*Random variable*", which is done in the following section.

6.2. RANDOM VARIABLE

Random variable helps us to obtain solutions in those situations, where the sample space large enough and it is highly difficult to write the same and calculate required probabilities. For example, sample space when two coins are tossed simultaneously or one coin tossed two times is **Ω = {HH, HT, TH, TT}**, where *H* represents head and *T* represents tail.

Similarly, if 3 coins are tossed:

$$\text{Sample space } = \Omega = \{\text{HHH, HTH, THH, TTH, HHT, HTT, THT, TTT}\}.$$

In this fashion, if we want to write the sample space for the experiment when we toss 10 or 15 coins, it is very time consuming and laborious. For example, if the distance is small, we can walk, but requires a vehicle if it is large. Similarly, the concept of random variable, helps like a vehicle, to solve large, laborious and difficult physically to write down sample spaces, to solve the required probabilities. In the above examples, if we introduce, a random variable X representing number of heads, then in two coins case sample space is $X = 0, 1, 2$. Similarly, in 3 coins case $X = 0, 1, 2, 3$. In this manner writing down the sample space in 10 coins is $X = 0, 1, 2, 3, 4, 5, 6, 7, 8, 9, 10$. And so on. X is called the *random variable* (*r.v.*), representing number of heads. We can also introduce another random variable Y representing number of tails. In this fashion, we can write sample spaces for 100 or 1000 coins also. Thus the random variable maps the sample space to the real line. Now we can calculate probabilities when two coins are tossed as : $P(X = 0) = 1/4$, $P(X = 1) = 2/4 = 1/2$ and $P(X = 2) = 1/4$ and the total $1/4 + 1/2 + 1/4 = 1$. Similarly, when 3 coins are tossed, $P(X = 0) = 1/8$, $P(X = 1) = 3/8$, $P(X = 2) = 3/8$ and $P(X = 3) = 1/8$ and the total of probabilities i.e. $1/8 + 3/8 + 3/8 + 1/8 = 1$. We can observe that these probabilities are un-equal to each other. This is the distribution of total probability 1 to different events by the random variable X. Random Variables (R.V.) are represented by capital letters like X, Y, Z and so on. The values that the random variable (*r.v.*) takes are denoted by small letter like x, y, z and so on. If we draw the distribution curve now, we cannot get a straight line as in Fig. (6.1.1) but a different shape as shown in the Figure (6.2.1).

Example (6.2.1): Write down various probabilities for different events when 3 coins are tossed and represent the distribution through a frequency curve.

Solution: The probability distribution of the R.V. X is given as follows.

R.V.X	0	1	2	3
Probabilities	1/8 = 0.125	3/8 = 0.375	3/8 = 0.375	1/8 = 0.125

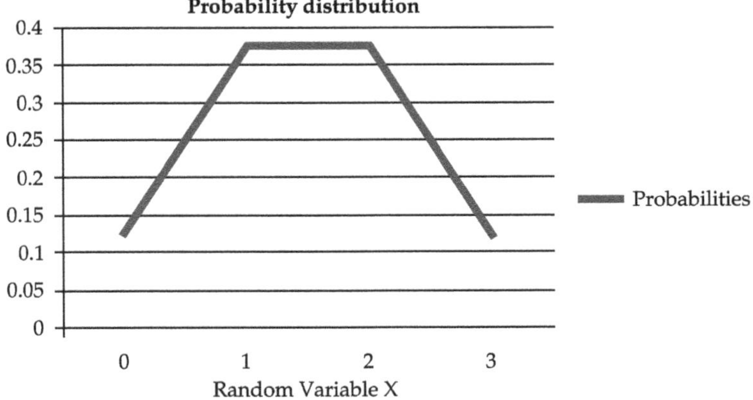

Fig. 6.2.1: *Probability distribution when three coins are tossed.*

6.2.1. Definition of a Random Variable

A *Random Variable* (R.V.) is defined as a real valued function defined on the sample space of a random experiment. In other words, random variable assigns a unique real number x to each one of the outcomes of a random experiment.

Random variables are of two types, namely:

(*a*) Discrete random variable and

(*b*) Continuous random variable.

6.2.2. Definition of Discrete Random Variable

A random variable is said to be discrete. If it takes only a finite or infinite but countable number of values.

Examples:

1. Number of heads occurred when coins are tossed.

$$X = 0, 1, 2, 3 .,.,., n.$$

2. Number of print mistakes in a page of news paper.

$$Y = 0, 1, 2, 3, .,.,., k.$$

3. Number of defective items produced from a machine.
4. Number of students in a class or university and so on.

6.2.3. Definition of Continuous Random Variable

A random variable is said to be continuous if it can take any value in an interval of two numbers a and b i.e. $[a, b]$.

Examples:

1. Weight of new born babies.
2. Height of a tree.
3. Length of a leaf.
4. Weight of a fish in a tank and so on.

Important results: To find $P(X \geq a) = 1 - P(X < a)$. (6.2.1)

Similarly, to find $P(X \leq a) = 1 - P(X > a)$. (6.2.2)

In order to find expected number of persons in a population of size N and having a particular character is $N.p$, where p is the probability of having that character.

6.3. BINOMIAL DISTRIBUTION

Binomial distribution is a discrete probability distribution which is obtained when the probability p of the happening of an even is same in all the trials and there are only two events in each trial. In other words, binomial distribution is to be applied when of an experiment are only 2 outcomes or events like, head or tail; success or failure; good or bad; defective or non defective; affected by a disease or not and so on. Let 'x' denote the R.V., representing number of heads or number successes, number print mistakes or number of affected persons from a disease or number of defective items produced from a machine and so on. Then, the R.V., X takes value, 0, 1, 2, 3, ... n times. Here n is a finite value say 100 or 200 or 5000 but n is a known value.

Let p = Probability of getting head (or) getting success > 0.

q = Probability of getting a tail or getting a defective

Such that

$$q = 1 - p \text{ or } p + q = 1.$$

We are assuming that the value of p and q should not change in the middle of the experiment that is, they are assumed as constants. Further, we assume that the number of trials 'n' is finite and the value of n is known.

We further assume that these 'n' trials are independently performed. If we add p and q, we have to get 1 i.e. $p + q = 1$.

6.3.1. Definition of Binomial Distribution

The random variable X is said to be a Binomial Random Variable. If the probability function is given by

$$P(X = r) = \binom{n}{r} p^r\, q^{n-r} \quad r = 0, 1, 2, ..., n. \tag{6.3.1}$$

The distribution of the R.V. X is known as binomial distribution. The values n and p are called *"parameters"* of the binomial distribution.

6.3.2 Properties of Binomial Distribution

1. Mean of the binomial distribution = np.
2. Variance of binomial distribution = npq.
3. Standard deviation of binomial distribution = $\sqrt{npq}$.
4. In binomial distribution mean is always greater than variance $np > npq$ i.e. Mean > Variance
5. n and p are called parameters of binomial distribution.
6. Since, $X = 0, 1, 2, 3 \ldots, n$, this distribution is known as discrete variable distribution.

Example (6.3.1): If 10 coins are tossed simultaneously, calculate the probability that there are (*a*) exactly 8 heads (*b*) at least 8 heads and (*c*) at most 3 heads. If the experiment is repeated 1000 times, estimate how many times we can expect exactly 8 head.

Solution:

Let the random variable X represents number of heads appear when 10 coins are tossed. Hence $X = 0, 1, 2, 3, 4, 5, 6, 7, 8, 9, 10$.

(*a*) here we have to find

$$P(X = 8) = \binom{10}{8}\left(\frac{1}{2}\right)^8\left(\frac{1}{2}\right)^{10-8} = 45/2^{10}$$

$$= 45/1024 = 0.04395.$$

(*b*) $P(\text{at least 8 heads}) = P(X \geq 8) = P(X = 8) + P(X = 9) + P(X = 10)$

$$P(X = 9) = \binom{10}{9}\left(\frac{1}{2}\right)^9\left(\frac{1}{2}\right)^{10-9} = 10/2^{10} = 10/1024 = 0.00977$$

And $P(X = 10) = 1/2^{10} = \mathbf{0.00098}$

$$P(X \geq 8) = 0.04395 + 0.00977 + 0.00098 = \mathbf{0.0547.}$$

(c) $P(\text{at most 3 heads}) = P(X \le 3) = P(X = 0) + P(X = 1) + P(X = 2) + P(X = 3)$.

$$P(X = 0) = 0.00098$$
$$P(X = 1) = 0.00977$$
$$P(X = 2) = 0.04395 \text{ and}$$
$$P(X = 3) = 120/1024 = \mathbf{0.11719.}$$

$P(\text{at most 3 heads})\ 0.00098 + 0.00977 + 0.04395 + 0.11719 = 0.17189$.

To estimate expected number of times exactly 8 heads turn up out of 1000 times is 1000(0.04395) = 439 times.

Example (6.3.2): Stating the suitable assumptions, calculate the probability that a family consisting of 6 children have 2 male and 4 female children.

Solution: Here we assume that the probability of having a male or female child is equal. The probability of a male child 'p' is equal to the probability of a female child 'q' i.e. $p = q = 1/2$. Let number of male children is denoted by the R.V. X. Here we have to consider $n = 6$ and $X = 2$. Thus it is required to calculate

$$P(X = 2) = \binom{6}{2}\left(\frac{1}{2}\right)^{2}\left(\frac{1}{2}\right)^{6-2} = 15/2^{6} = 15/64.$$
$$= 0.234375.$$

Aliter:
We can also consider number of female children as a random variable Y. Now we have to calculate $P(Y = 4)$. Proceeding on similar lines as above, we have:

$$P(Y = 4) = \binom{6}{4}\left(\frac{1}{2}\right)^{4}\left(\frac{1}{2}\right)^{6-4} = 15/64 = 0.234375.$$

It is interesting to note that whatever may be the R.V. representing male or female children, we get the same answer.

Example (6.3.3): From the past experience, it is known that Dr. Ravi complete the surgery successfully in 8 out of 10 cases. If 8 surgeries are to be done by him in a month, find the probability that (*a*) all the eight are successful (*b*) exactly 6 are successful (*c*) 4 are successful and 4 are failure.

Solution: Here we have to assume that the probability of a successful operation $p = 8/10 = 0.8$ and that it fails is $q = 1 - p = 2/10 = 0.2$, and $n = 8$.

Let the R.V. X denote number of successful surgeries.

Thus $X = 1, 2, 3, 4, 5, 6, 7, 8$.

(*a*) Here we have to find $P(X = 8) = \binom{8}{8}\left(\frac{8}{10}\right)^{8}\left(\frac{2}{10}\right)^{8-8} = 1.(0.16778).1$

$$= 0.16778$$

The probability that all surgeries is 0.0039.

(*b*) Here we have to find $P(X = 6) = \binom{8}{6}\left(\frac{8}{10}\right)^{6}\left(\frac{2}{10}\right)^{8-6}$

$$= 28(0.262144)(0.04) = 0.2936$$

(*c*) Here we have to find $P(X = 4) = \binom{8}{4}\left(\frac{8}{10}\right)^4\left(\frac{2}{10}\right)^{8-4}$

$= 70\ (0.4096)(0.0016) = 0.045875$

It is more probable that 6 operations are successful and 2 failure ones by comparing (*a*), (*b*) and (*c*).

Example (6.3.4): The incidence of occupational disease in an industry is such that the workers have 20% chance of suffering from it. What is the probability that out of randomly chosen six workers (*a*) all are suffering (*b*) none are suffering (*c*) exactly 4 are suffering from the disease.

Solution: Here $p = 20/100 = 1/5 = 0.2$ and $q = 1 - p = 1 - 0.2 = 0.8$ and $n = 6$.

Let the random variable X represents number of workers suffering from the disease.

(*a*) $P(X = 6) = \binom{6}{6}\left(\frac{1}{5}\right)^6\left(\frac{4}{5}\right)^{6-6} = 1.\ (1/5)^6 \cdot (4/5)^0 = 1/15625 = 0.000064.$

(*b*) $P(X = 0) = \binom{6}{0}\left(\frac{1}{5}\right)^0\left(\frac{4}{5}\right)^{6-0} = 1\ (1)(0.262144) = 0.262144.$

(*c*) $P(X = 4) = \binom{6}{4}\left(\frac{1}{5}\right)^4\left(\frac{4}{5}\right)^{6-4} = 15\ (0.0016)(0.64) = 0.01536.$

The probability that none suffering from the disease is more when compared to (*a*), (*b*) and (*c*).

6.4. POISSON DISTRIBUTION

Poisson distribution is a discrete variable distribution and was discovered by French Mathematician Simen Denis Poisson in the year 1837. He derived Poisson distribution as a limiting form of binomial distribution in which *n*, the number of trials become very large and *p*, the probability of success of the event is very, very, small such that '*np*' is a finite quantity and is a constant, not necessarily large.

Thus Poisson distribution is assumed as a limiting form of binomial distribution as $n \to \infty$ such that $n \cdot p = \lambda$ = Mean (a constant).

As number of trials '*n*' increases larger and larger the value of *p* will become (or) tends to zero (or) reaches to zero i.e. $p \to 0$, such that $n.p = \lambda$. The Poisson Random Variable X takes value 0,1,2,3..........∞. Poisson distribution is the most widely used distribution in many real life problems. Basic difference between Binomial distribution and Poisson distribution is that *n* is finite and a known value in the former one, where as *n* is very large and not possible to count practically. For example, total number of high way accident or total number of affected persons from a disease and so on. In these situations it is not possible to know the value of *n* exactly.

6.4.1. Definition of Poisson Distribution

The probability distribution of a random variable X is said to have a Poisson distribution it takes only non-negative values and if its distribution is given by:

$$P(X = x) = \frac{\lambda^x e^{-\lambda}}{x!} \quad x = 0, 1, 2, 3, \ldots, \infty.$$

Here, λ is the parameter and $e = 2.7183$.

6.4.2. Conditions Under which Poisson Distribution to be Used

1. The random variable X should be discrete.
2. A dichotomy of events should be present. That is happening or not happening of an event should be present.
3. Probability of happening of events should be very small. That is p should be nearer to zero.
4. Events should happen independently. That is happening of one event does not affect the happening of other event.

Thus Poisson distribution has equal mean and variance. λ is called parameter of the Poison distribution. Poisson distribution has large variety of application in real life.

6.4.3. Application of the Poisson's Distribution.

1. Number of accidents in a town in a unit of time.
2. Number of deaths from a diseases like heart attacks, cancer, AIDS.
3. Number of deaths due to snake bite.
4. Number of suicides reported in a city (or) town.
5. Number of defective items produced from a machine.
6. Number of printing mistakes in a page of the first proof of a book.
7. Number of air accidents in a unit of time in a city or in a town.
8. Number of defective spots on the skin.
9. Number of telephone calls coming to a switch board in 1 hour.
10. Number of vehicles coming to a petrol bunk.
11. Number of gamma rays (or) radioactive particles produced from a substance.
12. Number of alpha particles produced in one hour.
13. Number of bacteria developed in a region.
14. Number of births in a city or a town.
15. Number of defective needles or screws in a packet of 100 needles or screws.
16. Number of airplanes coming to an airport.
17. Number of cars passing through a highway, say N.H. 4 at time t.
18. Number of fragments received by a surface area, in an atom bomb explosion.
19. Flashing of number of lightings per second.
20. Number of runs or goals in a test series of cricket or football or hockey.

Above list of events explains that the probability of occurrence of an event is very small. Hence, Poisson distribution is also known as "Rare Events distribution".

6.4.4. Properties of Poisson Distribution

1. Poisson distribution is a discrete random variable distribution.
2. It depends mainly on the value of the mean λ, hence λ is known as the parameter of the distribution.
3. If n is large, and p is small, this distribution is a close approximation to binomial distribution.
4. Mean is equal to variance in Poisson distribution.
5. Poisson distribution is a positively skewed distribution. That is mean is larger than mode.
6. Happening of Poisson events in an interval are independent of the events happened prior to the interval. This is an important property and is known as **"memory less property"**.
7. Poisson distribution has only one parameter i.e. its mean λ.
8. The probability of happening more than one event in a very small interval is negligible.

Example (6.4.1): Suppose a book of 600 pages contains 48 typographical errors. If we assume that these errors are randomly distributed throughout the book, What is the probability that 10 pages selected at random have (*a*) zero errors (*b*) exactly 2 mistakes (*c*) more than 2 mistakes. (use $e^{-0.8} = 0.44933$).

Solution: In the problem, it is given that number of pages $n = 10$ and $P = 48/600 = 0.08$. Hence mean $= \lambda = n.p = 10(0.08) = 0.8$.

Let the random variable X represents number of typographical mistakes per page.

(*a*) We have to find $P(X = 0) = \dfrac{\lambda^x e^{-\lambda}}{x!} = \dfrac{(0.8)^0 e^{-0.8}}{0!} = e^{-0.8} = 0.44933.$

(*b*) Here we have to find $P(X = 2) = \dfrac{(0.8)^2 e^{-0.8}}{2!} = e^{-0.8}\,(0.64)/2 = 0.14379.$

(*c*) Here we have to find $P(X > 2) = 1 - [P(X = 0) + P(X = 1) + P(X = 2)]$

Now $P(X = 1) = \dfrac{(0.8)^1 e^{-0.8}}{1!} = e^{-0.8}\,(0.8) = 0.359464.$

$$P(X > 2) = 1 - (0.44933 + 0.359464 + 0.14379)$$
$$= 1 - 0.952584 = 0.047416.$$

Example (6.4.2): In a survey, on heart patients, it is found that the mortality rate 60 out of 10,000 patients. If 400 heart patients are randomly selected from a city, find the probability that there are (*a*) exactly two deaths (*b*) at least three deaths and (*c*) at most two deaths in the randomly selected sample. (it is given that $e^{-2.4} = 0.09072$)

Solution: In the problem it is given that $n = 400$ and $p = 60/10{,}000 = 0.006$.

Hence the mean $= \lambda = n.p = 400(0.006) = 2.4$.

Let X denote the random variable representing number of deaths.

(*a*) Here we have to find $P(X = 2) = \dfrac{(2.4)^2\, e^{-2.4}}{2!}$ $[(5.76) \cdot (0.09072)]/2$

$= 0.26127.$

(*b*) Here we have to find $P(\text{at least three deaths}) = P(X \geq 3) = P(X > 2)$
$= 1 - [P(X = 0) + P(X = 1) + P(X = 2)].$

$$P(X = 0) = \frac{(2.4)^0\, e^{-2.4}}{0!} = e^{-2.4} = 0.09072 \text{ and}$$

$$P(X = 1) = \frac{(2.4)^1\, e^{-2.4}}{1!} = (2.4)\, e^{-2.4} = 0.21772.$$

Hence $P(X > 2) = P(X \geq 3) = 1 - (0.09072 + 0.21772 + 0.26127)$
$= 1 - 0.56971 = 0.43029.$

(*c*) here we have to find $P(\text{at most two deaths}) = P(X \leq 2)$
$= P(X = 0) + P(X = 1) + P(X = 2) = 0.09072 + 0.21772 + 0.26127$
$= 0.56971.$

Example (6.4.3): In a Syringe needle manufacturing company, there is a small chance that 2 out of 1000 needles are defective needles. These manufactured needles are supplied in packets of 10. Using Poisson distribution, estimate approximate number of packets out of 10,000 consignment, consists of (*a*) No defective needles (*b*) one defective needle and (*c*) at most two defective needles. It is given that $e^{-0.02} = 0.980199$.

Solution: Here $N = 10{,}000$, $n = 10$ and $p = 2/1000 = 0.002$.

Hence, mean $= \lambda = n.p = 10(0.002) = 0.02$.

Let X denote the random variable representing number of defective needles in the packet of 10.

(*a*) We have to find $P(X = 0) = \dfrac{(0.02)^0\, e^{-0.02}}{0!} = e^{-0.02} = 0.980199.$

Therefore expected number of packets with zero defective needles are $N.p = 10{,}000(0.980199) = 9802$ packets (approx).

(*b*) On similar lines, $P(X = 1) = \dfrac{(0.02)^1\, e^{-0.02}}{1!} = (0.02)\, e^{-0.02} = 0.0196.$

Hence expected number of packets with 1 defective needle $= Np$
$= 10{,}000(0.0196) = 196$ packets (Approx.)

(*c*) Here we have to determine number of packets containing at most 2 defective needles $= NP(X \leq 2)$.

Thus $P(X \leq 2) = P(X = 0) + P(X = 1) + P(X = 2)$.

It is required to calculate $P(X = 2) = \dfrac{(0.02)^2\, e^{-0.02}}{2!} = [(0.02)^2\, e^{-0.02}]/2$

$= (0.0004)(0.980199)/2 = 0.000196.$

Therefore, $P(X \leq 2) = 0.980199 + 0.0196 + 0.000196 = 0.99999.$

Hence 10,000(0.99999) = 99999 packets consists of at most two defective needles. This implies that in one packet we can expect more than two defective needles.

6.5. NORMAL DISTRIBUTION

Normal distribution was first discovered by English Mathematician "De – Moivre" in year 1733. This distribution was also discovered by Laplace before 1774 due to some historical error the credit has gone to Gauss, who used this distribution in predicting the movement of planets in Astronomy.

The normal distribution of a variable, when represented graphically, takes the shape of a symmetrical curve known as the "Normal curve". Normal distribution can also be considered as the limiting form of binomial distribution under the following conditions.

1. Number of trials 'n' is infinitely large i.e. $n \to \infty$ and
2. Both p and q are nearly equal and are very small.

Normal distribution is a continuous random variable distribution and is having lot of Theoretical Importance and Applications. Earlier, normal distribution used to be called as "distribution of errors". This is because of the fact that errors usually follow normal distribution. Normal distribution is also known as "Gaussian distribution" named after Karl Friedrich Gauss, who used this distribution to describe the accidental errors of measurements involved in the calculation of orbit of heavenly bodies.

6.5.1. Definition of Normal Distribution and Standard Normal Distribution

A continuous random variable X is said to have normal distribution with mean μ and standard deviation σ if the probability density function is given by

$$f(x) = \frac{1}{\sigma\sqrt{2\pi}} e^{-\frac{1}{2}(x-\mu)^2/\sigma^2} \quad -\infty < x < \infty \tag{6.5.1}$$

where $e = 2.7183$ and $\pi = 22/7$.

The graph of normal distribution is given in the following figure.

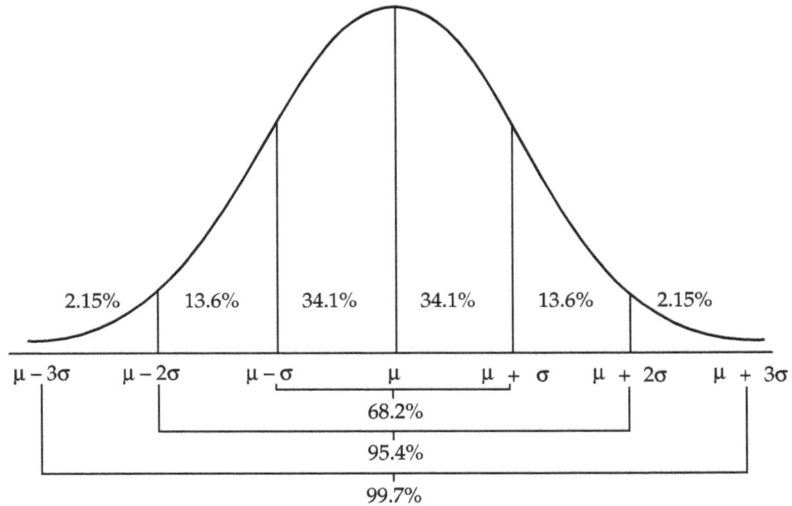

Fig. 6.5.1: *Distribution area of normal curve with mean μ and* S.D. σ.

In equation (6.5.1) if $\mu = 0$ and $\sigma^2 = 1$ then normal distribution is known as "Standard Normal Distribution" and is denoted by the random variable Z. It is important to note that whatever may be the distribution of the random variable X, the new variable Z = (x – Mean)/S.D. or $(X - \mu)/\sigma$ follows normal distribution with mean 0 and variance 1. That is Z follows standard normal distribution.

6.5.2. Definition of Standard Normal Distribution or Z-Distribution

A random variable z which has mean 0 and variance 1 is said to have a standard normal distribution if its probability density function is given by:

$$f(z) = \frac{1}{\sqrt{2\pi}} e^{-z2/2} \quad -\infty < z < \infty \qquad (6.5.2)$$

where $\pi = 22/7$. Z is called standard normal variable (S.N.V.)

The graph of probability density function of the standard normal variable is given as follows:

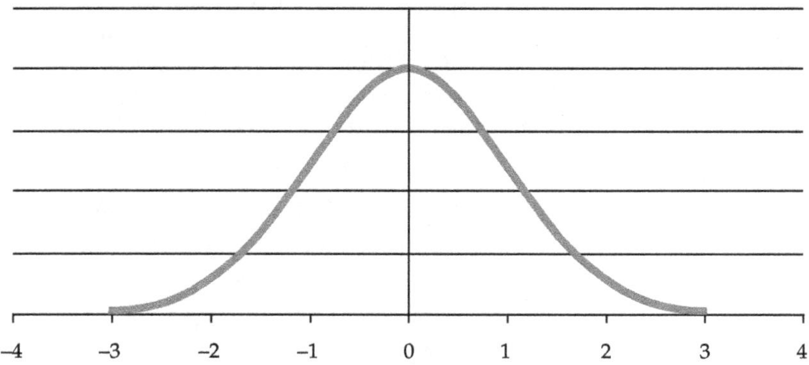

Fig. 6.5.2. *Graph of standard normal distribution mean = 0 and S.D. = 1*

6.5.3. Properties of Normal Distribution

Normal distribution has lot of theoretical importance in statistical analysis because of the following properties.

1. Normal distribution curve is a bell shaped curve.
2. In normal distribution Mean = Median = Mode.
3. The area covered under the left tail is exactly equal to the area under the right tail.
4. Length of the left tail = length of the right tail
5. If the curve is folded vertically at its mean both tails will exactly co-inside.
6. The two tails of the curve extended indefinitely and never touches the *x*-axis.
7. No portion of the curve lies below the *x*-axis because the area under the represents the probability and probabilities cannot be negative.

8. The total area under the normal curve is equal to one and the percentage of distribution of area under the normal curve is shown in Fig. (6.5.1) and is given as follows:
   (*i*) About 68% of the area falls between $\mu - \sigma$ and $\mu + \sigma$.
   (*ii*) About 95.5% of the area falls between $\mu - 2\sigma$ and $\mu + 2\sigma$.
   And (*iii*) About 99.73% of the area falls between $\mu - 3\sigma$ and $\mu + 3\sigma$.

6.5.4. Importance of Normal Distribution

Normal distribution is a very popular distribution having lot of theoretical importance. There are many theorems like central limit theorems, law of large numbers and so on using Normal approximations.

It plays a very vital role in large sample tests and non-parametric tests. Applications of normal distribution are listed below:

1. Normal distribution can be used to approximate the binomial and poisson distribution.
2. Normal distribution has extensive applications in the theory of sampling.
3. Normal distribution has wide applications in testing of hypothesis and large sample tests.
4. Normal distribution has variety of applications in the field of industry and statistical quality control.
5. In many statistical problems, we generally assume the normality in fairly large populations.
6. Normal distribution serves as guiding instrument in the analysis and interpretation of statistical data.

Note: It is important to note that to work out problems, we have to use standard normal table given in Appendix A-1. The numbers represent area under the curve from 0 to z and z ranges from 0 to 3. Total area is 1 and half of the area to the left is 0.5 and another half to the right is 0.5.

Example (6.5.1): It is known from the past experience that the average life time of bulbs produced from a company has 120 days and 20 days as standard deviation. An office installed 10,000 bulbs purchased from this company. Assuming that the life times of these bulbs follow normal distribution, calculate (a) How many bulbs will expire in less than 90 days.

(b) How many bulbs will expire after 149 days? (c) If the office manager has decided to replace all bulbs together, what interval should be allowed between replacements if not more than 10% should expire before each replacement.

Solution: Let R.V. X denote the life time of bulbs. It is given that mean of X is 120 days and S.D. is 20 days i.e. μ = 120 days and σ = 20 days. We have to convert X to Z where $Z(X - \mu)/\sigma = (X - 120)/20$ is a standard normal variable. To answer the given questions, we have to use the table of standard normal distribution given in Appendix (A – 1). Figures in the table represent area under the curve at different points.

(*a*) Here we have to find $P(X < 90) = P[Z < (90 - 120)/20] = P(Z < -1.5)$
$= 0.0668.$

The required area is represented as shaded portion under the curve in Fig. (6.5.1).

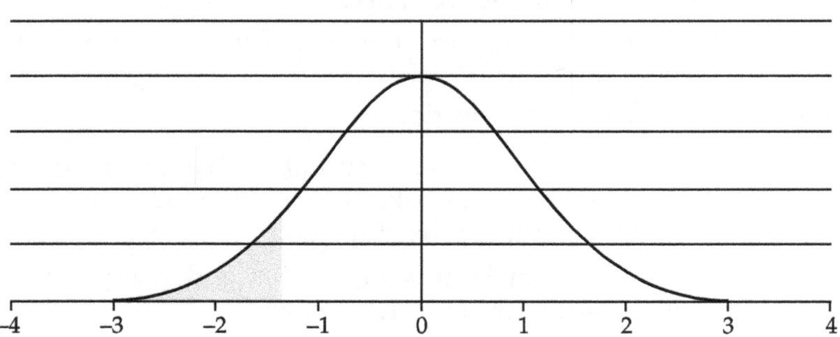

Fig. (6.5.3) Area of Z less than -1.5 under Standard Normal Curve.

Hence, out of 10,000 bulbs, expected number of bulbs fail before 90 days are $N.p = 10{,}000(0.0668) = 668$ bulbs.

(*b*) Here we have to find $P(X > 140) = P[Z > 140 - 120)/20] = P(Z > 1.00)$ $= 0.5 - 0.3413 = 0.1587$. Required area is shown in Fig. (6.5.2).

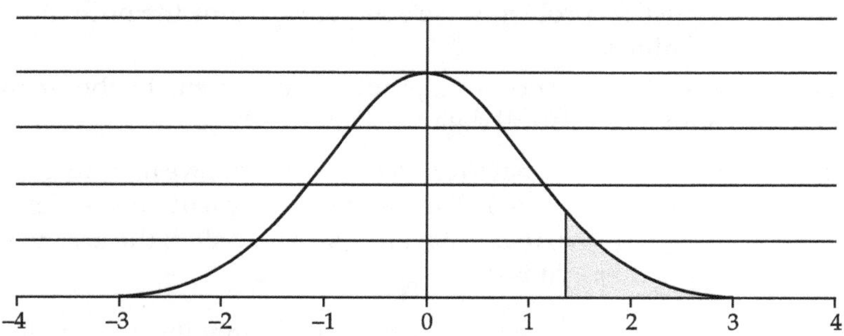

Fig. 6.5.4: *Area under S.N.V., above 1.*

Expected number of bulbs fail after 140 days are

$$N.p = 10{,}000(0.1587) = 1587 \text{ bulbs.}$$

(c) Here we have to find the value of X by determining Z i.e., we have to find X such that not more than 10% or 0.1 expire before replacement. Thus the value of Z to an area $0.5 - 0.1 = 0.4$ is 1.28. Thus the required area is that Z should be less than $- 1.28$ i.e. $(X - 120)/20 = -1.28$.

$$X = -1.28\,(20) + 120 = -25.6 + 120 = 94.4 \text{ or } 94 \text{ days (approx.)}$$

Thus the bulbs may be replaced after every 94 days. The interval between replacements must be 94 days.

Example (6.5.2): A survey is conducted to measure the height of 10th class male students and found that the average height is 68.22 cms with variance 10.8 cms and follows Nor. In a school, there are 800 students studying 10th class. Assuming that their heights are normally distributed with mean and variances mentioned above, estimate number of students in the school having more than 72 cms height.

Solution: Let X denote the random variable representing the height of the student. We assume that the distribution of X is normal with mean = 68.22 cms and variance = 10.8 cms. Hence, Standard deviation = $\sqrt{10.8}$ = 3.286 and it is given that $N = 800$.

Now we have to find

$$P(X > 72) = P[Z > (72 - 68.22)/3.286]$$
$$= P(Z > 3.78/3286 = 1.15) = 0.1251$$

That is area to the right of the coordinate at $z = 1.15$.

That is from the area under the curve 0 to ∞, i.e. 0.5 we have to subtract the area under the curve from 0 to 1.15. From the table of normal area, A – 1, we have the area under the curve, from 0 to 1.15 as 0.3749. Hence, area above 1.15 is (0.5 – 0.3749) = 0.1251. Hence the probability that height above 72 cms is 0.1251. Required area is shown in the following figure.

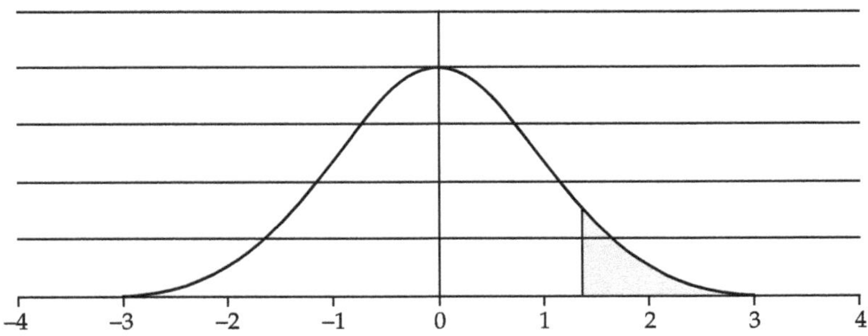

Fig. 6.5.5: *Area under S.N. Curve above 1.15.*

To estimate number of students having above 72 cms height is $N.p$ = 800 (0.1251) = 100.08 or 100 students (approx.)

We estimate that around 100 students will have height above 72 cms among 800 students in the school studying 10th class.

Example (6.5.3): In an agriculture field experiment, it was found that the mean yield for one acre plot is 662 kgs with a standard deviation of 32 kgs.

Assuming normal distribution for the yield of the crop, how many one acre plots in a batch of 10,000 plots expect yield (*a*) over 700 kgs (*b*) below 650 kgs and (*c*) What is the lowest yield of 1000 plots?

Solution: Here $\mu = 662$, $\sigma = 32$ and $N = 10{,}000$. Let R.V. X represents the yield of the crop per acre and the distribution of X is normal with mean 662 and S.D. 32. Standard normal variable $Z = (X - 662)/32$.

(a) here we have to find $P(X > 700) = P[Z > (700 - 662)/32] = P(Z > 38/32)$

$$= P(Z > 1.1875 \text{ or } 1.19) = 0.117.$$

To calculate the above area under the curve, we have to subtract the area from 0 to 1.19 = 0.383 (from A – 1) from the area from 0 to ∞ i.e. 0.5. Thus (0.5 – 0.383) = 0.117. Required area is shown in the following Figure.

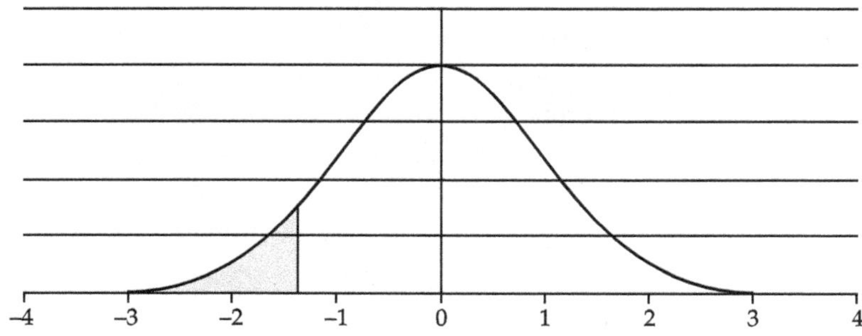

Fig. 6.5.6: *Area of S.N.V. greater than 1.19.*

Hence, estimated number of plots out of 10,000 given plots, giving yield over 700 kgs is $N.p$ = 10,000(0.117) = 1170 plots.

(b) Here we have to find $P(X < 650) = P[Z < (650 - 662)/32] = P(Z < -12/32)$

$P(Z < -0.375 \text{ or } -0.38) = 0.352$.

To calculate the area below – 0.38, we have to subtract the area from 0 to 0.38 = 0.148 from 0.5. i.e. (0.5 – 0.148) = 0.352.

Hence, expected number of plots giving the yield less than 650 kgs, among given 10,000 plots are $N.p$ =10,000(0.352) = 3520 plots.

Required area is shown in the figure.

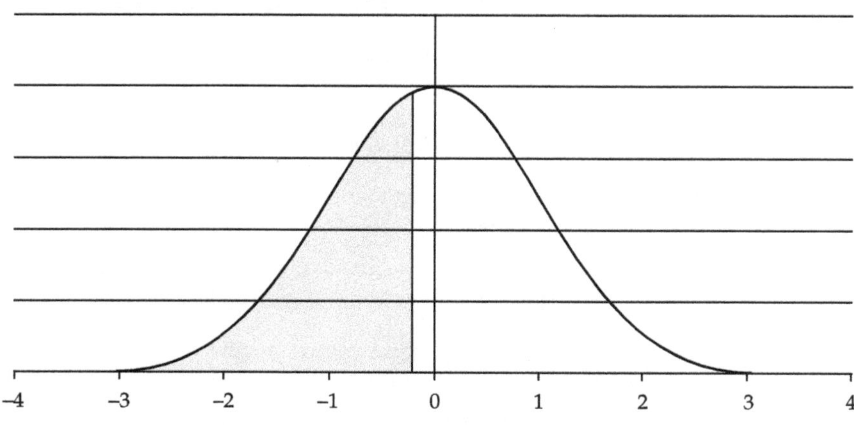

Fig. 6.5.7. *Area under S.N.V. less than –0.38.*

(c) We have to find the lowest yield in 1000 plots = 1000/10000 = 0.1. i.e. we have to find the value of Z such that the area is 0.1. From tables A – 1, we have area is 0.1 when z = 1.28. Thus we have to find X such that

$$z = 1.28 \text{ or } (X - 662)/32 = 1.28 \text{ or } X = 1.28(32) + 662 = 40.96 + 662$$

$$= 702.96 \text{ kgs or } 703 \text{ kgs (approx.).}$$

Example (6.5.4): Marks obtained in a competitive examination by 5,000 students, follow normal distribution with 45 and variance 100. Estimate the number of students who got (*a*) less than 40 marks (*b*) more than 60 marks (*c*) marks between 50 and 65.

Solution:

Let the R.V. X represents number of marks in the examination. It is given that X follows normal distribution with mean 45 marks and variance 100 marks. That is standard deviation = $\sqrt{100}$ = 10 marks and

$$N = 5{,}000 \text{ and } Z = (X - 45)/10.$$

(a) We have to find $P(X < 40) = P[Z < (40 - 45)/10]$

$= P(Z < -0.5)$ or $P(Z > 0.5)$ using symmetric property of normal distribution.

$= 0.5 - P(0 < z < 0.5) = 0.5 - 0.1915$ (from table A – 1) = 0.3085.

Required area is shown in the following figure.

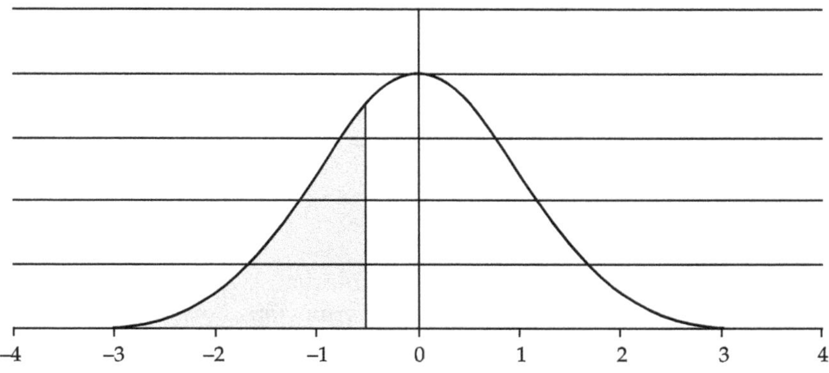

Fig. 6.5.8: *Area of S.N.V. less than –0.5.*

Hence expected number of students who got less than 40 marks out of 5000 students are $N.p = 5{,}000\ (0.3085) = 1542.5$ or 1543 students.

(b) Here we have to find $P(X > 60) = P[Z > (60 - 45)/10] = P(Z > 1.5)$

$= 0.5 - P(0 < Z < 1.5) = 0.5 - 0.4332$ (from tables $A - 1$) = 0.0668.

Hence, expected number of students who got more than 60 marks among 5,000 students appeared for the examination are $N.p = 5000(0.0668) = 334$ students. Required area is given in the following figure.

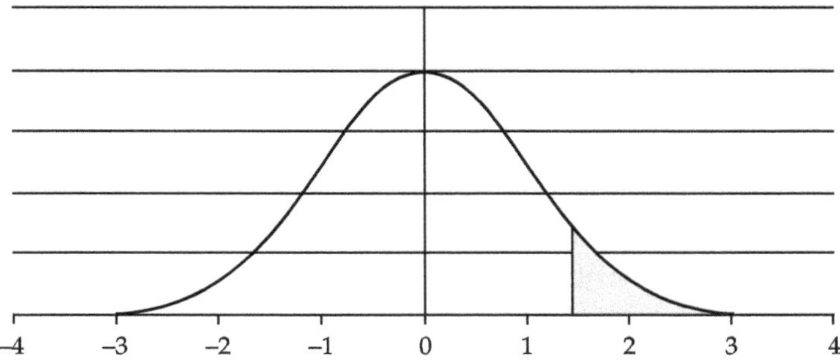

Fig. 6.5.9: *Area of S.N.V. greater than 1.5.*

(*c*) Here we have to find $P(50 < X < 65) = P[(50 - 45)/10 < Z < (65 - 45)/10]$
$= P(0.5 < Z < 2.0) = P(Z < 2.0) - P(Z < 0.5) = 0.4772 - 0.1915 = 0.2857.$

Hence, expected number of students who got marks between 50 and 65 are $N.P = 5000(0.2857) = 1428.5$ students or 1429 students (approx). Required area is shown in the following figure.

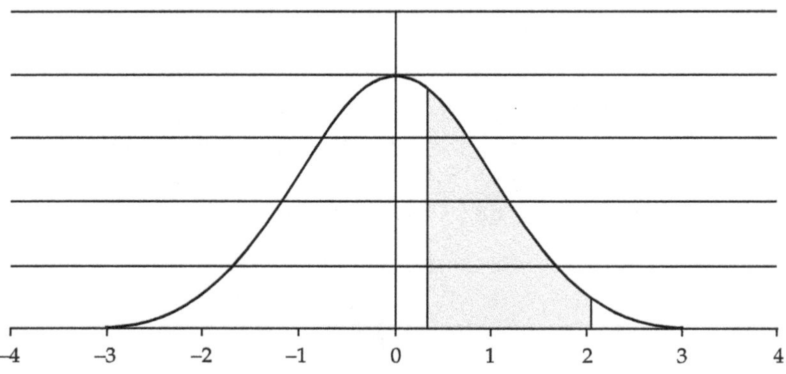

Fig. 6.5.10: *Area of S.N.V. between 0.5 to 2.0.*

6.6. EXPONENTIAL DISTRIBUTION

Exponential distribution is a continuous variable distribution used more popularly in many real life problems like Poisson distribution. Poisson distribution is a discrete variable distribution whereas, exponential distribution is a continuous variable distribution. In many life testing problems, queuing problems, survival problems and reliability problems, this distribution is very popularly used. This is because of the fact that this distribution represents life time distributions of many equipments or individuals. Exponential distribution is also known as '*Negative Exponential Distribution*" and is defined as:

Definition: A continuous random variable X is said to follow *exponential distribution* with mean μ, if it has the probability density function $f(x)$ if given by

$$f(x) = \mu e^{-\mu x} \text{ where, } \mu > 0 \text{ and } x > 0. \quad (6.6.1)$$
$$= 0 \text{ otherwise.}$$

μ is called the parameter of the exponential distribution.

6.6.1. Properties of Exponential Distribution

1. Mean of exponential distribution is $1/\mu$.
2. Variance of exponential distribution is $1/\mu^2$.
3. Standard deviation of exponential distribution is $1/\mu$.
4. In exponential distribution Mean = S.D.
5. Exponential distribution is a positively skewed distribution.
6. Exponential distribution has memory less property.

7. There exists a close relation between Poisson distribution and exponential distribution such that if occurrence of events follow Poisson distribution with mean μ, then the interval between two successive occurrences of events follow exponential distribution with mean 1/μ.

REVIEW QUESTIONS AND PROBLEMS

A. Objective Type Questions

1. In Binomial distribution mean is always --------- the variance.

(*a*) less than (*b*) equal to
(*c*) greater than (*d*) less than or equal to

2. In Binomial distribution with parameters n and p standard deviation is given by ------.

(*a*) $\sqrt{npq}$ (*b*) np
(*c*) npq (*d*) $(npq)^2$.

3. In a Binomial distribution mean = 10 and variance = 8 then n = -----.

(*a*) 500 (*b*) 50
(*c*) 5 (*d*) 150

4. In Poisson distribution mean is always ------- the variance.

(*a*) less than (*b*) equal to
(*c*) greater than (*d*) less than or equal to

5. Poisson distribution is a ---------- variable distribution.

(*a*) continuous (*b*) discrete
(*c*) uniform (*d*) uniformly continuous

6. Poisson distribution is also known as --------- events distribution.

(*a*) rare (*b*) normal
(*c*) common (*d*) frequently occurring.

7. Normal curve is a -------- shaped curve.

(*a*) *J*–shaped (*b*) *U*–shaped
(*c*) Z–shaped (*d*) Bell shaped.

8. Mean = Median = Mode in --------- distribution.

(*a*) normal (*b*) binomial
(*c*) Poisson (*d*) uniform.

9. Normal distribution with mean 0 and variance 1 is called ------- distribution

(*a*) standard normal (*b*) binomial
(*c*) Poisson (*d*) uniform

10. Mean of the exponential distribution is 1/μ, then variance is --------.

(*a*) $1/\mu$ (2) $1/\mu^2$

(3) $1/\sqrt{\mu}$ (4) μ^2

11. Let N represents the Poisson random variable with mean K.

Then interval between two successive Poisson events is an exponential distribution with mean -------.

(*a*) $1/K^2$ (*b*) $1/K$
(*c*) K^2 (*d*) $\sqrt{K}$.

12. -------------- distribution has memory less property.

(*a*) binomial (*b*) normal
(*c*) standard normal (*d*) exponential.

13. Normal distribution is a ------------- variable distribution.

(*a*) continuous (*b*) discrete
(*c*) uniform (*d*) uniformly continuous.

14. Mean = variance in ------------- distribution.

(*a*) normal (*b*) binomial
(*c*) Poisson (*d*) uniform.

15. Number of road accidents usually follow --------- distribution.

(*a*) normal (*b*) binomial
(*c*) uniform (*d*) Poisson.

16. Normal distribution is a --------- curve.

(*a*) skewed (*b*) symmetric
(*c*) asymmetric (*d*) non-symmetric.

B. Short Answer Questions

1. Define a random variable and give two examples of a random variable.
2. Distinguish discrete and continuous random variables with suitable examples.
3. Define binomial distribution and discuss its properties.
4. List out various applications of Poisson distribution.
5. Define Poisson distribution state the conditions under which this distribution is derived as a limiting form of binomial distribution.
6. Discuss the importance of normal distribution.
7. Define normal distribution and discuss its properties.
8. Define standard normal distribution and explain its role.
9. Define exponential distribution and discuss its applications.
10. Write short note on probability distributions.

C. Essay Type Questions

1. Write detailed notes on probability distributions discuss their applications.
2. Explain the role of a random variable and discuss its classification.
3. Explain why Poisson distribution is known as rare events distribution.
4. Write detailed notes on Poisson distribution.

5. Explain the normal curve and discuss its important properties.

6. There are 64 beds in a rose garden and 3 seeds of a particular type of rose are sown in each bed randomly. The probability of a rose being white is 2/5. Find the probability that number of beds with 0, 1, 2, 3 white roses.

   [**Hint:** Let the Binomial R.V. takes values 0, 1, 2, 3 and $n = 3$, $N = 64$, $p = 2/5$ and hence $q = 3/5$. To find number of beds with 1 white rose = $N \times P(X = 1)$]

7. If 10 coins are tossed 100 times, how many times would you expect 7 coins to fall tail upward?

   [**Hint:** $p = 1/2$, $q = 1/2$, $n = 10$, $N = 100$. Binomial R.V. takes values 0, 1, 2,.,., 10 and expected number of times 7 turns up = $N \times P(X = 7)$].

8. A manufacturer, who produces medicine bottles, finds that 0.1% of the bottles are defective. Manufactured bottles are packed in boxes containing 500 bottles. A drug manufacturer purchases 1000 such boxes from the above manufacturer of bottles. Using Poisson distribution, find how many boxes will contain (*a*) zero defective (*b*) two defectives and (*c*) at least two defective bottles.

   [**Hint:** Poisson variable X takes values in (*a*) $X = 0$, (*b*) $X = 2$ and (*c*) $X \geq 2$.

   Above probabilities are to be calculated by using Poisson distribution mass function]

9. It is known from the past experience that in a hospital there are on the average 4 deaths due to heart attacks per month. Find the probability that there will be less than 4 deaths due to heart attacks, in a randomly selected month. (it is given that $e^{-4} = 0.0183$)

   [**Hint:** Poisson R.V. X takes values 0, 1, 2,.,.,., using Poisson probability mass function find $P(X < 4) = P(X = 0) + P(X = 1) + P(X = 2) + P(X = 3)$]

10. Life time of C.T. scan tube produced from a company has a mean life time of 400 hrs and standard deviation of 45 hrs. Assuming the distribution of life time to be normal, find (*a*) percentage of C.T. scan tubes with life time of at least 470 hrs (*b*) number of C.T. scan tubes out of 10,000 having life times between 385 hrs and 415 hrs (*c*) the minimum lifetime of the best 10% of C.T. scan tubes.

    [**Hint:** Let X denote the lifetime of C.T. scan tubes. Using SNV density function $Z = (X - 400)/45$. Find $P(X \geq 470)$ (*b*) $10{,}000 \times P(385 < X < 415)$ and (*c*) find X such that $(X - 400)/45 = 0.1$].

11. In a survey, the waist measurements of 800 girls are normally distributed with mean 66 cms and standard deviation 5 cms. Find number of girls with waists (*a*) between 65 cms and 70 cms (*b*) greater than or equal to 72 cms (*c*) less than or equal to 60 cms.

    [**Hint:** Let X represent the measurement of waist. Find (*a*) $800 \times P(65 < X < 70)$ (*b*) $800 \times P(X \geq 72)$ and (*c*) $800\ P(X \leq 60)$]

12. In a survey, on the collection of human skulls, an index X is calculated based on length and breadth of the skull. Assuming that X follows normal distribution with mean 74.36 units with standard deviation 3.22 units, estimate number of human skulls in 1000, having index (*a*) greater than

70 units (*b*) less than or equal to 68 units (*c*) in between 65 units and 75 units.

[Number of skulls with index (*a*) 1000 × $P(X \geq 70)$ (*b*) 1000 × $P(X \leq 68)$ and (*c*) 1000 × $P(65 < X < 75)$].

References

1. Gupta S.P. 1990 "Statistical Methods". Sultan Chand & Sons, New Delhi.
2. Wayne W. Daniel 2008 Biostatistics, 9th edition, John Wiley & Sons. Inc. Newyork.
3. P.N. Arora *et al.* 2007 "Comprehensive Statistical Methods" Sultan Chand and company Ltd. First edn. New Delhi.
4. VK. Kapoor 1986 "Problems and solutions in Business statistics" Sultan Chand and sons New Delhi.

Answers to Objective Type Questions

1 – c; 2 – a; 3 – b; 4 – b; 5 – b; 6 – a; 7 – d; 8 – a; 9 – a; 10 – b; 11 – b; 12 – d; 13 – a; 14 – c; 15 – d; 16 – b.

CORRELATION AND REGRESSION

7.1. INTRODUCTION TO CORRELATION AND REGRESSION ANALYSIS

So far, we have discussed statistical tools and techniques, useful to take decisions by comparing two or more variables. In other words, we can compare with respect to Mean, or Median or Mode; with respect to variance or standard deviation or with respect to C.V., or skewness or kurtosis or with respect to probability and to take appropriate decisions.

Now, we shift our concentration for prediction or forecasting the value of the variable, and to take appropriate decisions. We can predict or forecast the behavior or value of a variable, using the known value is another closely related variable to the first variable. This method of prediction is done through the concept of '*Regression*'. First variable is usually called as dependent variable or main variable or '*the effect*' and the second variable is known as Independent variable or Concomitant variable or '*the cause*'. Hence, regression models are also known as **Cause and effect models.**

Before discussing the concept of regression and its models, first, we concentrate on the relation between the two variables. Namely relation between independent and dependent variables and the relationship between these two variables is known as "correlation". In many real life problems, we get number of variables, which are related to each other. For example, taller people will have higher weights as compared to persons of shorter height. Hence, there exists some relation between height and weight. Similarly, students who work hard and study more number of hours will get more marks in the examination than, those students, who study lesser number hours. Thus, number of study hours and marks in the examination are related. On similar lines, supply and price of a commodity; temperature of the soil and germination time of a seed, food intake and calories of energy obtained by a person; rain fall and yield of a crop also have some relation between them. If change in one variable brings the corresponding change in the other variable on an average, then we say that two variables are related and we can measure this relation or '*correlation*'. Correlation is denoted by small letter '*r*'.

Before going to discuss the concept of correlation, there is a need to understand the concept of 'covariance' between two quantitative variables X and Y. Let (x_1, y_1), (x_2, y_2), (x_3, y_3).,., (x_n, y_n) are pairs of n observations on the variables X and Y. Then, covariance between X and Y is denoted by Cov(X, Y) and is defined as:

$$\text{Cov}(X, Y) = \frac{1}{n}[(x_1 - \bar{x})(y_1 - \bar{y}) + (x_2 - \bar{x})(y_2 - \bar{y}) + (x_3 - \bar{x})(y_3 - \bar{y})$$

$$+,,,,,,, + (x_n - \bar{x})(y_n - \bar{y})]$$

$$= \frac{1}{n}\Sigma(x_i - \bar{x})(y_i - \bar{y}) = \Sigma XY - \frac{\Sigma Y \Sigma Y}{n}. \qquad (7.1.1)$$

Here $\bar{x}$ = Arithmetic mean of the variable X = $\sum x_i/n$ and

$\bar{y}$ = Arithmetic mean of the variable $Y = \sum y_i/n$.

Example (7.1.1): Calculate covariance for the following data collected in pairs on the variables *X* and *Y*.

X:	4	5	6	7	8	12
Y:	16	14	12	10	8	6

Solution: Mean of $X = 42/6 = 7$ and mean of $Y = 66/6 = 11$.

$(X - 7) = x = -3 -2 -1 \quad 0 \quad 1 \quad 5$

$(Y - 11) = y = 5 \quad 3 \quad 1 \quad -1 \quad -3 \quad -5$

$x \cdot y = -15 \quad -6 \quad -1 \quad 0 \quad -3 \quad -25$ Sum = –50.

Therefore Cov (*X*, *Y*) = – 50/6 = 8.33333.

In the above formula, calculation of covariance is complicated in the data is large in size. Now we discuss a shortcut method which is explained as follows:

Step – 1: Calculate $x_i = (X_i - A)$ and $y_i = (Y_i - B)$

Step – 2: Calculate the sum of *X* i.e. Σx_i and sum of *Y* i.e. Σy_i.

Step – 3: Calculate the product of *X* and *Y* i.e. $\Sigma x_i \cdot y_i$

Step – 4: Calculate the difference $\Sigma x_i \cdot y_i - (\Sigma x_i \Sigma y_i)/n$

Step – 5: Divide the quantity obtained in step–3 by *n* to get the covariance between *X* and *Y*.

Example (7.1.2): Calculate the covariance between *X* and *Y* using short-cut method.

X:	65	66	67	68	69	70	71	72
Y:	60	65	68	68	70	78	80	88

Solution: Calculate the required sums as shown in the following table.

X	Y	$X - A = x$	$Y - B = y$	$x \cdot y$
65	60	–3	–8	24
66	65	–2	–3	6
67	68	–1	0	0
68 = A	68 = B	0	0	0
69	70	1	2	2
70	78	2	10	20
71	80	3	12	36
72	88	4	20	80
Sum		4	33	168

$$\text{Cov}(X, Y) = \text{Cov}(x, y) = [\Sigma x_i \cdot y_i - (\Sigma x_i \, \Sigma y_i)/n]/n$$
$$= [168 - (4 \times 33)/8]/8 = (168 - 132/8)/8 = (165 - 16.5)/8$$
$$= 18.5625.$$

Using the concept of covariance, we can calculate correlation just dividing the covariance with the product of standard deviations of X and Y. Thus correlation analysis is a statistical procedure, by which we can determine the degree of association or relationship between two variables. If we consider only two variables, X, Y then the correlation if *'simple correlation'* and if we consider more than two variables, then it is known as *'multiple correlation'*. Simple correlation is again divided into of two categories, namely:

1. Positive correlation and
2. Negative correlation.

7.1.1. Positively Correlated Variables

If one variable increases then the other variable also increases on an average, or if one variable decreases on an average the other variable also decreases, then we say that two variables are *'positively correlated variables'*. For example, if number of study hours increases, marks obtained in the examination also increase hence, number of study hours and marks in the examination are positively correlated. Similarly, intake of food and energy gained; demand and price of an item; height and weight of a person; sugar intake and blood sugar levels; cholesterol levels and risk of heart attacks; are positively correlated variables.

7.1.2. Negatively Correlated Variables

On the other hand, of one variable decreases the other variable increases on an average or vice-versa, then we say that two variables are *'Negatively Correlated Variables'*. For example, temperature of the soil and the germination time of the seed; supply and price of a commodity; number of hours of usage and remaining energy in the battery, number of working hours of a worker and remaining energy in the worker; and so on are negatively correlated variables.

7.2. SCATTER DIAGRAM METHOD

To know whether two variables are related? or not? We use scatter diagram method, which is explained as follows.

Consider one variable on X-axis and other variable on Y-axis. Then plot each pair of observations by choosing suitable scale. The resultant figure is called scatter diagram. Scatter diagram explains the scatter of or spread of pairs of observations in the graph and hence, it is known as *'Scatter Diagram'* and determining whether two variables are related? Or not? Is known as 'scatter diagram method', which is explained as follows:

Example (7.2.1): Draw scatter diagram for the following data representing number of study hours per week, denoted by the R.V. X and marks obtained in the examination denoted by the R.V. Y.

X	2	5	8	10	14	18	20	22	24	28	30	32
Y	12	16	20	25	32	45	50	62	70	80	86	95

Solution:

Consider number of study hours (independent variable) on x–axis and number of marks obtained in the examination (dependent variable) on y–axis and plot the points as shown in the figure. The scatter of the points on the graph explains the correlation between the two variables under consideration. The resultant figure is called scatter diagram and is as shown in the following figure.

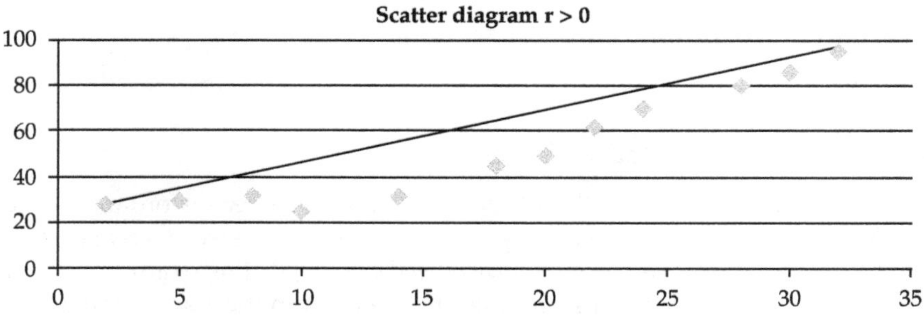

Fig. 7.2.1: *Scatter diagram explaining the relation between number of study hours and marks obtained in the examination.*

Number of study hours/week

Example (7.2.2): Represent the following data through scatter diagram.

X	2	5	8	10	14	18	20	22	24	28	30	32
Y	92	86	72	65	53	45	40	36	27	18	6	2

Solution: Consider the random variable X on x-axis and the random variable Y on y-axis and draw points for each pair. Through a straight line, join first and last plotted points.

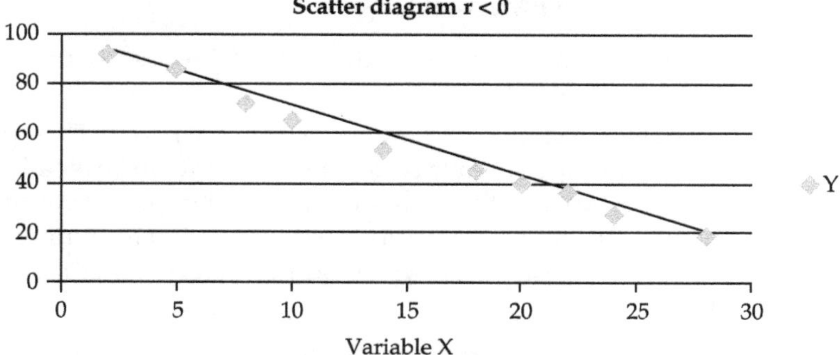

Fig. 7.2.2: *Scatter diagram for negative correlation.*

Example (7.2.3): Represent the following through a scatter diagram.

X	2	5	8	10	14	18	20	22	24	28	30	32
Y	92	16	72	25	82	95	85	62	27	68	18	95

Solution:

Consider the random variable X on x–axis and the random variable Y on y–axis and draw points for each pair.

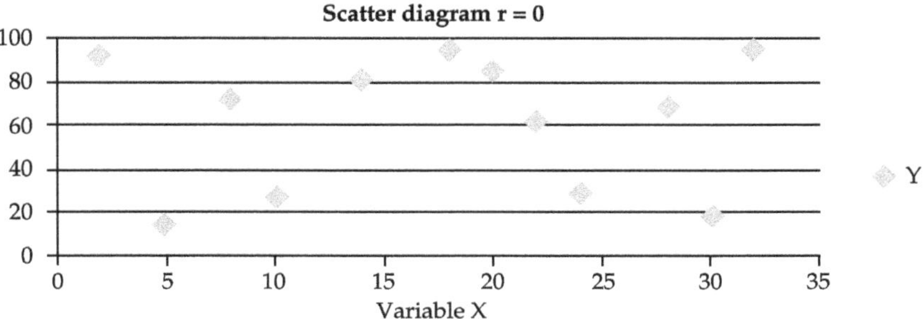

Fig. 7.2.3: *Scatter diagram for independent variables*

Example (7.2.4): Construct the scatter diagram for the following data.

X	2	3	8	10	15	18	20	22	24	28	30	32
Y	10	15	40	50	75	45	100	110	120	140	150	160

Solution: Consider the variable X on x–axis and the variable Y on y–axis and plot the points. Join the first and last points with a straight line.

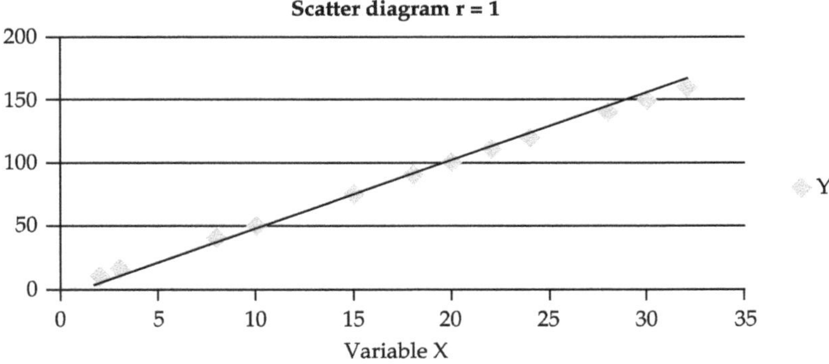

Fig. 7.2.4: *Scatter diagram for perfect positively correlated variables.*

Example (7.2.5): Draw the scatter diagram for the following data.

X	1	2	3	4	5	6	7	8	9	10	11	12
Y	100	95	90	85	80	75	70	65	60	55	50	45

Solution: Consider the random variable X on x–axis and the random variable Y on y–axis and draw points for each pair.

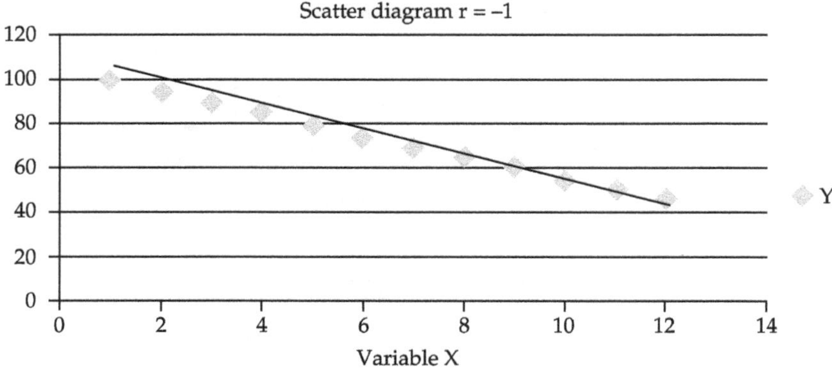

Fig. 7.2.5: *Scatter diagram for perfect negatively correlated variables.*

If the scatter of the points shows the trend as shown in figure (7.2.1). We say that two variables are positively correlated and hence, the correlation $r > 0$ in figure (7.2.1).

If the scatter of the points shows the trend as shown in fig (7.2.2), we say that X and Y are negatively correlated. Thus $r < 0$ in figure (7.2.2).

If the scatter of the points is evenly distributed throughout the space as shown in figure (7.2.3). We say that two variables X and Y are independent, then $r = 0$.

If all the points fall on a straight line as shown in figure (7.2.4), we say that two variables X and Y are perfectly positively correlated. Then $r = +1$.

If all the points fall on a straight line as shown in figure (7.2.5), we say two variables are perfectly negatively correlated, then $r = -1$.

Thus correlation coefficient always lies in between –1 and +1. If it is near to '0' it is assumed that the relationship is weak. If the correlation coefficient $r = 0$ we say that two variables are independent.

7.2.2. Limitations of Scatter Diagrams

In scatter diagrams, we can consider at a time two variables only. Another disadvantage of scatter diagram is that it only explains whether two variables are related or not but we can't calculate or measure exactly the relationship which is necessary in statistical analysis. Karl Pearson suggested a method with the help of which one can calculate or measure the correlation coefficient between two variables. Hence, this method is known as Karl Pearson correlation coefficient method, which is explained in the following section.

7.3. KARL PEARSON'S METHOD

In Scatter diagram method, we can only know whether two variables are related or not? But this information is not enough to use in predicting the value of an un-known variable. Since, our ultimate aim is to predict the un-known value of a dependent variable, if independent variable is known or given. Karl Pearson, (1857 – 1936) was a great Bio-statistician and suggested a mathematical formula to measure the degree of relation between two variables.

Karl Pearson's Correlation Coefficient is denoted by r_{XY} and is given as follows:

$$r_{XY} = \frac{Cov\,(X, Y)}{\sqrt{\text{var}\,(X) \cdot \text{var}\,(Y)}} = \frac{Cov\,(X, Y)}{S.D.(X) \cdot S.D.(Y)} \quad (7.3.1)$$

$$= \frac{\Sigma\, XY - \dfrac{\Sigma\, Y\, \Sigma\, Y}{n}}{\sqrt{\text{var}\,(X) \cdot \text{var}\,(Y)}} \quad (7.3.2)$$

Where $\text{Cov}\,(X, Y) = \Sigma XY - \dfrac{\Sigma Y\, \Sigma Y}{n}$

$\text{Var}\,(X) = \Sigma\, X^2 - (\Sigma\, X)^2/n$

$\text{Var}\,(Y) = \Sigma\, Y^2 - (\Sigma\, Y)^2/n$

and $n =$ Number of pairs of observations.

Example (7.3.1): Calculate Karl Pearson's correlation coefficient for the following data, where X represents marks in bio-statistics and Y marks in zoology.

X:	10	12	60	60	70
Y:	15	20	20	20	50

Solution: Calculate the required sums as in the following table.

X	Y	X^2	Y^2	$X \cdot Y$
10	15	100	225	150
12	20	144	400	240
60	20	3600	400	1200
60	20	3600	400	1200
70	50	4900	2500	3500
Total 212	125	12344	3925	6290

$$r_{XY} = \frac{[6290 - (212)(125)/5]}{\sqrt{\{[12344 - (212)^2/5][3925 - (125)^2/5]\}}}$$

$$= (6290 - 5300)/\sqrt{\{[12344 - 8988.8][3925 - 3125]\}}$$

$$= 990/\sqrt{(3355.2)(800)} = 990/1638.3406 = 0.60427$$

Correlation between X and Y is positive and is equal to 0.60427.

If the data is large in size, above explained procedure, is a cumbersome and time consuming hence a short cut method is explained as follows:

Step – 1: Calculate $x_i = (X_i - A)$ and $y_i = (Y_i - B)$

Step – 2: Calculate the sum of X i.e. $\Sigma\, x_i$ and sum of Y i.e. $\Sigma\, y_i$.

Step – 3: Calculate the product of X and Y i.e. $\Sigma\, x_i \cdot y_i$

Step – 4: Calculate the difference $\Sigma\, x_i \cdot y_i - (\Sigma\, x_i\;\; \Sigma\, y_i)/n$

Step – 5: Divide the quantity obtained in step – 3 by n to get the covariance between X and Y.

Step – 6: To calculate the correlation coefficient divide the quantity obtained in step–6 by the product of S.D.(X).S.D.(Y). This is given in the formula (7.3.2).

7.3.1. Properties of Correlation Coefficient

1. Correlation coefficient r always lies between –1 and +1. That is $-1 \leq r \leq 1$.
2. If X and Y are 'independent variables' then the correlation coefficient $r = 0$. But converse is not true.
3. Correlation coefficient if independent of change of origin and scale of measurements.
4. Absolute value of correlation coefficient is always less than or equal to 1. That is $|r| \leq 1$.
5. If X and Y are independent, they are un-correlated but it does not imply that if $r = 0$, X and Y are independent.

Example (7.3.2): Calculate Karl Pearson's correlation coefficient for the following data. The random variable X represents temperature measured in centigrade of the soil and the random variable Y represents the flowering time measured in days.

Temperature X	50	42	40	38	43	45	42	44	40	46
Flowering time Y	14	26	30	41	29	27	27	19	18	19

Solution:

From the given data we have to calculate sums of different columns as shown in the following table.

X	Y	$x = X - A$	$y = Y - B$	xy	x^2	y^2
50	14	10	–13	–130	100	169
42	26	2	–1	–2	4	1
40 = A	30	0	3	0	0	9
38	41	–2	14	–28	4	196
43	29	3	2	6	9	4
45	27 = B	5	0	0	25	0
42	27	2	0	0	4	0
44	19	4	– 8	– 32	16	64
40	18	0	– 9	0	0	81
46	19	6	– 8	– 48	36	64
		30	– 20	– 234	198	588

Thus Karl Pearson's correlation coefficient r_{XY} is given using the formula (7.3.2) as :

$$r_{XY} = \frac{[-234 - (30)(-20)/10]}{\sqrt{[(198 - (30)^2/10)(588 - (-20)^2/10)]}} = \frac{[-234 + 60]}{\sqrt{[(198 - 90)(588 - 40)]}}$$

$$= -174/\sqrt{(108)(548)} = -174/243.27762 = -0.715232 = -0.7 \text{ (approx).}$$

Hence the relation between the temperature of the soil and the flowering time are negatively related and correlation coefficient is – 0.7.

That is if temperature is more, flowering time reduces and vice-versa.

7.4. SPEARMAN'S METHOD

Karl Pearson's method can be used only when we have quantifiable or measurable variables like temperature, marks, B.P., blood sugar, height, weight, calories of energy gained and so on. Always, it is not possible to measure the variables for example, response to a stimulus treatment, skin color, eye color, pain, response of a psychological patient to a shock treatment, honesty, sincerity, punctuality and so on. Sometimes, we can compare and give *'ranks'* or *'scores'* in such situations. Then it is not possible to use Karl Pearson's method to calculate correlation coefficient. Spearman was a psychologist, and suggested another formula used when the data is in the form of ranks or scores. Finding correlation coefficient using the formula suggested by Spearman is known as 'spearman's rank correlation' or simply, rank correlation coefficient, denoted by the symbol ρ_{xy} and is given by the formula :

$$\rho_{XY} = \frac{6\Sigma D^2}{n(n^2-1)} \tag{7.4.1}$$

Where, D^2 = square of difference of corresponding ranks of X and Y and

n = Number of pairs of observations on X and Y.

We can use above formula if no ties are there in the given data.

Example (7.4.1): Calculate Spearman's rank correlation coefficient for the following data.

X:	89	78	57	97	59	79	68	69
Y:	137	125	108	156	107	136	123	112

Solution: In the first step we have to give ranks to X and Y. One can give 1st rank to height data item in the series, next rank to the next height data item and last rank to the smallest item and calculate the required sums as shown in the following table.

X	Y	Rank of X R1	Rank of Y R2	Difference D = R1 – R2	D^2
89	137	2	2	0	0
78	125	4	4	0	0
57	108	8	7	1	1
97	156	1	1	0	0
59	107	7	8	–1	1
79	136	3	3	0	0
68	123	6	5	1	1
69	112	5	6	–1	1
Total				$\Sigma D = 0$	$\Sigma D^2 = 4$

Spearman's Rank correlation

$$\rho_{xy} = \frac{6\Sigma D^2}{(n^2-1)} = 1 - 24/[8(64-1)] = 1 - 24/504 = 1 - 0.047619.$$

$$= 0.952381.$$

Remarks: Spearman's method is an easy method when compared to Karl Pearson's Method and give same result if no ties are there in the data as in the above example.

If ties are present in the data, i.e., if two or more data items are equal to each other, then giving ranks will become a difficult one. This problem of repeated ranks is called 'A Tie'. When tie exists among the data items, we have to give average rank of those ranks if they are distinct. For example, two data items are equal i.e., 68 and 68 and ranks to be allotted to these items are 4 and 5 say. Then the average rank 4.5 is to be allotted for both the data items. Since, we have converted the discrete variable (ranks) in to continuous variable and hence a correction $\frac{1}{12}(m^3-m)$, where m is the size of the tie or number of observation in a tie is to be made to ΣD^2. This correction is to be made for every tie. Like that, every tie is to be resolved and correction is to be added to ΣD^2. Thus the formula given in (7.4.1) is to be modified as follows:

$$\rho_{xy} = 1 - \frac{6\left[\Sigma D^2 + \frac{1}{12}(m_1^3 - m_1) + \ldots, + \frac{1}{12}(m_k^3 - m_k)\right]}{n\,(n^2-1)} \qquad (7.4.2)$$

Here m = Number of observations in a tie with repeated ranks and

k = Number of ties in the given data or problem.

Example (7.4.2): Calculate Spearman' correlation coefficient for the following data.

X	35	23	48	17	10	42	10	6	28	42
Y	48	34	54	20	14	48	12	4	31	48

Solution: In the given data there are three ties which are explained as follows:

Tie - 1 : In X series two numbers are equal to 42. Hence this is a tie with size $m = 2$. Hence rank 2.5 is allotted for both. This is an average of 2nd and 3rd ranks. Next rank allotted should be 4.

Tie – 2 : In X series two numbers are equal to 10. Hence, this is another tie with size $m = 2$. Average rank of 8 and 9 i.e. 8.5 is allotted to both observations.

Tie – 3: In Y series, three numbers are equal to 48. Hence, this is another time of size $m = 3$. Average of ranks 2, 3 and 4 i.e. 3 is allotted to all the three observations. Next rank allotted should be 5.

Thus in the given problem, we have three ties and corrections are to be made three times in the formula (7.4.2). Thus $k = 3$.

X	Y	Rank of X	Rank of Y	Difference	D^2
		R1	R2	R1 – R2 = D	
35	48	4	3	1	1
23	34	6	5	1	1
48	54	1	1	0	0
17	20	7	7	0	0
10	14	8.5	8	0.5	0.25
42	48	2.5	3	–0.5	0.25
10	12	8.5	9	–0.5	0.25
6	4	10	10	0	0
28	31	5	6	–1	1
42	48	2.5	3	–0.5	0.25
Total					4

Spearman's Correlation

$$\rho_{xy} = 1 - \frac{6\left[4 + \frac{1}{12}(2^3 - 2) + \frac{1}{12}(2^3 - 2) + \frac{1}{12}(3^3 - 3)\right]}{10(10^2 - 1)}.$$

$$= 1 - [6 \times (4 + 0.5 + 0.5 + 2)]/990 = 1 - 42/990 = 1 - 0.042424$$

$$= 0.95758.$$

There exists positive correlation between X and Y and the rank correlation is 0.958 which is nearer to 1. Hence a high positive relation exists between X and Y variables.

Example (7.4.3): There are 10 competitors in a beauty contest, who were ranked by three judges in the following manner.

S.No.	:	1	2	3	4	5	6	7	8	9	10
1st Judge	:	1	6	5	10	3	2	4	9	7	8
2nd Judge	:	3	5	8	4	7	10	2	1	6	9
3rd Judge	:	6	4	9	8	1	2	3	10	5	7.

Are the three judges similar in thinking about the concept of Beauty? If not which judges rankings coincide with each other?

Solution: The data represents ranks assigned by three different judges to 10 competitors in a beauty contest. Let $R12$ represent the rank correlation between judges 1 and 2. Similarly, $R13$ represent rank correlation between judges 1 and 3; and $R23$ represents rank correlation between judge 2 and judge 3. Let $R1$, $R2$ and $R3$ represent ranks by judges 1, 2 and 3 respectively.

R1	R2	R3	D12 = R1 – R2	D13 = R1 – R3	D23 = R2 – R3	$(D12)^2$	$(D13)^2$	$(D23)^2$
1	3	6	–2	–5	–3	4	25	9
6	5	4	1	2	1	1	4	1
5	8	9	–3	–4	–1	9	16	1
10	4	8	6	2	–4	36	4	16
3	7	1	–4	2	6	16	4	36
2	10	2	–8	0	8	64	0	64
4	2	3	2	1	–1	4	1	1
9	1	10	8	–1	9	64	1	81
7	6	5	1	2	1	1	4	1
8	9	7	–1	1	2	1	1	4
Sum						200	60	214

$R12 = 1 - (6 \times 200)/ 990 = 1 - 1200/990 = 1 - 1.21212 = - 0.21212$
$R13 = 1 - (6 \times 60)/990 = 1 - 360 / 990 = 1 - 0.36363 = 0.63636$
$R23 = 1 - (6 \times 214)/990 = 1 - 1284/990 = 1 - 1.29697 = - 0.29697.$

Based on the rank correlations, we conclude that there is negative relation between judges 1 and 2 but, positive thinking or similar thing between judges 1 and 3. Hence judge 1 and judge 3 ranks coincide than judge 2 towards understanding of the concept of beauty in the competition.

Example (7.4.4): Following data is collected from a jute industry in West Bengal, in which the length *X* (in cm.) of green plants and the weight of the dry jute fiber *Y* (in grm).

X	148	172	183	162	160	141	150	190	176	180
Y	2.3	6.4	4.7	3.5	4.1	2.9	2.8	6.6	5.2	6.2

Calculate (*i*) Karl Pearson's and (*ii*) Spearman's correlation coefficients and comment on your answers.

Solution: (*i*) Calculation of Karl Pearson's correlation coefficient:

X	Y	x = X – A	y = Y – B	x^2	y^2	x . y
148	2.3	–12	–2.4	144	5.76	28.8
172	6.4	12	1.7	144	2.89	20.4
183	4.7 = B	23	0	529	0	0
162	3.5	2	–1.2	4	1.44	–2.4
160 = A	4.1	0	–0.6	0	0.36	0
141	2.9	–19	–1.8	361	3.24	34.2
150	2.8	–10	–1.9	100	3.61	19.0
190	6.6	30	1.9	900	3.61	57.0
176	5.2	16	0.5	256	0.25	8.0
180	6.2	20	1.5	400	2.25	30.0
		62	2.3	2834	23.41	195

Karl Pearson's correlation coefficient is given by:

$$r_{xy} = \frac{[195 - (62)(-2.30)/10]}{\sqrt{[(2834 - (62)^2/10)(23.41 - (-2.3)^2/10)]}}$$

$$= \frac{[195 + 14.26]}{\sqrt{[(2834 - 384.4)(23.41 - 0.529)]}} = 209.26/\sqrt{(2449.6)(22.881)}$$

$$= 209.26/236.7473 = 0.883896 \text{ or } 0.89 \text{ (approx)}.$$

(*ii*) Calculation of Spearman's correlation coefficient.

X	Y	Rank of X = R1	Rank of Y = R2	R1 – R2 = D	D^2
148	2.3	9	10	–1	1
172	6.4	5	2	3	9
183	4.7	2	5	–3	9
162	3.5	6	7	–1	1
160	4.1	7	6	1	1
141	2.9	10	8	2	4
150	2.8	8	9	–1	1
190	6.6	1	1	0	0
176	5.2	4	4	0	0
180	6.2	3	3	0	0
Total					26

Spearman's Rank correlation $= 1 - 6(26)/10[(10)^2 - 1] = 1 - 156/990$

$= 1 - 0.15757 = 0.8424 = 0.84$ (approx).

Thus comparing both answers, we conclude that both Karl Pearson's method and Spearman's method will give approximately same results if there are no ties in the given data. Based on the nature of data we can use any method to measure the degree of association or strength of relation between two variables X and Y. It is important to note that above measures the linear relation between variables X and Y.

If there exists curvilinear relation, we have to study such relations through "non-linear" correlations. This topic is out of the scope of this book. Since, correlation measures only linear relations, the concept of correlation is also known as '*Linear correlations*'.

If we consider more than two variables and measure the association among them then it is called 'multiple correlation'. This topic is out of the scope of this book hence, not discussed here. Now we concentrate on the concept of 'regression' in the following section.

7.5. REGRESSION LINES AND REGRESSION COEFFICIENTS

We know that correlation discussed earlier measures only linear relations, the related regression models are also known as '*Linear Regression Models*'. Here we deal only linear models of the type:

$$Y = a + bX \tag{7.5.1}$$

where '*a*' is known as the 'intercept' and '*b*' is known as the slope of the equation which are constants and *X* and *Y* are dependent and independent variables respectively. The equation is a straight line equation and hence is known as '*regression line* '. Here, we consider the problem of prediction or estimation of the value of the dependent variable *Y* from a known value of the other independent variable *X*, which is closely related to the dependent variable *Y*.

Regression means, to return or to back towards the mean value. The tendency or force presenting in the variable going toward its mean or average is known as 'Regression'. The term regression was first used by Sir Francis Galton in the problem of heredity. He found that 'tall fathers have tall sons and short fathers have short sons'. If the average height of sons of tall fathers is × above the general height, the average height of their sons is (2/3) × above the general height. The recession in the average height was described by Galton as regression to the average height or regression to the mediocrity. This concept of regression is used in many fields in recent times particularly in biological sciences, business forecasting, medical fields, economics and so on, where, the tendency to regress or set back to the general average nature is present.

Regression shows a relationship between the average values of two variables *X* and *Y*. Hence, the concept regression is very useful in forecasting or predicting or estimating the average value of one variable *Y* for a given value of another closely related known value of the variable *X* using line of regression given in (7.5.1). The independent variable *X* in the equation (7.5.1) is also known as 'regressor' or 'predictor' or "explanatory' or 'cause' variable and the dependent variable *Y* is also known as "regressed' or 'explained' or 'effected' variable. There are two types of regression lines, namely:

(*i*) Regression line of *Y* depending on *X* and

(*ii*) Regression line of *X* depending on *Y*.

7.5.1. Need of Studying Two Regression Lines

In many real life problems our interest lies on two types of enquiries, namely, (*a*) What is the expected behavior or value of the variable '*Y*' when the value of the dependent variable '*X*' is known or given. Similarly, (*b*) for what value of '*X*' we get the required result of the dependent variable '*Y*'. These two questions seem to be alike but are entirely different in the enquiry which is explained with some examples as follows:

A student is interested to know (*a*) the number of marks that he can expect if he/she reads daily 4 hours? or (*b*) if he/she want to get 85 per cent in the examination how many hours he/she has to study per day? Similarly, a doctor wants to know (*a*) how many mg/dl of blood sugar will be reduced if increase the insulin dosage from 15 ml to 20 ml? or (*b*) if we want to control post prandial blood sugar from 224 mg/dl to normal range i.e., 80 – 140 mg/dl, how many units of insulin is to be injected? Similarly, in market research, a business analyst want to predict (*a*) expected price of a product or share, for a given demand for that product or share or (*b*) if we increase or decrease the price a product/share, what will be expected demand for that product/share?

Similarly, a business man wants to (*a*) estimate the increased business if he spends Rs. 5,000/- on advertisements? or (*b*) if he wants to increase the business from 10 lakhs to 15 lakhs, how much amount he has to spend on advertisements?. Thus there exist numerous instances, where our interest of enquiries lies in two ways as explained above. To answer these two queries, we need two regression lines namely : (*a*) regression line of *Y* on *X* and (*b*) regression line of *X* on *Y* which are defined as follows:

7.5.2. Regression Line and Regression Coefficient of Y on X.

The regression line of *Y* on *X* gives the best estimate of the dependent variable Y for any given value of the independent variable X and is defined as:

$$(Y - \bar{y}) = r \frac{S.D.(y)}{S.D.(x)} (X - \bar{x})$$

$$= r \frac{\sigma(y)}{\sigma(x)} (X - \bar{x}) \tag{7.2.1}$$

Where Y = Dependent variable

X = Independent variable

r = Correlation coefficient between X and Y.

$\bar{y}$ = Arithmetic mean of Y

$\bar{x}$ = Arithmetic mean of X

S.D. $(y) = \sigma(y)$ = Standard deviation of X and

S.D. $(x) = \sigma(x)$ = Standard deviation of Y.

By substituting various values of statistics and after simplification, the equation (7.2.1) will become :

$$Y = a + bX \tag{7.2.2}$$

The quantity $b = r\dfrac{\sigma(y)}{\sigma(x)}$ is called the 'regression coefficient of *Y* on *X*' and is denoted by b_{yx}.

7.5.3. Regression Line and Regression Coefficient of X on Y

The regression line of *X* on *Y* gives the best estimate of the independent variable *X* for any given value of the dependent variable *Y* and is defined as:

$$(X - \bar{x}) = r \frac{S.D.(x)}{S.D.(y)} (Y - \bar{y})$$

$$= r \frac{\sigma(x)}{\sigma(y)} (Y - \bar{y}) \tag{7.2.3}$$

Where Y = Dependent variable

X = Independent variable

r = Correlation coefficient between X and Y.

$\bar{y}$ = Arithmetic mean of Y

$\bar{x}$ = Arithmetic mean of X

S.D. $(y) = \sigma(y)$ = Standard deviation of X and

S.D. $(x) = \sigma(x)$ = Standard deviation of Y.

By substituting various values of statistics and after simplification, the equation (7.2.2) will become :

$$X = c + dY \tag{7.2.4}$$

The quantity $d = r\dfrac{\sigma(x)}{\sigma(y)}$ is called the 'regression coefficient of X on Y' and is denoted by b_{xy}.

7.5.4. Properties of Regression Coefficients

1. The correlation coefficient is the geometric mean of both regression coefficients i.e. $r = \sqrt{b_{xy} \cdot b_{yx}}$.

   Proof: We know that, by definition of regression coefficients,

   $$b_{yx} = r\frac{\sigma(y)}{\sigma(x)} \text{ and } b_{xy} = r\frac{\sigma(x)}{\sigma(y)}$$

   If we multiply both regression coefficients, we have :

   $$b_{xy} \times b_{yx} = r\frac{\sigma(x)}{\sigma(y)} \times r\frac{\sigma(y)}{\sigma(x)} = r^2.$$

   Hence $r = \sqrt{b_{xy} \cdot b_{yx}}$.

   [Geometric mean of two numbers a and b is the square root their produce i.e., geometric mean of a and b is $\sqrt{a \cdot b}$]

   Hence, correlation coefficient is considered as the geometric mean of both the regression coefficients i.e. b_{xy} and b_{yx}. Hence the proof.

2. If one regression coefficient if greater than 1 then the other regression coefficient must be less than 1.

   Proof: We know that correlation coefficient lies in between –1 and +1. Hence r^2 must be less than 1, that is $r^2 \leq 1$.

   Hence $r^2 = b_{xy} \times b_{yx} \leq 1$.

   If anyone regression coefficient is greater than 1 the other one must be less than 1. Hence the proof.

3. Arithmetic mean of both regression coefficients is always greater than the correlation coefficient r.

4. Both regression coefficients must have same sign. That is both must be positive or both must be negative. If both are negative, correlation coefficient r should be considered as negative. If both regression coefficients

are positive, then the correlation coefficient r must be considered as positive. This implies that it is impossible that one regression coefficient is positive and one is negative.

5. Regression coefficients are independent of change of origin but not scale.

7.5.5. Properties of Regression Lines

1. The two regression lines always intersect at their means. That is the intersect point is always $(\bar{x}, \bar{y})$.
2. Both regression coefficients and correlation coefficients have same sign.
3. If $r = 0$ then regression coefficients are also equal to 0. That is $b_{xy} = 0$ and $b_{yx} = 0$.
4. The regression lines become identical if $r = \pm 1$.

7.6. FITTING OF REGRESSION LINES

To fit regression lines for any given data, we use a powerful mathematical tool known as '*Method of Least Squares*' through which one can fit the best fitted regression line. Using the method of least squares one can obtain the regression equation best to a given set of observations. This method is based on the assumption that sum of the squares of differences between the estimated values and the actual observed values of the dependent variable, is minimum. This method is used in obtaining the equation for fitting a regression line. The method is mainly based on a system of equations known as '*Normal equations*'. These normal equations are to be solved and the values of constants are to be obtained and are to be substituted in the regression line. This fitted regression line useful to predict or estimate or forecast the required value of the variable. Method of fitting of regression lines is explained as follows:

7.6.1. Method of Least Squares for Fitting of the Regression Line of Y on X

The regression line of Y on X to be fitted is given by:

$$Y = a + bX. \tag{7.6.1}$$

In order to fit above line, we have to determine the values of 'a' and 'b' using the information or data. To do this, first we have to write the "*Normal equations*' as follows:

$$\Sigma y = Na + b\,\Sigma x \tag{7.6.2}$$

$$\Sigma xy = a\,\Sigma x + b\,\Sigma x^2 \tag{7.6.3}$$

Where, Σy = Sum of the dependent variable y.

Σx = Sum of the independent variable x.

Σx^2 = Sum of squares of independent variable x.

Σxy = Sum of the product of x and y.

N = Number of pairs of observations in the data (X, Y).

After substituting the required sums calculated from the data, in normal equations (7.6.2) and (7.6.3) the constants '*a*' and '*b*' are to be evaluated because the problem is a two un-known's with two equations.

The evaluated constants are denoted by $\hat{a}$ and b. To obtain the fitted Regression line of *Y* on *X*, substitute the evaluated constants in equation (7.6.1) that is

$$y = a + bx. \tag{7.6.4}$$

This fitted equation will help to predict or estimate or forecast the value of *Y* when *X* is given or known. If we substitute the known value of *x* in (7.6.4) we obtain the estimated value of the variable *Y*.

7.6.2. Method of Least Squares for Fitting of the Regression Line of X on Y

The regression line of *X* on *Y* to be fitted is given by:

$$X = c + dY \tag{7.6.5}$$

In order to fit above line, we have to determine the values of '*a*' and '*b*' using the information or data. To do this, first we have to write the "*Normal equations*' as follows:

$$\Sigma x = Nc + d\Sigma y \tag{7.6.6}$$

$$\Sigma xy = c\Sigma x + d\Sigma y^2 \tag{7.6.7}$$

Where, Σy = Sum of the dependent variable *y*.

Σx = Sum of the independent variable *x*.

Σy^2 = Sum of squares of independent variable *x*.

Σxy = Sum of the product of *x* and *y*.

N = Number of pairs of observations in the data (*X*, *Y*).

After substituting the required sums calculated from the data, in normal equations (7.6.6) and (7.6.7) the constants '*c*' and '*d*' are to be evaluated because the problem is a two un-known's with two equations.

The evaluated constants are denoted by c and d. To obtain the fitted Regression line of *Y* on *X*, substitute the evaluated constants in equation (7.6.5) that is:

$$x = c + dy \tag{7.6.8}$$

This fitted equation will help to predict or estimate or forecast the value of *X* when *Y* is given or known. If we substitute the known value of *y* in (7.6.8) we obtain the estimated value of the variable *X*.

Using the above explained procedures of fitting of regression lines. Now we work out some examples.

Example (7.6.1): Following data represents temperature (*X*) and the germination of a particular variety of rice (*Y*) measured in days is collected. Fit both regression lines and (*a*) estimate the germination time when temperature is 48° (*b*) if the germination time is to be made 25 days, what temperature is to be maintained in the field?

Temperature (X)	52	42	40	38	43	45	42	44	40	46
Germination time (Y)	14	26	30	41	29	27	27	19	18	19

Solution: From the given data calculate the required sums by changing the origin of X to $x = X - A$ and Y to $y = Y - B$, were $A = 40$ and $B = 27$, as shown in the following table:

X	Y	x = X – A	y = Y – B	xy	x^2	y^2
50	14	10	–13	–130	100	169
42	26	2	–1	–2	4	1
40	30	0	3	0	0	9
38	41	–2	14	–28	4	196
43	29	3	2	6	9	4
45	27	5	0	0	25	0
42	27	2	0	0	4	0
44	19	4	–8	–32	16	64
40	18	0	–9	0	0	81
46	19	6	–8	–48	36	64
Total		30	–20	–234	198	588

(*a*) To estimate the germination time Y, when $X = 48$, we have to fit the Regression line of Y on X. i.e.

$$Y = a + bX \tag{7.6.9}$$

Normal equations for the equation are:

$$\sum y = Na + b\sum x \tag{7.6.10}$$

$$\sum xy = a\sum x + b\sum x^2 \tag{7.6.11}$$

Substituting above calculated sums in equations (7.6.10) and (7.6.12) we have:

$$-20 = 10\,a + 30\,b \tag{7.6.12}$$

$$-234 = 30\,a + 198\,b \tag{7.6.13}$$

First eliminate a in equations (7.6.12) and (7.6.13). To do this, multiply equation (7.6.12) with 3 and equation (7.6.13) with 1. Then subtract equation (7.6.13) from equation (7.6.12). That is

$$[-20 = 10\,a + 30\,b] \times 3 \tag{7.6.14}$$

$$[-234 = 30\,a + 198\,b] \times 1 \qquad (7.6.13)$$

$$60 = 30\,a + 90\,b \qquad (7.6.14)$$

$$234 = 30\,a + 198\,b \tag{7.6.15}$$

$$174 = 0 - 108\,b.$$

Hence, $\qquad b = -174/108 = -1.61111.$

To determine the value of a, substitute the calculated value of b in equation (7.6.12) and solve. Thus we have:

$$a = (-20 - 30 \times -1.61111)/10 = 28.3333/10 = 2.833 \text{ (approx.)}$$

Thus fitted regression line of Y on X is given by:

$$y = 2.83333 - 1.61111x \tag{7.6.16}$$

the equation (7.6.16) is in x and y, i.e., change of scale variable which are to be converted back to X and Y. Thus we have:

$$(Y-27) = 2.83333 - 1.61111\,(X-40)$$

i.e. $$Y = +27 + 2.83333 - 1.61111\,X + 40\,(1.61111)$$

i.e. $$Y = 29.8333 + 64.444 - 1.61111\,X$$

i.e. $$Y = 94.2773 - 1.61111\,X \qquad (7.6.17)$$

Equation (7.6.17) is the required equation used for forecasting or predicting the value of Y when X is given i.e., $X = 48$. Substitute the value of $X = 48$ in (7.6.17) and solve for Y, we have, estimated value of Y denoted by Y:

$$Y = 94.2773 - 1.61111(48) = 16.9445 = 17 \text{ days (approx.)}$$

Thus if the temperature is maintained at 48 degrees centigrade, we expect the germination on the average as 17 days.

(b) To estimate the required temperature X for given germination $Y = 25$, we have to fit the regression line of X on Y, to do this, we require the normal equations as:

$$\Sigma x = Nc + d\,\Sigma y \qquad (7.6.18)$$

$$\Sigma xy = c\,\Sigma x + d\,\Sigma y^2 \qquad (7.6.19)$$

By substituting the calculated total in the table, in the above equations (7.6.18) and (7.6.19) we have:

$$30 = 10\,c - 20\,d \qquad (7.6.20)$$

$$-234 = -20c + 588d \qquad (7.6.21)$$

Multiply equation (7.6.20) by 2 and equation (7.6.21) by 1 and adding equations (7.6.20) and (7.6.21) we have:

$$60 = 20c - 40d$$

$$-234 = -20c + 588\,d.$$

Thus we have $d = -174/548 = -0.31752$. Substituting the value of d in (7.6.20) and solving $-174 = 548d$ for c we have $c = (30 + 20 \times 0.31752)10 = 3.635$.

Fitted regression equation of X on Y is: $x = 3.635 - 0.31752y$ (7.6.22)

In terms of X and Y we have $X - 40 = 3.635 - 0.31752\,(Y - 27)$ i.e.

$X = 3.635 + 40 - 0.31752\,Y + 8.57304 = 52.20804 - 0.31752Y$ (7.6.23)

By substituting $Y = 25$ in equation (7.6.23) we have:

$X = 52.20804 - 0.31752\,(25) = 44.27004 = 44°$ (approx.).

Hence, to get the seed to be germinated in 25 days, we have to maintain 44 degrees temperature (approx.).

Example (7.6.2): Following data represents the dosage of insulin X measured in units/day where a unit = (1/100)th of an ml, and fasting blood glucose levels Y measured in mg/dl among diabeties mellitus patients.

X	10	12	14	18	20	22	26	30
Y	140	132	130	125	115	100	90	75

(*a*) Estimate the fasting blood glucose level if insulin is taken as 24 units/day.

(*b*) If we want to maintain fasting blood glucose at 80 mg/dl, what dosage of insulin is to be suggested?

(*c*) Using both regression coefficients calculate the correlation coefficient between Insulin dosage and fasting blood glucose in diabeties mellitus patients.

Solution:

(*a*) To estimate fasting blood glucose levels Y when the insulin dosage X = 24 ml/day, we have to fit the regression line of Y on X. To do this, first we have to calculate required sums from the given data. We can change the origin of X and Y by considering A =18 and B = 100. i.e. $x = X - 18$ and $y = Y - 100$ in the following table.

X	Y	x = X – A	y = Y – B	x^2	y^2	x . y
10	140	–8	40	64	1600	– 320
12	132	– 6	32	36	1024	– 192
14	130	– 4	30	16	900	– 120
18 = A	125	0	25	0	625	0
20	115	2	15	4	225	30
22	100 = B	4	0	16	0	0
26	90	8	– 10	64	100	– 80
30	75	12	– 25	144	625	– 300
Total		8	107	344	5099	– 982

Normal equations for fitting Y on X are:

$$107 = 8\,a + 8\,b \qquad (7.6.24)$$

$$-982 = 8\,a + 344\,b \qquad (7.6.25)$$

Subtracting (7.6.25) from (7.6.24) we have:

$$875 = -336\,b \text{ i.e. } b = -875/336 = -2.6042.$$

Substituting the value of b in (7.6.24) and solving for 'a' we have:

$$a = [107 - 8(-2.6042)]/8 = 127.8336/8 = 15.9792.$$

Fitted regression line of y on x is given by:

$$y = 15.9792 - 2.6042\,x \qquad (7.6.26)$$

Hence converting (7.6.26) into Y and X we have:

$$(Y - 100) = 15.9792 - 2.6042\,(X - 18)$$

i.e. $$Y = 15.9792 + 100 + 46.8756 - 2.6042X.$$

The fitted regression line of Y on X is $Y = 162.8548 - 2.6042X$ (7.6.27)

Equation (7.6.27) is used to predict Y when X = 24. Put X = 24 in (7.6.27), we have the predicted value of Y denoted by $\hat{Y}$ is given by:

$$\hat{Y} = 162.8548 - 62.5008 = 100.354 \text{ or } 100 \text{ mg/dl (approx.)}$$

(*b*) Fitting regression line of X on Y to predict the value of X when $Y = 80$.

Normal equations required for fitting of this equations are:

$$8 = 8c + 107d \tag{7.6.28}$$

$$982 = 107c + 5099d \tag{7.6.29}$$

To eliminate c multiply equation (7.6.28) by 107 and the equation (7.6.29) by 8. Thus we have:

$$856 = 856c + 11449d \tag{7.6.30}$$

$$-7856 = 856c + 40792d \tag{7.6.31}$$

$$7000 = -29343d$$

Hence $\qquad d = -7000/29343 = -0.23856.$

Substituting the value of '*d*' in equation (7.6.28) and solving for '*c*' we have $c = [8 - 107(-0.23856)]/8 = 33.52592/8 = 4.19074$

Hence, the regression line of x on y is:

$$x = 4.19074 - 0.23856\, y.$$

The fitted regression line of X on Y is given by:

$$(X - 18) = 4.19074 - 0.23856(Y - 100)$$

i.e. $\qquad X = 4.19074 + 18 + 23.856 - 0.23856\, Y$

or $\qquad X = 46.04674 - 0.23856\, Y \qquad (7.6.32)$

Substitute $Y = 80$ in equation (7.6.32) we have the predicted value of X denoted by $\hat{X}$ and is given by $X = 46.04674 - 0.23856\,(80)$

$= 26.96194$ ml/day $= 27$ units/day (approx.).

(c) We know that the regression coefficient of Y on X, that is

$b_{yx} = -2.6042$ and the regression coefficient of X on Y, that is

$b_{xy} = -0.23856$. [Note that the regression coefficients satisfies the properties listed in (7.5.4)]. Now the correlation coefficient

$$r = \sqrt{b_{xy}\, b_{yx}} = \sqrt{(-2.6042)\,(-0.23856)}$$

$$= -0.788199 = 0.79 \text{ (approx.)}.$$

The regression lines help in predicting or estimating the value of one variable with the help another closely related variable. It is important to note that the estimated values are averages the corresponding variables. Thus decisions can be taken based on these estimated or forecasted values of the required variables. The correctness of these estimated is based on the relation or degree of the relation between the variables X and Y under consideration. If these variables are strongly related, our estimates or forecasts are also correct. If they are weakly related, our estimates are also erroneous.

REVIEW QUESTIONS AND PROBLEMS

A. Objective Questions

1. The degree of relation between two variables is studied Through the concept of ----------- .
   (*a*) averages (*b*) regression
   (*c*) correlation (*d*) skewness.

2. The range of correlation coefficient is ------------- .
   (*a*) –1 to +1 (*b*) 0 to 1 (3) –1 to 0
   (*c*) –10 to +10 (*d*) – 5 to + 5.

3. Scatter diagram is useful to know the ------------- between two variables.
   (*a*) regression (*b*) kurtosis
   (*c*) relation (*d*) skewness.

4. If X and Y are independent the correlation coefficient between them is ---------- .
   (*a*) – 1 (*b*) + 1
   (*c*) 0.5 (*d*) 0

5. If correlation coefficient between X and Y is equal to – 1 the variables are known as ----------------.
   (*a*) perfectly independent
   (*b*) perfectly negatively correlated
   (*c*) perfectly positively correlated
   (*d*) weakly correlated.

6. Both regression lines intersect at their -----------.
   (*a*) medians (*b*) modes
   (*c*) geometric means (*d*) means.

7. Regression lines are useful for ---------------.
   (*a*) prediction (*b*) calculate relations
   (*c*) degree of relation (*d*) strength of relation.

8. If both the regression coefficients are negative, then correlation is ----.
   (*a*) 0 (*b*) –1
   (*c*) +1 (*d*) negative.

9. If one regression coefficient is 0.738 the other one must be ---------.
   (*a*) less than 1 (*b*) equal to 0
   (*c*) greater than 1 (*d*) –1.

10. Regression line of Y on X is useful to predict ------- variable.
    (*a*) X (*b*) Y
    (*c*) both X and Y (*d*) X on Y.

B. Short Answer Questions

1. Write short notes on Scatter diagrams method.
2. Explain the term correlation and its types with suitable examples.
3. Explain the properties of correlation.
4. What are regression lines? Explain.
5. Define regression coefficients and discuss their properties.
6. Explain the method of least squares and discuss its application.
7. Draw scatter diagram for the following data.

X:	50	42	56	60	30	46	92
Y:	46	26	62	55	26	38	68

8. Explain the need for studying two regression lines with suitable examples.
9. Explain the method of fitting of regression line of *Y* on *X*.
10. Explain various properties of regression lines.

C. Essay Type Questions

1. Distinguish between Karl Pearson's and Spearman's method of finding correlation coefficient.
2. Explain in detail the scatter diagram method of finding correlation coefficient along with its limitations.
3. Explain the method of fitting of both the regression lines through the method of least squares.
4. Calculate Karl Pearson's method of correlation coefficient for the following data representing marks in bio-statistics *X* and marks in biology *Y*.

X	77	54	27	52	14	35	90	60
Y	35	58	60	40	50	40	35	42

5. A medical department gives training to its employees which is followed by a test. It is decided to terminate the service of any employee who does not do well in the test. The following data represents test scores *X* and assigned scores *Y* based on their service and performance in the test.

X	14	19	24	21	26	22	15	19	20	25
Y	31	36	48	37	50	45	33	39	32	48

Calculate Spearman's rank correlation between X and Y.

6. Calculate (*a*) Karl Pearson's and (*b*) Spearman's correlation coefficients between price *X* and the demand *Y* for a newly introduced drug to control Hepatitis-*B*.

X in Rs.	80	100	150	170	200	220	240	250
Y in '000	20	30	32	35	37	40	42	45

7. Fit both regression lines for the following data. Also estimate (*a*) the value of *Y* when *X* 25 and (*b*) the value of *X* when *Y* = 55′

X:	10	14	15	28	35	48
Y:	74	61	50	54	43	46

8. The following table gives the age of cars of the certain make and annual maintenance cost measured in 1000's (X). (If the car is age of 2 cost is 1000). (*a*) Estimate the maintenance cost of the age of the car is 12 years. (*b*) If the owner wants to dispose the car when the maintenance cost become more than 50,000 at what age he has to sell the car? (or) how many years he has to wait to sell the car ?.

X:	2	4	6	8	10
Y:	10	20	25	30	35

9. Following data represents heights of fathers *X* and their eldest sons *Y* measured in cms. Estimate (*a*) the height of the son whose father's height is 168 cms. (*b*) If Ravi's height is 164 cms, predict Ravi's father height.

X	167	170	162	163	166	167	170	171	172	168	165	170
Y	170	175	160	165	167	169	168	168	175	170	160	169

10. The following data represents rainfall X measured in cms., and yield of paddy per hector measured in kgs. (*a*) Predict the yield of paddy in the rainfall is 135 cms. (*b*) Similarly, predict the rainfall if the yield of paddy is 22 kgs per plot.

X	112	114	113	85	98	116	90	100	110	120
Y	17.8	20.8	20.8	15.2	17.5	22.6	16.8	19.4	20.6	21.7

References

1. Gupta S.P. 1990 "Statistical Methods". Sultan Chand & Sons, New Delhi.
2. Wayne W. Daniel 2008 Biostatistics, 9th edition, John Wiley & Sons. Inc. Newyork.
3. P.N. Arora *et al.* 2007 "Comprehensive Statistical Methods" Sultan Chand and Company Ltd. First edn. New Delhi.
4. VK. Kapoor 1986 "Problems and solutions in Business statistics" Sultan Chand and Sons New Delhi.

Answers to Objective Questions

1 – c; 2 – a; 3 – c; 4 – d; 5 – b; 6 – d; 7 – a; 8 – d; 10 – b.

8 TESTING OF HYPOTHESES — LARGE SAMPLE TESTS

8.1. INTRODUCTION TO TESTING OF HYPOTHESES

A 'Hypothesis' is a statement made by the experimenter or researcher or by a businessman, or scientist, or a common man, made based on his/her own belief or past experience. That is, a hypothesis is a conclusion which is tentatively drawn on logical basis. For example, 'if we increase the dosage of insulin by 2 ml, blood glucose will be reduced to 75mg/dl' or 'if temperature is 4 degrees higher than present, germination of the seed will be reduced to 10 days' or 'if bank rate of Interest increased by 3%, savings will increased to 20%' or 'to solve the present financial crises, inflation is to be controlled to 2 percent' or 'if I write the examination I am sure of getting distinction' or 'if supply of the rice is increased to 5% the price will come down to Rs. 800 per bag'. 'There are water deposits on the Moon', 'after death good people will go to Heaven' and so on. All above mentioned statements are hypotheses but not statistical hypothesis? A statement may be true or false. If the validity of a hypothesis is judged based on the results of a random experiment, such hypothesis alone is known as "statistical hypothesis". A statistical hypothesis is a tentative conclusion that specifies the properties of a distribution of a random variable. In other words, a statistical hypothesis is some assumption of statement, which may or may not be true, about a population or a probability distribution characterizing the distribution.

The procedure of judging the validity of a hypothesis through a random experiment or statistical experiment is known as "testing of hypothesis". In other words, testing of hypothesis is a procedure that helps us to ascertain the formed hypothesis is true of false, based on the results of a random experiment. Judging the truth in a statistical hypothesis based on the evidence from a random sample or based on the results of a random experiment is known as "testing for statistical validity". To have 'statistical validity' for any statement or a research finding, one has to verify through an appropriate statistical test. Only statistically valid statements are alone have acceptability in scientific studies or enquiries in this world.

Usually, testing of hypotheses are applied in the following two situations, namely:

Situation – I: To test sample characteristics or statistics with that of population characteristics or parameters. For example, sample mean with population mean or to test sample proportion with population proportion or to test sample variance with population variance of sample correlation coefficient with population correlation coefficient and so on.

Situation – II: Two test significant difference between two sample characteristics or statistics. For example, significant difference between two sample means or to test significant difference between two sample variances, to test significant difference between two sample proportions and so on.

These statistical testing of hypotheses used in both situations are broadly classified as follows:

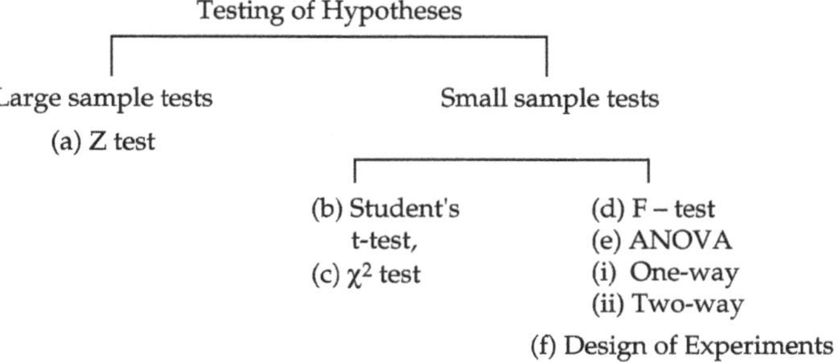

Fig. 8.1.1: *Classification of tests of hypotheses*

In this chapter 8 we concentrate on large sample tests and other sample tests are discussed in Chapter–9. Before we discuss these tests, it is necessary to introduce some fundamental concepts and definitions used in 'Testing of Hypotheses' which is done in the following section.

8.2. SOME FUNDAMENTAL DEFINITIONS AND CONCEPTS USED IN TESTING OF HYPOTHESIS

Statistical hypotheses are broadly classified into two categories, namely:

1. Null-hypothesis and
2. Alternative hypothesis.

8.2.1. Null-Hypothesis

The hypothesis which makes no significant difference between the statistic and the parameter (in situation–I) or no significant difference between two sample statistics (situation–II) is known as Null-hypothesis and is denoted by the symbol H_0. Since it always assumes 'no significant difference' or 'nil difference' or 'insignificant difference', it is known as 'null-hypothesis'. Under this hypothesis, any small or insignificant differences are attributed to random errors or sampling errors or errors due to un-controllable factors which are numerous in number. It is not possible to control all of them and the difference is very, very small or negligible. For example, changes in the body temperature from time to time in a day may be attributed to many causes like out-side temperature, room coolness, body resistance power, work load on the body and so on. Under these situations, the body temperature will change slightly which is negligible. If there is viral fever in the body, then also body temperature changes from time to time but large or significant changes in the temperature we can observe. This is because of 'viral fever'. Such variations are called "significant differences" and we can find a cause for such significant variation in the variable under consideration. Null-hypothesis always assumes such insignificant changes, and we assume that these differences are ignorable and consider the data consists of no significant variations.

Null-hypothesis always plays a neutral role in testing of hypothesis like a judge in the court or an umpire in the fields of cricket or hockey. They should play very neutral and should give un-biased judgments or decisions. Similar way, null-hypothesis plays neutral role or gives un-biased judgment in the field of testing of statistical hypotheses. Prof. R.A. Fisher, Father of Statistics, remarked, 'the null-hypothesis is the hypothesis which is to be tested for possible rejection under the assumption that it is true'. Some examples of null-hypothesis are:

$\mathbf{H_0}$: There is no significant difference between the sample mean and the population mean. That is $\bar{x} = \mu$.

$\mathbf{H_0}$: There is no significant difference between two sample means. That is $\bar{x} = \bar{y}$.

$\mathbf{H_0}$: There is no significant difference between two sample variances. That is $V(x) = V(y)$.

$\mathbf{H_0}$: The two attributes or variables under consideration are independent. That is sample correlation coefficient $r = 0$.

$\mathbf{H_0}$: The two sample proportions are equal or there is no significant difference between two sample proportions. That is $p_1 = p_2$.

$\mathbf{H_0}$: There is no significant difference between sample proportion and the population proportion. That is $p = P$.

8.2.2. Alternative Hypothesis

Alternative hypothesis is opposite to null-hypothesis, where we assume there is significant difference between statistics and parameters.

In other words the hypothesis which is not a null-hypothesis is called 'alternative hypothesis' and is denoted by the symbol H_1. For example, if we want to test the hypothesis that "average height of students joined in a medical college is 168 cm". The null-hypothesis to be considered is:

$\mathbf{H_0}$: Average height of students studying in the medical college is equal to 168 cms, i.e., $\mu = 168$ cms $(= \mu_0)$, and the alternative hypothesis could be any one of the following:

1. $H_1 : \mu \neq \mu_0$. That is $\mu > \mu_0$ $\mu < \mu_0$. or
2. $H_1 : \mu > \mu_0$ or
3. $H_1 : \mu < \mu_0$.

Thus there can be more than one possible alternative hypotheses for a given situation. But there will be only one possible null-hypothesis. Always any test is conducted between H_0 and H_1.

Based on the alternative hypothesis, we can classify the tests as two categories. Namely:

1. One-tailed tests and
2. Two tailed tests.

8.2.3. One-tailed and Two-tailed Tests

In the previous section we have discussed that alternative hypothesis can be any one of the three forms. Depending on the situation, we have to choose any one of the forms for alternative hypothesis H_1. In some situations, both cases are possible. For example, we are comparing two patients A and B, with respect to their body weight. In this situation, H_0: $A = B$ with respect to body weight. Alternative hypothesis to be considered should be $H_1 : A \neq B$. This is because of the fact that A may be having lesser weight than B or B may be lesser weight than A if null-hypothesis is not true. i.e. $A < B$ or $A > B$ with respect to their body weights. Both situations are possible. Such tests are called "Two tailed tests". In some situations, both are not possible but only one situation is possible.

For example, consider an exercise or drinking of Complan or Boost or any other drink for the increase of height in children. If this exercise or drink is effective, height will increase otherwise not. But the height of the child will not decrease because of the exercise or drink. Similarly, if we introduce a new teaching method, may increase the knowledge of the student but it will not decrease the knowledge already the student has. Under these situations, we have to consider only one possibility but not both. That is if $\bar{x}$ represent the average height of the child before taking the beverage or an exercise and $\bar{y}$ represent the average height of the after doing the exercise for one year or taking the beverage for 6 months then $\bar{x} < \bar{y}$ is possible but $\bar{x} > \bar{y}$ is not possible. Hence in this situation we have to consider $H_1 = \bar{x} < \bar{y}$ only.

Hence this is a 'one-tailed test'. Similarly, in some situations, other case $\bar{x} > \bar{y}$ is possible, but not $\bar{x} < \bar{y}$.

Suppose we have given a medicine to reduce B.P. or blood sugar. Let $\bar{x}$ represent average of B.P. or blood sugar before giving the medicine or treatment and $\bar{y}$ represent the average of the character after giving the medicine or treatment. Then, $H_0 = \bar{x} = \bar{y}$ and $H_1 = \bar{x} > \bar{y}$. These are one-tailed tests.

Two-tailed tests:	One-tailed tests:	
$H_1 = \bar{x} \neq \bar{y}$	$H_1 = \bar{x} < \bar{y}$;	$H_1 = \bar{x} > \bar{y}$
$H_1 = V(x) \neq V(y)$	$H_1 = V(x) < V(y)$;	$H_1 = V(x) > V(y)$
$H_1 = \mu \neq \mu_0$	$H_1 = \mu < \mu_0$;	$H_1 = \mu > \mu_0$
$H_1 = P \neq p$	$H_1 = P < p$;	$H_1 = P > p$.

8.2.4. Type – I and Type – II Errors

Now we concentrate on 'errors' that occur in testing of hypothesis. Basically, why an error should occur? is to be understood. In testing of hypothesis, we accept or reject the null-hypothesis based on experimental results or sample results. Sometimes, sample results may give wrong information or we may be misleading, by sample results. This is explained with an example as follows:

Consider a basket of 100 apples which are to be purchased by taking a sample of 10 apples randomly from the selected basket. Among these selected apples, if more than two apples are rotten apples, we reject the basket. Otherwise we purchase the basket. In this process, sometimes, selected sample will give misleading results as follows: For example let us think that in basket, there are 10 good apples and remaining 90 are rotten apples. In the sample, we got all the good 10 apples and since, number of rotten apples in the sample are nil, according to our rule, we have purchased the box, where all the remaining apples are rotten in the box. This is one situation. Similarly, consider another situation, where there are 97 good apples and only 3 rotten apples in a box. While selecting the sample of size 10, the three rotten apples were selected and we have rejected the lot as a bad lot. Here, all remaining apples are good one in the rejected box. In these two situations, we have committed error because in the first case we have purchased all rotten apples and in the second case, we have rejected even though the box contains all good ones. Similar situations can occur in testing of hypothesis. Usually the following four situations can occur in testing of hypothesis, which are listed as follows:

1. When H_0 is true, we accepted H_0. [Correct]
2. When H_0 is true we reject H_0. [Type – I error]
3. When H_0 is wrong, we accept H_0 [Type – II error] and
4. When H_0 is wrong, we reject H_0. [Correct]

Among the above four cases, case 1 and case 4 are correct decisions. Case 2, i.e. rejecting H_0, when it is true is called "Type – I error" and Case 3, i.e. accepting H_0, when it is false is called "Type –II error". That test is the best test in which above two errors are not possible. But, such tests do not exist, because, sampling is a must and one has to depend on the sample. It is not possible to get information from all units in the sample. For example, if we want to know, blood sugar, it is impossible to test all the blood in the patient body in the laboratory. If is enough a sample of 2 ml of blood from the patient body is testes in the laboratory. Similarly, in many life testing experiments, we have to depend on the sample, but not on every individual in the population. Hence, sampling is a must. Under the above situation, we try to suggest tests, which have lesser errors. We calculate the probabilities, for each type of error and minimize in a particular fashion.

Let probability of committing Type – I error is denoted by the symbol α and the probability of committing Type – II error is denoted by the symbol β. i.e., P [type – I error] = α and P[Type –II error] = β.

8.2.5. Some Important Definitions

(i) Size of the test : The probability of committing type – I error is known as size of the test and is denoted by P [type – I error] = α. It is also known as *'level of significance'* **(los)**. Thus the level of significance is the maximum probability of making type – I error. Thus $(1 - \alpha)$ gives the probability of making correct decision. We usually fix the level of significance at 5% (0.05) or 1% (0.01) which means that there is a chance of rejecting good items or boxes of apples 5 out of 100 times (5%) or 1 out of 100 times (1%).

(ii) Critical region or rejection region

Critical region is the region under standard normal curve, corresponding to a pre assigned value of α (usually 0.05 or 0.01). If the sample point falls in this region, we reject the null hypothesis H_0, hence, this region is also known as *'rejection region'*. In the sample space, other than this region is known as *'acceptance region'* and is denoted by (1 – α). That is the region under the standard normal Z-distribution curve as shown in the flowing figure:

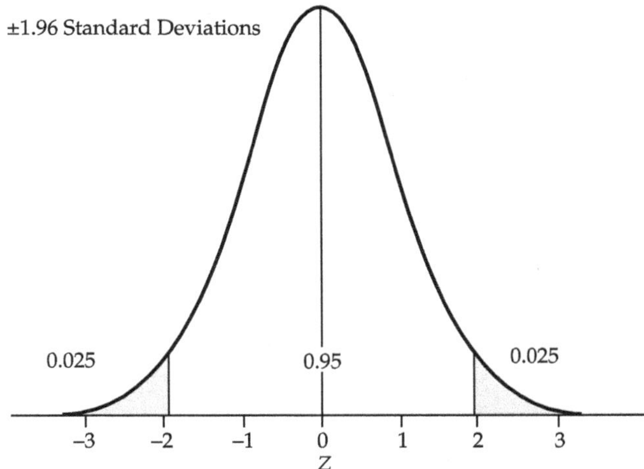

Fig. 8.2.1: *Critical region and acceptance region when* $\alpha = 0.05$.

In the figure, shaded area is critical region and un-shaded area is the acceptance region.

(*iii*) Critical value: The value of the sample statistic that defines, the region of acceptance and rejection is called the *Critical value.* In the figure (8.2.1.) –1.96 and 1.96 on the x–axis are critical values. Critical value divides the sample space into two parts i.e. Acceptance region and Rejection region. Critical value at α is denoted by $Z\alpha$. Rejection region is on both sides which means that the test is the test is a two tailed test. For one-tailed test, we have to consider only one side and the area is $\alpha/2 = 0.05/2 = 0.025$. This implies that in one tailed test $\alpha = 0.025$, means that $\alpha = 0.05$ in two-tailed test. Similarly, if $\alpha = 0.1$ in two tailed test, then $\alpha = 0.05$ in one tailed test. Based on the critical region, one tailed tests are again divided in to two categories. Namely (*a*) right tailed tests in which the critical region is on the right side of the curve and (*b*) left tailed tests in which the critical region is on the left side of the curve. In two-tailed tests, critical region is on both sides of the curve as shown in the fig. (8.2.1.).

(*iv*) Power of the test: Probability of not committing type – II error is called the power f the test. That is (1 – β) is called *"power of the test"*. As β decreases, i.e., probability of committing type – II error decreases, power of the test (1 – β) will be increased. All the tests discussing in this book are having maximum power and hence are known as *'Most Powerful Tests'* (MPT's).

(*v*) Sampling distribution and standard error: Let 't' is a statistic i.e. a function of sample observations. We get different samples from the same population. That is if we want to select a sample of size 'n' from a population of size 'N', we can select $\binom{N}{n}$ different samples. We can get different values of the test statistic–'t' from different samples. Thus the test statistic is a function of sample observations taking different values for different samples. The distribution this statistic is known as 'sampling distribution'. The standard deviation of this statistic 't' is called standard error of 't' and is denoted by S.E. (t). **Thus the standard deviation of the sampling distribution of 't', is called "standard error" of 't'.**

***(vi)* Large sample and small sample tests:** If the sample size n is greater than 30, then the test is known as 'large sample test' and we assume standard normal distribution to determine the critical value. In this case we use standard normal distribution which is known as Z–distribution. The critical values of Z–distribution at various values of α to be considered in large sample tests ($n > 30$) are as follows:

(8.2.1) Table of critical values for large sample tests ($n > 30$).

α values	10% or 0.1	5% or 0.05	1% or 0.01
Two Tailed Test	$\lvert Z\alpha \rvert = 1.645$	$\lvert Z\alpha \rvert = 1.96$	$\lvert Z\alpha \rvert = 2.58$
Right Tailed Test	$Z\alpha = 1.28$	$Z\alpha = 1.645$	$Z\alpha = 2.33$
Left Tailed Test	$Z\alpha = -1.28$	$Z\alpha = -1.645$	$Z\alpha = -2.33$

When the sample size n is less than 30, then the tests are known as 'small sample tests'. Student's t, F and chi-square tests are small sample tests. In the present chapter we discuss large sample tests.

***(vii)* Z – statistic:** In large sample tests, as the sample size n is > 30, we use Z – statistic which is defined as follows :

$$Z = \frac{t - E(t)}{S.E.(t)} \sim N(0, 1) \text{ as } n \to \infty. \qquad (8.2.1)$$

Where, t is the statistic and S.E. (t) is the standard error of the statistic t.

We know that $N(0, 1)$ is the standard normal distribution with mean zero and variance 1. It is also known as Z-distribution and t-test is known as Z-test.

8.3. LARGE SAMPLE TEST PROCEDURE

A common test procedure useful for testing in large sample cases involve the following steps:

Step – 1. Frame null-hypothesis H_0 and alternative H_1 for the given problem.

Step – 2. Determine one-tailed test or two-tailed test based on alternative hypothesis H_1.

Step – 3. Calculate the statistic 't' and $E(t)$ and S.E.(t) from the given data.

Step – 4. Calculate test statistic under $H_0 = Z_{cal} = \dfrac{t - E(t)}{S.E.(t)}$.

Step – 5. Determine the critical value at $\alpha = 0.05$ or 0.01 level denoted by Z_α.

Step – 6. If $Z_{cal} \leq Z_\alpha$ we accept the null hypothesis H_0. If $Z_{cal} > Z_\alpha$ we reject the null hypothesis H_0.

The values of t, $E(t)$ and S.E. (t) values changes from problem to problem.

8.4. TESTS FOR PROPORTIONS

Here we concentrate on attribute data. In attributes we count number of persons having the attribute and number of persons not having the attribute and calculate the respective proportions for each category. Thus when we have to deal attribute data, proportions are used. For example, proportion of persons suffering from a disease, proportion of male and female births, proportion of persons having color blindness, proportion of patients susceptible to penicillin injection and so on.

(a) Testing sample proportion with population proportion

Here we consider the phenomenon or characteristic, which are not capable of direct quantitative measurement, but we can only study the presence or absence of a particular quality or attribute in a group of individuals. For example, color blindness, deafness, honesty, beauty, satisfaction, skin color, eye color, pain and so on. Here, it is not possible to measure the magnitude of the deafness or color blindness or pain or eye color, but we can get it quantitatively by counting the number of persons who have the attribute of our interest and those who do not have. Thus, in a phenomenon, where we can study only presence or absence of a particular characteristic or attribute. In such situations, we consider proportion of the population having some attribute and proportion of the population not having the attribute, under the study.

Let a population consists of N units, of which X units having certain attribute and remaining $N - X$ units are not having the attribute. Then the proportion of units having the attribute denoted by $P = X/N$ and the proportion of units not having the attribute is denoted by $Q = 1 - P = 1 - X/N = (N - X)/N$. Let a sample of n units are drawn from N units randomly and x sampled units are having the attribute and $n - x$ sampled units are not having the attribute. Then the sample proportion of units having the attribute is denoted by $p = x/n$ and the number of sampled units not having the attribute, denoted by $q = 1 - p = 1 - x/n = (n - x)/n$. Under the above circumstances, the random variable X follows binomial distribution with its mean $= E(X) = NP$, $\text{Var}(X) = NPQ$ and standard deviation $\sqrt{NPQ}$.

Now we calculate

$$E(P) = E(X/N) = E(X)/N = NP/N = P.$$

$$\text{Var}(P) = \text{Var}(X/N) = [NPQ]/N^2 = PQ/N \text{ (because } \text{Var}(X/a) = [V(X)]/a^2)$$

Hence the standard error of the statistic P is $\sqrt{PQ/N}$. On similar lines, we can show that S.E.$(p) = \sqrt{pq/n}$. Using these information, the test statistic Z for testing proportions is given by:

$$Z_{cal} = \frac{t - E(t)}{\text{S.E.}(t)} = [p - P]/\sqrt{PQ/N} \sim N(0, 1) \text{ as } N \to \infty. \qquad (8.4.1)$$

If P and Q are not known, S.E.(P) is estimated by using sample standard deviation $\sqrt{pq/n}$. Thus we have:

$$Z_{cal} = [p - P]/\sqrt{pq/n} \sim N(0, 1) \text{ as } n \to \infty. \qquad (8.4.2)$$

The 99.73 confidence limits or most probable limits for p are $p \pm 3$ S.E.(p) and 95 % confidence limits are $p \pm 1.96$ S.E.(p). Similarly, 99% confidence limits are $p \pm 2.58\ \text{S.E.}(p)$ where $\text{S.E.}(p) = \sqrt{pq/n}$. (8.4.3)

Example (8.4.1): In a hospital there are 480 male and 520 female births in a month. Test whether the data supports that the male and female births are equally probable, or not?

Solution: Let P is the population proportion and p is the sample proportion.

H_0 = Male and female births are equally probable. i.e. $p = P$ or there is no significant difference between p and P.

H_1 = Male and female births not equally probable i.e. $p \neq P$ or there is significant difference between p and P.

This is a two tailed test because, male births may be more than female births or female births may be more than male births. Both situations are possible. Hence this is a two tailed test. Let p is the proportion of male births. And q = Proportion of female births.

Here $P = Q = ½ = 0.5$ and sample size $n = 480 + 520 = 1000$,

$p = 480/1000 = 0.48$ and $q = 520/1000 = 0.52$.

Standard error of p = S.E.(p) = $\sqrt{(0.48)(0.52)/1000}$ = 0.0157987.

$Z_{cal} = (0.48 - 0.5)/0.0157987 = 1.126593$.

Z_{tab} at $\alpha = 0.05$ is 1.96 i.e. $Z_\alpha = 1.96$. [from table (8.2.1) for a two-tailed test]

Since $Z_{cal} = 1.126$ is less than $Z_\alpha = 1.96$ we accept H_0 and conclude that both male and female births are equally probable.

Example (8.4.2): A coin is tossed 500 times and found that head turns up for 290 times. Based on this information can we conclude that the coin is unbiased?

Solution: Let P is the population proportion and p is the sample proportion.

H_0 : The coin is unbiased i.e. $p = P$. or, There is no significant difference between p and P.

H_1 : The coin is biased $p \neq P$. or There is significant difference between p and P.

This is a two-tailed test. i.e. $p > P$ or $p < P$.

From the sample, we have $p = 290/500 = 0.58$. Hence, $q = 0.42$.

$$\text{S.E. }(p) = \sqrt{[(0.58)(0.42)]/500} = 0.02207.$$

$$Z_{cal} = (0.58 - 0.5)/0.02207 = 3.62483$$

Z_{tab} at $\alpha = 0.05$ is 1.96 i.e. $Z_\alpha = 1.96$. [from table (8.2.1) for a two-tailed test]

Since, Z_{cal} is larger than $Z_\alpha = 1.96$, we reject H_0. That is the coin is a biased coin.

Example (8.4.3): From a large population, 500 people are selected randomly and found that 65 persons are suffering from kidney failure and undergoing dialysis. Show that the standard error of persons suffering from kidney failure is 0.015. Also estimate the 95% confidence limits for the percentage of people undergoing dialysis is between 10.06 to 15.94.

Solution: It is given that $n = 500$ and $x = 65$. Hence the sample proportion of kidney failures is $p = 65/500 = 0.13$ and $q = 1 - 0.13 = 0.87$. Hence, standard error of P is given by :

$$\text{S.E.}(p) = \sqrt{(0.13)(0.87)/500} = 0.01504 \text{ or } 0.015 \text{ (approx.)}$$

Hence estimated proportion in the population is $P = p = 0.17$ and $Q = q = 0.87$. Using (8.3.3) we have $p \pm$ S.E. $(p) = 0.13 \pm 1.96\ (0.015) = 0.13 \pm 0.0294$ i.e. the confidence limits are (0.1006, 0.1594). Hence if we express the limits in terms of percentages, we have (10.06,15.94). This implies that in any random sample from the given population approximately, 10% to 16% people are suffering from kidney problem and undergoing dialysis. This statement if true 95% true.

Example (8.4.4): There are 16,000 families living in a colony of a metropolitan city. From these, 860 families are selected randomly and found that 215 families are suffering from waterborne diseases. Find (*i*) 1% and (*ii*) almost certain probability limits, for persons suffering from waterborne diseases in that colony.

Solution: It is given that $N = 16{,}000$, $n = 860$, x = Persons suffering from waterborne diseases = 215. Hence, $p = x/n = 215/860 = 0.25$. Therefore, $q = 1 - p = 1 - 0.25 = 0.75$ and $\text{S.E.}(p) = \sqrt{(0.25)(0.75)/860} = 0.014766$. 1% confidence interval (C.I) = $p \pm 2.58$ S.E.$(p) = 0.25 \pm 0.038$. That is 1% C.I. = (0.212, 0.288). To get number of families suffering from waterborne diseases, these probability limits are to be multiplied by 16,000. Thus we have 1% C.I. of families is (3392, 4608).

That is, estimated number of families suffering from waterborne diseases in the colony lies between 3392 and 4608. This statement is 99% true.

To find almost certain probability limits we have to consider 3 instead of 2.58 as multiplicative constant to S.E.(p). Thus we have : $0.25 \pm 3\ (0.014766) = 0.25 \pm 0.044298$. Thus almost certain C.I. for probability is given by (0.2057, 0.2943). Thus estimated number of families suffering from waterborne diseases in the colony are between 3291 and 4709. This statement is almost certain i.e., probability of this statement being true is 0.9973.

(b) Testing the difference two sample proportions:

Let two samples are drawn with sizes n_1 and n_2. Let x_1, x_2 represent number of units having a specific attribute in the selected samples respectively. Then $p_1 = x_1/n_1$ and $p_2 = x_2/n_2$. We want to test whether these two samples came from the same population or from two different populations. i.e., $p_1 = p_2$ or $p_1 \neq p_2$. The test procedure to test the significant difference between two sample proportions is given as follows:

Step – 1: Frame the hypotheses H_0: $p_1 = p_2$ and $H_1 : p_1 \neq p_2$ or $p_1 > p_2$ or $p_1 < p_2$.

Step – 2: Determine whether the test is a one-tailed or two-tailed test.

Step – 3: Calculate the required quantities from the given data.

Step – 4: The test statistic under H_0 is given by:

$$Z_{cal} = \frac{p_1 - p_2}{S.E.(p_1 - p_2)} = \frac{p_1 - p_2}{\sqrt{PQ\left(\frac{1}{n_1} + \frac{1}{n_2}\right)}} \tag{8.4.4}$$

Where, $p = (n_1 p_1 + n_2 p_2)/(n_1 + n_2)$.

$Q = 1 - p$.

Step – 5: Determine Z_α value at $\alpha = 5\%$ or 1% from table (8.2.1).

Step – 6: If Z_{cal} is less than or equal to Z_α we accept H_0 at $\alpha\%$ level of significance If Z_{cal} is greater than Z_α we reject H_0 at $\alpha\%$ level of significance.

Example (8.4.5): A sample survey results show that out of 800 males, 480 and out of 600 females, 350 are attacked by a viral fever in a town. (*a*) Test whether there exists any significance difference between proportions of male and female persons suffering from viral fever?

(*b*) Can we conclude that male is suffering more than female from this viral fever, in that town?

Solution: It is given in the problem that n_1 = male = 800 and

n_2 = female = 600. $n = n_1 + n_2 = 800 + 600 = 1400$ people.

X_1 = male sufferers = 480, x_2 = female sufferers = 350.

Let p_1 = proportion of male sufferers = 480/800 = 0.6

And p_2 = proportion of female sufferers = 350/600 = 0.583.

(a) Frame the hypothesis:

H_0 : There is no significant difference between proportions of male and female sufferers from viral fever, or $p_1 = p_2$.

H_1 : There is significant difference between proportions of male and female sufferers from viral fever, or $p_1 \neq p_2$.

This is a two-tailed test and the test statistic is:

$$Z_{cal} = \frac{p_1 - p_2}{S.E.(p_1 - p_2)} = \frac{p_1 - p_2}{\sqrt{PQ\left(\frac{1}{n_1} + \frac{1}{n_2}\right)}} \sim N(0, 1).$$

Where, $\hat{P} = (n_1 p_1 + n_2 p_2)/(n_1 + n_2)$ and $\hat{Q} = 1 - \hat{P}$.

Now $\hat{P} = (480 + 350)/1400 = 0.5929$ and $\hat{Q} = 1 - 0.5929 = 0.4071$.

Hence $Z_{cal} = (0.6 - 0.583)/\sqrt{(0.5929)(0.4071)(0.00125 + 0.00167)}$

$= 0.017/\sqrt{0.000704} = 0.017/0.0265 = 0.6415.$

Now Z_α when $\alpha = 0.05$ is 1.96 [from table (8.2.1)] . Here $Z_{cal} < Z_\alpha$.

Hence, we accept the null hypothesis that there is no significant difference between proportions of male and female sufferers. Both male and female sufferers are equal statistically. The difference in number of sufferers, occur because of sampling fluctuations.

(b) Here we have to frame hypothesis as:

H_0 : There is no significant difference between proportions of male and female sufferers from viral fever, or $p_1 = p_2$.

H_1 : Proportions of male are more than female sufferers from viral fever, or $p_1 > p_2$.

This is a one-tailed test in particular, is a right tailed test. The test is a one tailed test or two-tailed test, Z_{cal} value will be the same i.e. Z_{cal} = 0.6415 but Z_α will change. Here we have to see the table value at 0.1 l.o.s. This is because of the fact that, if we use two-tailed test at 10% which means that this is 10/2 = 5% in one tailed test. We can observe that 10% values in two-tailed test is equal to 5% values on one-tailed test in table (8.2.1). Hence Z_α = 1.645.

Since $Z_{cal} < Z_\alpha$ we accept the null hypothesis and conclude that both male and female are suffering equally from viral fever in the town. In other words, survey results reveal that, there is no statistical evidence that male are suffering more than female, with viral fever.

Example (8.4.6): In a sample of 600 person of a village-1, 400 are suffering from chicken-guinea. In a sample of 900 person in another village-2, there are 450 persons suffering from chicken-guinea. Based on this data, can we conclude that (a) both villages do not differ statistically significant with respect to the proportion of persons suffering from chicken-guinea? (b) Proportion of persons in village-1 are suffering from more statistically than proportion of persons in village-2 suffering from chicken-guinea.

Solution: It is given in the problem that $n_1 = 600$, $n_2 = 900$ and $n = n_1 + n_2 = 600 + 900 = 1{,}500$, $x_1 = 400$, $x_2 = 450$, $p_1 = 400/600 = 0.667$ and $p_2 = 450/900 = 0.5$.

(a) Frame the hypothesis as follows:

H_0 : There is no significant difference between proportions of sufferers of village-1 and village-2, from chicken-guinea, or $p_1 = p_2$.

H_1 : There is significant difference between proportions of suffers of village-1 and village-2 from chicken-guinea, or $p_1 \neq p_2$.

This is a two tailed test. Now calculate the test statistic as follows:

$$\text{The test statistic is } Z_{cal} = \frac{p_1 - p_2}{S.E.(p_1 - p_2)} = \frac{p_1 - p_2}{\sqrt{PQ\left(\frac{1}{n_1} + \frac{1}{n_2}\right)}}$$

Where, $\hat{P} = (n_1 p_1 + n_2 p_2)/(n_1 + n_2)$ and $\hat{Q} = 1 - \hat{P}$.

Hence, $\hat{P} = (400 + 450)/1500 = 0.5667$ and $\hat{Q} = 1 - \hat{P} = 1 - 0.5667 = 0.4333$.

$$Z_{cal} = (0.667 - 0.5)/\sqrt{(0.5667)(0.4333)(0.00166 + 0.00111)}$$

$$= 0.167/\sqrt{0.00068} = 0.167/0.026 = 6.4231 \quad \text{(approx.)}$$

Z_α, $\alpha = 0.05$ is given by 2.58. i.e. $Z_\alpha = 2.58$. Since $Z_{cal} > Z_{0.01}$ we reject H_0 at 1% l.o.s. Which means that, both villages are statistically different with respect to the proportion of persons suffering from chicken-guinea.

(*b*) Frame hypotheses as follows:

H_0 : There is no significant difference between proportion of suffers of village – 1 and village – 2 from chicken-guinea, or $p_1 = p_2$.

H_1 : The proportion of persons suffering in village – 1 are more than sufferers in village 2 from chicken-guinea, or $p_1 > p_2$.

This is a one-tailed test in particular a right tailed test.

Here Z_α , $\alpha = 0.01$, is 2.33. i.e. $Z_\alpha = 2.33$. Here $Z_{cal} > Z_{0.01}$ hence, we reject the null-hypothesis. That is, the proportion of persons in village-1 is statistically more than the proportion of persons in village – 2 suffering from chicken-guinea.

8.5. TESTS FOR MEANS

Now, we concentrate on variable data. When we deal variable data, mean and variance are two important statistics which helps to take decision. In the present section, we concentrate means and in the next section we deal with variances.

(a) Testing sample mean $\bar{x}$ with population mean μ:

Let $x_1, x_2,.,.,., x_n$ are random sample observations taken from the population of size N with mean μ and variance σ^2

i.e. $$\mu = (X_1 + X_2 +.,.,., + X_N)/N \text{ and } \sigma^2 = \frac{1}{n}\Sigma(X - \bar{X})^2 \quad (8.5.1)$$

Test procedure explained in six steps explained in the previous section 8.3, are same except the difference that the test statistic Z_{cal} will change as follows:

$$Z_{cal} = (\bar{X} - \mu)/S.E.(\bar{X}) = (\bar{X} - \mu)/(\sigma/\sqrt{n}) \quad (8.5.2)$$

And instead of proportions, mean $\bar{X}$ and S.D. σ are to be calculated from the data or from the information given in the problem.

Example (8.5.1): The mean I.Q. of 1,600 children studying 10th class in Andhra Pradesh is 99. Is it likely that this was a random sample from the population with mean I.Q. 100 and standard deviation 15.

Solution: From the data given, we know that sample size n = 16,000, mean = $\bar{x}$ = 99, population μ = 100 and σ = 15.

H_0 : There is no significant difference between the sample mean and the population mean. i.e. $\bar{x} = \mu$.

H_1 : There is significant difference between the sample mean and the population mean. i.e. $\bar{x} \neq \mu$.

This is a two-tailed test. Substituting the values in the test statistic given in (8.4.2) we have:

$$Z_{cal} = (99 - 100)/(15/\sqrt{1,600}) = -1/(15/40) = -40/15 = -2.67.$$

Now Z_α when α = 0.05 is 1.96. [from table (8.2.1)]. Here $|Z_{cal}| > Z_\alpha$.

Hence, we reject H_0 at 5% l.o.s. and conclude that the sample is not taken from the population with mean I.Q. 100 and S.D. 15. This means that the conclusion drawn is true in 95 times out of 100 times and may fail 5 out of 100 times.

Example (8.5.2): The mean life of a sample of 400 fluorescent lights, used in operation theatre, produced form an electronic company was found to be 1570 hours with a standard deviation of 150 hours. Test the hypothesis that the mean lifetime of the bulbs produced by this company is 16,000 hours against that it is greater than 16,000 hours at 1% l.o.s.

Solution: From the given problem, we can observe that the sample size n = 400, mean = $\bar{x}$ = 1570 hrs, population μ = 16,000 hrs and σ = 150 hrs.

H_0 = The mean life of bulbs is 16,000 hrs. i.e. $\bar{x} = \mu$ = 16,000 hrs.

$H_1 = \mu >$ 16,000 hrs. Hence, this is one-tailed test in particular a right tailed test. The test statistic is given by:

$$Z_{cal} = (1570 - 16000)/(150/\sqrt{400}) = -30/(150/20) = -4.00.$$

Now Z_α when $\alpha = 0.01$ is 2.33. [from table (8.2.1)] . Here $|Z_{cal}| > Z_\alpha$.

Hence, we reject the null-hypothesis and conclude that the mean life of fluorescent lamps used in the operation theatre is more than 16,000 hours.

Example (8.5.3): A sample of 400 medical students of a college was found to have a mean height of 171.38 cms. Can it be regarded as a sample from large population of medicos with mean height 171.17cms and standard deviation of 3.30 cms?

Solution: From the problem we have $n = 400$, mean = $\bar{x}$ = 171.38 cms, population $\mu = 171.17$ hrs and $\sigma = 3.30$ cms.

H_0 : There is no significant difference between sample mean $\bar{x}$ and the population mean μ. i.e. $\bar{x} = \mu = 171.7$ cms.

H_1: $\bar{x} \neq \mu$. This is a two-tailed test. Now calculate the test statistic:

$$Z_{cal} = (171.38 - 171.17)/(3.3/\sqrt{400}) = 0.21/(3.3/20) = 0.21/0.165$$
$$= 1.27.$$

Now Z_α when $\alpha = 0.05$ is 1.96. [from table (8.2.1)] .

Here $|Z_{cal}| < Z_\alpha$.

Thus we accept the null-hypothesis H_0 at 5% l.o.s. This implies that the sample of 400 medicos are drawn from the large population of medicos whose mean height is 171.17 cms and standard deviation 3.3 cms.

(*b*) Testing the significant difference between two sample means.

Let A and B be two populations with means μ_1 and μ_2 and variances $\sigma_1{}^2$ and $\sigma_2{}^2$ respectively. Let us take two independent samples of size n_1 and n_2 from these two populations. $\bar{x}$ and $\bar{y}$ be corresponding sample means. Our problem is to test the significant difference between these two sample means $\bar{x}$ and $\bar{y}$ i.e. $\bar{x} - \bar{y}$. The test procedure explained in six steps explained 8.3 is same except the test statistic, which is defined as follows:

$$Z_{cal} = (\bar{x} - \bar{y})/S.E.(\bar{x} - \bar{y}) \qquad (8.5.3)$$

where $$\text{S.E.}(\bar{x} - \bar{y}) = \sqrt{(\sigma_1^2/n_1) + (\sigma_1^2/n_2)}$$

If the populations variances are not known then we can substitute unbiased estimators of these variances. That is we can substitute sample variances $s_1{}^2$ and $s_2{}^2$ in the place of $\sigma_1{}^2$ and $\sigma_2{}^2$ respectively in equation (8.4.3).

Example (8.5.4): The research unit in the medical university wishes to determine whether scores on the scholastic aptitude test conducted for male and female doctors differs significantly or not? A sample of 399 female doctors got 502.1 with S.D. 86.2. Another sample of 204 male doctors, got 510.5 with S.D. 90.4. Determine, whether there exists any statistical evidence that male doctors have more scholastic aptitude than female doctors.

Solution: From the given problem, it is known that :

n_1 = female doctors = 399 ; n_2 = male doctors = 204.

Means: $\bar{x} = 502.1$ $\qquad \bar{y} = 510.5$

S.D.s : $\sigma_1 = 86.2$ $\qquad \sigma_2 = 90.4$

H_0 : There is no significant difference between male and female doctors with respect to scores on the scholastic aptitude test. i.e. $\bar{x} = \bar{y}$.

H_1 : $\bar{x} < \bar{y}$. This is a one-tailed test particularly a left tailed test.

Substituting these values (8.4.3) we have:

$$Z_{cal} = (502.1 - 510.5)/\sqrt{(86.2^2/399) + (90.4^2/204)}$$

$$= -8.4/\sqrt{7430.44/399 + 8172.16/206} = -8.4/\sqrt{18.62 + 40.06}$$

$$= -8.4/7.66 = -1.097.$$

$Z_\alpha = -1.645$ at $\alpha = 0.05$ l.o.s. Here $|Z_{cal}| < Z_\alpha$. Hence, we accept the null-hypothesis. Hence, we conclude that there is no significant difference between male and female Doctors with respect to scores on the scholastic aptitude test.

Example (8.5.5): A sample of 100 plots from the district – A results the mean yield of wheat of 210 kgs and standard deviation 12 kgs. In another sample of 150 plots from the district – B results the mean yield as 220 kgs with standard deviation 11 kgs. Test whether yield of wheat differ significantly with respect to mean in districts *A* and *B* at 1% level of significance (l.o.s.).

Solution: It is given in the problem that $n_1 = 100$ plots and $n_2 = 150$ plots.

Means: $\bar{x} = 210$ kgs $\qquad \bar{y} = 220$ kgs.

S.D.s : $s_1 = 12$ kgs $\qquad s_2 = 11$ kgs.

Frame the hypotheses:

H_0: There is no significant difference between mean yields of wheat in both the districts *A* and *B*. i.e. $\bar{x} = \bar{y}$

H_1: $\bar{x} \neq \bar{y}$. This is a two-tailed test. Substituting these in equation (8.4.3) we have:

$$Z_{cal} = (210 - 220)/\sqrt{(12)^2/100 + (11)^2/150} = -10/\sqrt{1.44 + 0.8067}.$$

$$= -10/1.4989 = 6.6715.$$

Now Z_α when $\alpha = 0.01$ is 2.33. [from table (8.2.1)] . Here $|Z_{cal}| > Z_\alpha$.

Hence, we reject the null-hypothesis at 1% l.o.s. and conclude that there is significant difference between mean yields of wheat per plot in both the districts *A* and *B*.

8.6. TEST THE SIGNIFICANT DIFFERENCE BETWEEN TWO SAMPLE STANDARD DEVIATIONS (S.D.'s)

When we deal with variable data, along with the means, we have to compare variances. Comparing variances is equivalent with comparing standard deviations. Thus in this section, we propose the test procedure to test the significant difference between two sample standard deviations s_1 and s_2. The test procedure is explained already in section 8.3. in six steps. To recollect once again, we explain them as follows:

Step – 1: Frame the null-hypothesis H_0: There is no significant difference between two sample standard deviations, i.e. $s_1 = s_2$.

Step – 2: Frame the alternative hypothesis H_1: $s_1 \neq s_2$ or $s_1 < s_2$ or $s_1 > s_2$ and determine whether the test is two-tailed test or one-tailed.

Step – 3: Calculate sample sizes n_1, n_2, sample variances and standard deviations s_1, s_2 and population variances σ_1^2 and σ_2^2 from the given data or problem.

Step – 4: Test statistic $Z_{cal} = \dfrac{s_1 - s_2}{S.E\,(s_1 - s_2)}$

$$= \frac{s_1 - s_2}{\sqrt{(\sigma_1^2/2n_1) + (\sigma_2^2/2n_2)}} \sim N(0, 1) \qquad (8.6.1)$$

Step – 5: Determine Z_α value at $\alpha = 0.05$ or 0.01 based on the requirement from table (8.2.1).

Step – 6: If $Z_{cal} \leq Z_\alpha$ value, we accept H_0. Otherwise, i.e. if $Z_{cal} > Z_\alpha$ we reject H_0 at α % level of significance (l.o.s.).

Example (8.6.1): A sample of 100 plots from the district – *A* results the mean yield of wheat of 200 lbs per acre and standard deviation 10 lbs per acre. In another sample of 150 plots from the district – *B* results the mean yield as 220 lbs with standard deviation 14 lbs. Test whether yield of wheat differ significantly with respect to S.D.s in districts *A* and *B* at 1% level of significance (l.o.s.) assuming that standard deviation of the entire state has 11 lbs as standard deviation.

Solution: It is given in the problem that $n_1 = 100$ plots and $n_2 = 150$ plots.

Means: $\bar{x} = 200$ kgs $\qquad \bar{y} = 220$ kgs.

S.D.s : $s_1 = 10$ kgs $\qquad s_2 = 14$ kgs.

Population S.D. $\sigma_1 = 11$ lbs and $\sigma_2 = 11$ lbs.

Frame the hypotheses:

H_0 : There is no significant difference between the S.D.s of yields of wheat in both the districts *A* and *B*. i.e. $s_1 = s_2$.

H_1: There is significant difference between two sample standard deviations $s_1 \neq s_2$.

This is a two-tailed test. Substituting these in equation (8.6.1) we have:

$$Z_{cal} = (10 - 14)/\sqrt{(11)^2/2 \times 100 + (11)^2/2 \times 150} = -4/\sqrt{0.605 + 0.4033}.$$

$$= -4/1.004 = -3.98406.$$

Now Z_α when $\alpha = 0.01$ is 2.33. [from table (8.2.1)] . Here $|Z_{cal}| > Z_\alpha$.

Hence, we reject the null-hypothesis at 1% l.o.s. and conclude that there is significant difference between S.D.s of yields of wheat per plot in both the districts *A* and *B*. The selected samples does not show any consistency because S.D.s show significant difference. This implies that their variances also show significant difference. Hence, selected samples are in-consistent with each other.

Example (8.6.2): A medical college conducts both day and night classes intended to be identical. A sample of 100 day students yield examination results as $\bar{x} = 72.4$ and $s_1 = 14.8$. Another sample of 200 night college students were selected and yields examination results as $\bar{y} = 72.4$ and $s_1 = 18.8$. Can we conclude that both day college students and night college students are consistent with respect to their marks in the examination?

Solution: In the problem it is given that:

$$n_1 = 100 \text{ and } n_2 = 200.$$
$$\bar{x} = 72.4 \quad \text{and } s_1 = 14.8$$
$$\bar{y} = 72.4 \quad \text{and } s_1 = 18.8.$$

H_0 : There is no significant difference between the day college and night college students. i.e. $s_1 = s_2$.

H_1 : There is significant difference between two sample standard deviations $s_1 \neq s_2$.

This is a two-tailed test. Substituting these in equation (8.6.1) we have:

$$Z_{cal} = (14.8 - 18.8)/\sqrt{(14.8)^2/2 \times 100 + (18.8)^2/2 \times 150}$$

$$= -4/\sqrt{1.0952 + 1.178133} = -4/2.27333 = -1.759533.$$

Now Z_α when $\alpha = 0.05$ is 1.96. [from table (8.2.1)] . Here $|Z_{cal}| < Z_\alpha$.

Hence we accept the null-hypothesis H_0. Hence we concluded that both day college and night college students are consistent in securing marks in the examination. Thus there is no significant difference between day college and night college students in securing marks.

Thus testing hypothesis gives, statistical validity for decisions made based on the experimental results. Now a days in this scientifically advanced and technologically developed society, only statistically valid statements alone are acceptable because, they have more validity i.e., the probability of the statistically valid statements being true is 0.95 or 0.99. In other words, the probability of statistically valid statement being false is 0.05 or 0.01. i.e. 5 out of 100 times or 1 out of 100 times.

Hence testing hypothesis is a very important statistical method of measuring the truth behind any statement made by scientist or researchers based on the results of Random Experiment. In all the above situations, we have considered large samples ($n > 30$). But in many scientific enquiries, getting so much large samples is not possible. In such situations we use small sample tests like chi-square, Student – t and F – tests, which are discussed in chapter IX.

REVIEW QUESTIONS AND PROBLEMS

A. Objective Questions

1. In large sample tests sample size 'n' will be -----------------.

   (*a*) less than 30 (*b*) less than or equal to 30
   (*c*) greater than 30 (*d*) greater than or equal to 30.

2. In large sample test we use --------------- distribution.

   (*a*) binomial distribution (*b*) Z-distribution
   (*c*) F–distribution (*d*) Poisson distribution.

3. If $Z_{cal} = 6.78$, we ------------------ .
   (*a*) accept H_0 (*b*) reject H_1
   (*c*) reject H_0 (*d*) reject both H_0 and H_1.

4. If $Z_{cal} = 0.578$, we ------------------ hypothesis.
   (*a*) accept H_0 (*b*) reject H_1
   (*c*) reject H_0 (*d*) reject both H_0 and H_1.

5. Under H_0 we consider ----------------- difference between two sample proportions.
   (*a*) significant (*b*) large
   (*c*) not significant (*d*) considerable

6. If $|Z_{cal}| > Z_\alpha$ we --------------------------
   (*a*) accept H_0 (*b*) reject H_1
   (*c*) reject H_0 (*d*) reject both H_0 and H_1.

7. If $|Z_{cal}| < Z_\alpha$ we ---------------------------.
   (*a*) accept H_0 (*b*) reject H_1
   (*c*) reject H_0 (*d*) reject both H_0 and H_1.

8. Probability of committing type –I error is called -----------------.
   (*a*) critical region (*b*) power of the test
   (*c*) sample space (*d*) level of significance.

9. $1 - \beta$ is called ------------------------------.
   (*a*) critical region (*b*) power of the test
   (*c*) sample space (*d*) level of significance.

10. When a sample point falls in a critical region we ---------------.
    (*a*) accept H_0 (*b*) reject H_1
    (*c*) reject H_0 (*d*) reject both H_0 and H_1.

B. Short Answer Questions

1. Explain briefly various steps involved in a large sample test.
2. Write short notes on large sample tests.
3. What is meant by standard error? Explain with an example.
4. Explain type – I error and type – II error.
5. Distinguish between one-tailed and two tailed tests.
6. Explain the role of null hypothesis in testing of hypotheses.
7. Explain briefly, what is meant by a statistical hypothesis?
8. Write short notes on level of significance.
9. Explain briefly, a large sample test procedure to test the significance difference between sample proportion and population proportion.
10. Explain the large sample test procedure to test the significance difference between two sample standard deviations.

C. Essay Type Questions

1. What are large sample tests? Explain the test procedure to test the significance difference between two sample means.
2. Explain the terms (*i*) critical region (*ii*) statistical hypothesis (*iii*) null-hypothesis (*iv*) one-tailed test and (*v*) two-tailed test.
3. Explain the terms (*i*) level of significance (*ii*) standard error (*iii*) power of the test (*iv*) alternative hypothesis and (*v*) test statistic.
4. Explain large sample tests for testing proportions.
5. Explain large sample tests for testing of means.
6. A random sample of 700 vaccine filling bottles were selected from a large consignment, purchased by a pharmaceutical company, found that 200 were found to be defective. Based on this information, (*a*) can we conclude that purchased lot of bottles contains 30% of defective bottles or more? (*b*) Obtain 95% and 99% confidence interval for defective vaccine filling bottles in a consignment of 2000 vaccine filling bottles.

   [**Hint:** (*a*) Here, p = 200/700 = 0.2857 and q = 0.7143 and P = 0.3 and $H_0: p = P, H_1 = p \geq P$. This is a one-tailed test and Z_{cal} = 0.0143/0.017= 0.8412. Hence we accept H_0. (b) C.I. $p \pm 1.96$ S.E. (p)]
7. An X-ray machine produced 20 defective X–ray photos out of 400 samples. After overhauling the equipment, it produced 10 defective photos in a random sample of 300 photos. (a) Can we conclude that the overhauling improved the performance of the equipment or not? Test at 5% l.o.s.

   [**Hint:** P_1 = 0.05 and p_2 = 0.033 and $|Z_\alpha|$ = 1.134]
8. The mean I.Q. of 256 medicos in an university has 96. Can we conclude that in general, students from that university contains mean I.Q. is 102 and standard deviation 20? Test the statement at 1% l.o.s.

   [**Hint:** $\bar{x}$ = 96, μ = 102, σ = 20 and n = 2,500. Z_{cal} = –6/1.25 = – 4.8]
9. A random sample of male nurses in a city is taken and the mean number of hours of absenteeism for the year is found to be 50 hours. A similar sample of 50 female nurses has mean of 66 hours. Can we conclude that in general, the population from which these male and female nurses taken has the same mean with S.D. 10 hours?

   [**Hint:** $H_0 : \mu_1 = \mu_2$ and $H_1 : \mu_1 \neq \mu_2$ and $Z_{cal} = 63 - 66/\sqrt{(100/50 + 100/50)}$ = –3/2 = –1.5]
10. The Standard Deviation of the height of 100 medicos of a college 4.5 cms. Another sample of 50 medicos from another college has an S.D. of 3.5 cms with respect to their height. Assuming that population S.D. σ = 4.0 cms. Test the significant difference between the S.D.s of two samples. Can we conclude that both samples are consistent? Test at 5% l.o.s.

    [**Hint:** $H_0 : \sigma_1 = \sigma_2, H_1 : \sigma_1 \neq \sigma_2$ and Z_{cal} = 2.04]
11. Two stimulants, *A* and *B* were tested for effect on two random samples, each of 50 psycho-patients. One stimulant was administered to each group and the effect was measured by an *X* value on *A* and *Y* value on *B*. The results are as follows:

Stimulant A : $\Sigma X = 1{,}750$ $\Sigma X^2 = 62{,}520$

Stimulant B : $\Sigma Y = 1{,}980$ $\Sigma Y^2 = 85{,}610$

Does the sample evidence suggest that stimulant B is more effective than stimulant A? use the 1% l.o.s.

[**Hint:** $H_0: \mu_1 = \mu_2$ and $H_1 : \mu_1 < \mu_2$ and

$Z_{cal} = (39.6 - 35)/\sqrt{(25.4/50 + 144/50)} = 2.5 > 2.33$. Hence reject H_0]

12. Intelligent test given to two groups of male and female medicos gave the following results.

Female medicos : Mean marks = 78 S.D. = 12 $n = 80$

Male medicos : Mean marks = 75 S.D. = 14 $n = 120$

(*a*) Is there any significant difference between mean marks?

(*b*) Is there any significant difference between standard deviations?

[Answers: (*a*) $Z = 1.565$ (*b*) $Z = 2.212$]

13. A team of young surgeons has developed new techniques for a risky operation. Under the old method it is known that 30% of the patients who undergone this operation will be recovered. It is found that out of 225 operations using the new technique 90 have recovered. Can we say that the new technique is better than the old one? Use 5% level of significance.

[**Hint:** $H_0: p = 0.30$ $H_1 : p > 0.30$ $Z = 2.38$, H_0 rejected]

References

1. Gupta S.P. 1990 "Statistical Methods". Sultan Chand & Sons, New Delhi.
2. Wayne W. Daniel 2008 Biostatistics, 9th edition, John Wiley & Sons. Inc. Newyork.
3. P.N. Arora *et al.* 2007 "Comprehensive Statistical Methods" Sultan Chand and company Ltd. First edn. New Delhi.
4. VK. Kapoor 1986 "Problems and solutions in Business statistics" Sultan Chand and sons New Delhi.

Answers to Objective Questions

1 – c; 2 – b; 3 – c; 4 – a; 5 – c; 6 – c; 7 – a; 8 – d; 9 – b; 10 – c.

9 TESTING OF HYPOTHESIS — SMALL SAMPLE TESTS

9.1. INTRODUCTION

Large sample tests discussed in the previous Chapter are always not preferable, particularly in many scientific enquiries, where, laboratory experiments are involved. In laboratory experiments, there exists many situations, where, repeating the experiment itself is very costly, and time consuming. For example, conducting experiments on the surface of the Moon or in the space or on the Mars are very costly and requires years together, even to send a missile into the space and requires millions of rupees or U.S. dollars. Thus conducting a single time the experiment is so costly and requires large time. In such situations, we cannot expect the sample size is large in size like in large sample cases. We have observations, not larger than 30. In such situations, it is not reasonable to assume normality and apply standard normal distribution i.e., *Z*–distribution, in making decisions. If we use this distribution, our conclusions, or decisions may go wrong, because our basic assumption or normality may not hold good. Thus there is need to develop tests suitable for laboratory experiments, bases on small samples where, sample sizes are less than or equal to 30. The tests used in large samples are different from small samples. There are three such tests used, when sample size $n \leq 30$. They are:

(*i*) For attribute data: Chi-square test or χ^2 - test.
(*ii*) For variable data: (*a*) Student's *t* - test and (*b*) *F*-test.

In small sample tests, we use a new concept called 'degrees of freedom' (d.o.f) which is explained as follows:

9.1.1. Degrees of Freedom

The concept of degrees of freedom (d.o.f) is highly useful in small sample test procedures because of which we generalize our experimental results to the entire population, even though the sample size is small. "Degrees of Freedom" is defined as the number of data items in the given form of series of variables, which can be calculated independently or which can take independent values. The concept of degrees of freedom, denoted by 'v', is useful to make the results un-biased. This is explained with an example as follows :

Example (9.1.1): Consider that there are 15 students for a practical examination in which 15 practical problems, are to be distributed such that practical problem is to be assigned to each student. If this assignment is done by the regular teacher, who has done this practical, knowingly or un-knowingly his personal bias will act and results will be biased. He may assign easy problem to some candidates, whom he wants to do favor and difficult one to some candidates and so on. Instead of that, if we want to make the results un-biased, write these practical problem number or title in different identical chits or slips and after folding them properly, each student can come and select one slip and has to do the problem in that chit. Thus problems are allotted randomly to students and now the bias of the teacher is eliminated and the results are un-biased. In this process, first candidate has choice to select any one from the available (say 15) problems. Similarly, second student also has freedom to select the problem from the remaining 14 problems and so on. Continuing on similar lines, 14th student also has freedom to choose his problem from the remaining two chits. But last student has no freedom to choose and he must do the practical compulsorily the problem in the remaining one slip i.e. 15th slip. Thus this one candidate lost his freedom among 15 students. Thus out of 15 students only 14 students has freedom to choose the problem but not the 15th student. Thus degrees of freedom here is 14. In general, if we have n items or individuals or units we have $n - 1$ as degrees of freedom.

Thus degrees of freedom help us to make the results un-biased. Only un-biased results obtained from a sample can be generalized to entire population, so that our conclusions or inferences about the population have more statistical validity. This concept of d.o.f., is used in all small sample tests, to determine the critical values for the test statistic under consideration, for a required 'α%' level of significance.

9.2. CHI-SQUARE TEST OR χ^2 – TEST

The Chi-Square test is usually written as χ^2 – test, which is used for (*a*) comparing experimentally results with those expected theoretically and based on the hypothesis – this test is known as 'testing the goodness of fit' and (*b*) testing the independence of attributes – this test is known as 'testing the independence of attributes'. Chi-Square test statistic is given by the formula:

$$\chi^2_{cal} = \sum_{i=1}^{N} \left[\frac{(O_i - E_i)^2}{E_i} \right] \sim \text{ as } \chi^2 \text{ with } N - 1 \text{ d.o.f} \qquad (9.2.1)$$

where, O_i = Observed frequency of the ith event,

E_i = Expected frequency of the ith event and

N = Number of frequencies.

To determine the critical value of χ^2_α at α% level of significance (l.o.s) we have to use χ^2 – distribution values given in appendix, table $A - 2$, for various values of degrees of freedom (d.o.f). χ^2 – test procedure is explained as follows:

Step – 1: Frame the null-hypothesis as follows:

(*a*) In testing goodness of fit: H_0: The given fit is a good fit to the data and H_1: The given fit is bad fit to the data.

(*b*) In testing independence of attributes: H_0: Given two attributes are independent and H_1: Given attributes are dependent.

Step – 2: Calculated expected frequencies denoted by E_i. Observed frequencies in the given problem are denoted by O_i.

(*a*) Expected frequency = NP(Event of interest under H_0)

(*b*) Expected frequency $(Rix\ Cj)/G$. (9.2.2)

Where $Ri = i^{th}$ row total, $Cj = j^{th}$ column total and G = Grand total.

Step – 3: Calculate the difference $(O_i - E_i)$ and their squares i.e. $(O_i - E_i)^2$.

Step – 4: Calculate sum of $(O_i - E_i)^2$, for $i = 1, 2,.,.,.,N$. The calculated sum is the required χ^2_{cal} value.

Step – 5: Determine d.o.f 'v' and l.o.s. 'α' and determine critical value of $\chi^2_{v,\alpha}$ from tables $A - 2$. In case (*a*) d.o.f. = $v = N - 1$ and in case (*b*) d.o.f. = $(r - 1)(c - 1)$, where r = number of rows and c = number of columns in the given contingency table. A contingency table is a two-way frequency table for both attributes under consideration.

Step – 6: If χ^2_{cal} is less than or equal to $\chi^2_{v,\alpha}$, we accept H_0. Otherwise, we reject H_0.

It is important to note that χ^2_{cal} is always positive because each pair is squared deviation between O_i and E_i $i = 1, 2$ ..,.,., N. Hence χ^2 distribution is a positively skewed distribution. In χ^2 – distribution we always assume that O_i or E_i values are must always be more than 5 in frequency for every value of $I = 1, 2$,.,., N. In any case, if we get less than 5, we have to merge that class to the immediate preceding or succeeding class along with the frequencies. So that the new merged class frequencies are greater than 5.

Example (9.2.1): In a survey, of 320 families, with 5 children, the following data is obtained.

Number of Boys:	5	4	3	2	1	0
Number of Girls:	0	1	2	3	4	5
Number of Families:	14	56	110	88	40	12

Is this data consistent to conclude that male and female births are equally probable?

Solution:

Null hypothesis: H_0: Male and female births are equally probable.

Alternative hypothesis: H_1: Male and female births are no equally probable.

Here we have two outcomes namely, a male birth or a female birth and under H_0 we have P(male birth) ½ and P(female birth) = ½. Here we have to use binomial probabilities by considering the r.v. $X = 0, 1, 2, 3, 4, 5$. Thus $P(X = x)$ for various values of x are (1/32, 5/32, 10/32, 10/32, 5/32, 1/32), or under H_0 we have $(\frac{1}{2} + \frac{1}{2})^i$ $i = 0, 1, 2, 3, 4, 5$. Thus to get expected number of male births in 320 families are 320(1/32, 5/32, 10/32, 10/32, 5/32, 1/32) or 10, 50, 100, 100, 50, 10 families.

Thus we have the following table for calculation of χ^2_{cal}. In the table O = Observed frequencies and E = Expected frequencies

O_i	E_i	$(O_i - E_i)$	$(O_i - E_i)^2$	$(O_i - E_i)^2/E_i$
14	10	4	16	1.60
56	50	6	36	0.72
110	100	10	100	1.00
88	100	–12	144	1.44
40	50	10	100	1.00
12	10	2	4	0.40

		Total of $(O_i - E_i)^2/E_i = \chi^2_{cal} = 6.16$.		

Here, degrees of freedom 'v' is $n - 1 = 6 - 1 = 5$ and let $\alpha = 0.05$. From tables, $A - 2$, we can observe that χ^2 value at $v = 5$ and $\alpha = 0.05$ is 11.07. Here $\chi^2_{cal} < \chi^2_{v,\alpha}$. Hence we accept null hypothesis H_0 and conclude that male and female births are equally probable. The variations observed in the data are due to random causes and the difference among them can be ignored.

Example (9.2.2): The following data represents number of road accident cases admitted in 98 days into a super-speciality hospital on different days of a week. Find whether road accidents are uniformly distributed over the week.

Day of the week:	Sun	Mon	Tue	Wed	Thu	Fri	Sat
Number of accidents:	13	18	10	22	11	10	14

Solution: Frame the hypothesis as H_0: Road accidents are uniformly distributed throughout the week on all days.

H_1: Road accidents are not uniformly distributed throughout the week.

Under the H_0, if accidents are uniformly distributed throughout the week then P(Road accident on any day) = 1/7. Thus to get expected frequencies, we have to multiply total frequency $N = 92$ by the corresponding probability. Thus expected number of accidents per day are 98/7 = 14 cases per day.

$$\chi^2_{cal} = \Sigma(O_i - E_i)^2/E_i = [(13 - 14)^2/14 + (18 - 14)^2/14 + (10 - 14)^2/14 + (22 - 14)^2/14 + (11 - 14)^2/14 + (10 - 14)^2/14 + (14 - 14)^2/14]$$

$$= 1/14[1 + 16 + 16 + 64 + 9 + 16 + 0] = 122/14 = 8.7142.$$

$$\chi^2_{v,\alpha} = 12.59. \text{ [d.o.f. } v = 7 - 1 = 6 \text{ and } \alpha = 0.05 \text{ from table } A - 2.]$$

Here $\chi^2_{cal} < \chi^2_{v,\alpha}$. Hence we accept null hypothesis H_0 and conclude that number of road accident are uniformly distributed throughout on all days of the week. The variation observed in the number of cases admitted on these days is due to random variations and hence can be ignored.

Example (9.2.3): In a group of hospitals there are 200 doctors working on heart by-pass surgeries. Among them, for 150 doctors, a special training is given on the surgery using the new introduced electronic device. Among trained doctors, 100 doctors show good performance while performing surgeries. Similarly, among untrained doctors 36 doctors showed poor performance. Based on this information can we conclude that the training used has any effect in improving the performance of the doctors while performing the surgery. Test at 1% l.o.s.

Solution: From the given data first form the contingency table as follows:

	Good performance	Poor performance	Total
Trained doctors	100	50	150 = R1
Un-trained doctors	14	36	50 = R2
Total	120 = C1	80 = C2	200 = G

Now frame hypothesis H_0: Training and performance are independent.

Alternative hypothesis H_1: Training and the performance are dependent.

Now calculate expected frequencies as follows by using (9.2.2):

	Good performance	Poor performance	Total
Trained doctors	(150 × 120)/200 = 90	(150 × 80)/200 = 60	150 = R1
Un-trained doctors	(120 × 50)/200 = 30	(80 × 50)/200 = 20	50 = R2
Total	120 = C1	80 = C2	200 = G

$$\chi^2_{cal} = \Sigma(O_i - E_i)^2/E_i = (100-90)^2/90 + (50-60)^2/60 + (14-30)^2/30$$
$$+ (36-20)^2/20 = 100/90 + 100/60 + 256/30 + 256/20.$$
$$= 1.11111 + 1.66667 + 8.53333 + 12.8 = 24.1111.$$

In the given contingency table there are two rows and two columns. Hence number of rows = $r = 2$ and number of columns = $c = 2$. Therefore, d.o.f. $v = (r-1)(c-1) = 1 \times 1 = 1$ and $\alpha = 0.01$. From the table $A-2$, we have $\chi^2_{v,\alpha} =$ 3.84. Here $\chi^2_{cal} > \chi^2_{v,\alpha}$. Hence we reject the null hypothesis H_0. This implies that the training has significant effect on the performance of doctors while performing surgery on heart patients. This is stated at 1% level of significance. This means that conclusion drawn based on the data available, is 99 times true out of 100 cases and may fail 1 time out of 100 cases.

Example (9.2.4): In an experiment on immunization of from tuberculosis, an anti-bacterium was tested for its effect. This anti-bacteria was administered on 100 persons of them, 26 persons got affected from tuberculosis. In another batch of 100 persons, where this anti-bacteria was not used, 58 persons got affected. Based on this data, can we conclude that this anti-bacteria has any effect in controlling the tuberculosis? Test the hypothesis at 1% l.o.s.

Solution: From the given information, prepare the contingency table as follows:

	Affected	Unaffected	Total
Anti-bacteria used:	26	74	100 = R1
Anti-bacteria not used:	68	32	100=R2
Total:	94	106	200=G

Frame hypotheses as follows:

H_0: Anti-bacteria and affect from tuberculosis are independent.

H_1: Anti-bacteria and affect from tuberculosis are dependent or Anti-bacteria controls tuberculosis.

Now calculate expected frequencies using the equation (9.2.2) as follows:

	Affected	Unaffected	Total
Anti-bacteria used:	(100 × 94)/200 = 47	(100 × 106)/200 = 53	100 = R1
Anti-bacteria not used:	(100 × 94)/200 = 47	(100 × 106)/200 = 53	100=R2
Total:	94	106	200=G

$$\chi^2_{cal} = \Sigma(O_i - E_i)^2/E_i = (26-47)^2/47 + (74-53)^2/53 + (68-47)^2/47$$
$$+ (32-53)^2/53 = 441/47 + 441/53 + 441/47 + 441/53$$
$$= 9.3829 + 8.3207 + 9.3829 + 8.3207 = 35.4072.$$

Here, $r = 2$ and $c = 2$ and d.o.f. $v = (r-1)(c-1) = 1 \times 1 = 1$ and $\alpha = 0.01$. From the table $A-2$, we have $\chi^2_{v,\alpha} = 3.84$. Here $\chi^2_{cal} > \chi^2_{v,\alpha}$. Hence we reject the null hypothesis H_0. This implies that the anti-bacteria has effect in controlling the tuberculosis disease. This state is true in 99 persons out of 100. In other words, this anti-bacteria is not controlling the tuberculosis in one person out of 100. This implies that the effect of anti-bacteria is statistically proved its effect and is significantly controlling the tuberculosis disease.

9.3. STUDENT'S t-TEST

To test the significant difference between sample mean and the population mean or significant difference between two sample means we use the most popular and very frequently used test known as 'student's t-test'. There is a small history behind this test which explains the reason for deriving its name. This is briefly explained as follows. Before the introduction of this test, people use to apply z-test only irrespective of the sample size. But a student got doubt on the application of z-test when the sample size is small i.e. $n < 30$. Basically the assumption of normality may not hold good in small sample case.

Afraid of expressing his doubt in the class, he wrote his doubt on a small paper and pushed it into his professor's room and could not reveal his name, because of fear and wrote 'A Student'. Based on the doubt, expressed by the student, Prof. W.S. Gosset introduced this distribution in early 1900 and named this distribution as 'student's t-distribution'. The test procedure which uses this distribution is known as Student's t-test. Student's t-distribution is similar to normal distribution shorter than normal distribution. As degrees of freedom increases, to more than 30 student's t-distribution will become standard normal distribution. Student's t-distribution is also a symmetrical distribution. Thus this t-distribution is to be used when the sample size is less than or equal to 30. The t-test statistic is defined as :

(*a*) For testing the significant difference between sample mean and the population mean:

$$t = \frac{(\bar{X} - \mu)}{S} x\sqrt{(n-1)} \qquad (9.3.1)$$

Where $S = \sqrt{S^2}$

$$S^2 = \frac{1}{n-1}\Sigma(X - \bar{X})^2 = \frac{1}{n-1}[\Sigma D^2 - (\Sigma D)^2/n] \qquad (9.3.2)$$

here $D = X - A$, where A = Assumed mean and $\bar{X}$ is the sample mean and n = sample size and $n - 1$ is the degrees of freedom.

It is important to note that S^2 given in (9.3.2) is an un-biased estimate of the population variance σ^2. Only difference between this formula and the formula discussed in the previous chapter is that $n - 1$ is considered in the denominator than 'n'. In small sample case, variance is to be calculated by considering $n - 1$ in the denominator. In large sample case whether we put n or $n - 1$ that does not make any difference in the answer. But it is not the case with small samples. Here we have to consider the degrees of freedom $n - 1$ in the denominator. This is because variation will be produced by those elements which are free to take any value. Thus $n - 1$, elements only produce variance in the given data.

(*b*) For testing significant difference between two sample means:

$$t_{cal} = \frac{\bar{X}_1 - \bar{X}_2}{S}\sqrt{(1/n_1 + 1/n_2)} \qquad (9.3.3)$$

Where $\bar{X}_1$ = mean of the first sample

$\bar{X}_2$ = mean of the second sample

n_1 = number of observations in the first sample

n_2 = number of observations in the second sample

and $$S = \sqrt{[\Sigma(X_1 - \bar{X}_1)^2 + \Sigma(X_2 - \bar{X}_2)^2]/(n_1 + n_2 - 2)}. \qquad (9.3.4)$$

Or $$S = \sqrt{[(n_1 - 1)\, s_1^2 + (n_2 - 1)\, s_2^2]/(n_1 + n^2 - 2)} \qquad (9.3.5)$$

Here we assume that the two samples are taken from two populations whose variances are same. In t-test we are testing the differences between two sample means, with the assumption that the two sample's are drawn from populations with same variance. This condition on variances is known as 'Homo-scedasticity' condition. Test procedure is same except the difference that the test statistic is to be considered as explained in (9.3.1) or (9.3.3). Here, $(n_1 + n_2 - 2)$ is to be considered as degrees of freedom 'v'. The $t_{v,\alpha}$ can be noted from Student's t-table given appendix $A - 3$.

Example (9.3.1): A knee-caps manufacturing company was distributing special knee-caps through a large number of retail medical shops. Before a heavy advertisement campaign in a T.V. channel, the mean sale per medical shop was 14 dozens. After the campaign a sample of 26 shops taken and the mean sales figure 14.7 dozens with standard deviation 1.6 dozens. Can you consider that this data supports the statement that after the release of the advertisement in the T.V. channel sales for knee-caps were increased?

Solution: In the given problem, sample size = n = 26, sample mean = $\bar{X}$ = 14.7 dozens and standard deviation = 1.6 dozens. Population mean μ = 14 dozens.

H_0: There is no significant difference between sample mean and the population mean. i.e. $\bar{X} = \mu$.

H_1: After the release of the advertisement, sales of knee-caps increased. i.e. $\bar{X} > \mu$.

This is a one tailed test. The test statistic is given by:

$$t_{cal} = (\bar{X} - \mu)/S.E.(\bar{X}) = (14.7 - 14)/[1.6/\sqrt{26-1}] = 0.7/0.32 = 2.18.$$

Now t-critical value at α = 0.05 at d.o.f. = v = 25 denoted by $t_{0.05,25}$ = 1.708 (for one-tailed test). (From table $A-3$)

Since, $t_{cal} > t_{0.05,25}$, we reject H_0 at 5% l.o.s and conclude that the release of advertisement in the T.V. channel has increased sales significantly.

There is significant difference in the sales of knee-caps before and after the advertisement in T.V. channel. This statement is true in 95 cases out of 100 cases.

It is statistically proved that the advertisement in T.V. channel helped in increasing the sales of knee-caps.

Example (9.3.2): The owner of a private fishing pond says that the average length of fish in his pond is not less than 15 inches. A sample of 17 fish are caught randomly, from various locations in the pond resulted mean as 10.7 inches and standard deviation 4.8 inches. Do the data support the claim of the owner? Test at 1% level of significance (l.o.s).

Solution: Here sample size = n = 17, sample mean = $\bar{X}$ = 10.7 inches and standard deviation = 4.8 inches. Population mean μ = 15 inches.

H_0: There is no significant difference between sample mean and the population mean. i.e. $\bar{X} = \mu$.

H_1: $\bar{X} < \mu$.

This is a one tailed test. The test statistic is given by:

$$t_{cal} = (\bar{X} - \mu)/\text{S.E.}(\bar{X}) = (10.7 - 15)/[4.8/\sqrt{17-1}] = 4.3/1.2 = 3.583.$$

Now t-critical value at α = 0.01 at d.o.f. = v = 16 denoted by $t_{0.01,16}$ = 2.583 (for one-tailed test). (From table $A-3$)

Since, $t_{cal} > t_{0.01,16}$ we reject H_0 at 1% l.o.s. and conclude that the population mean length is less than 15 inches. Thus the claim made by the owner of the fishing pond is false. That average length of the fish in the tank is not more than 15 inches. This statement is true 99 times out of 100 times.

Example (9.3.3): Certain pesticide is packed into bags by a machine. A random sample of 10 bags is drawn and their contents are measured and found that they weigh 50, 49, 52, 44, 45, 48, 46, 45, 49 and 45 kgs respectively. Based on this sample information, can we conclude that the packing average weight is 50 kgs?

Solution: Frame the hypothesis as follows.

H_0: μ = 50 kgs. i.e., the average packing weight is 50 kgs.

H_1: $\mu \neq 50$. This is a two-tailed test.

Now, we have to calculate the sample mean and the standard deviation from the given data. Let X is the random variable representing the weight of the bag.

X:	50	49	52	44	45	48=A	46	45	49	45	Sum
D = X = 48:	2	1	4	–4	–3	0	–2	–3	1	–3	–7
D^2:	4	1	16	16	9	0	4	9	1	9	69

$$\text{Mean} = \bar{X} = 48 + -7/10 = 47.3 \text{ kgs.}$$

An unbiased estimate the population variance is given by:

$$S^2 = \frac{1}{n-1}\Sigma(X-\bar{X})^2 = \frac{1}{n-1}[\Sigma D^2 - (\Sigma D)^2/n] \quad \text{[from (9.3.2)]}$$

$$= (1/9)\,[69 - (-7)^2/10] = (69 - 4.9)/9 = 64.1/9 = 7.1222.$$

Hence $S = 2.6687$.

$$t_{cal} = (\bar{X} - \mu)/\text{S.E.}(\bar{X}) = (47.3 - 50)/[2.6687/\sqrt{10-1}]$$

$$= -2.7/0.889 = -3.0371.$$

Now t-critical value at $\alpha = 0.05$ at d.o.f. $= v = 9$ denoted by $t_{0.05,9} = 2.262$ (from table A – 3). Since $|t_{cal}| > t_{0.05,9}$ we conclude that H_0 is rejected at 5% level of significance and conclude that 'it is not a statistically valid statement that the pesticide bag average weight is 50 kgs,. In fact it is less than 50 kgs.

Example (9.3.4): To test the effect of fertilizer on rice production 24 plots of similar size were selected and made randomly into two groups A and B consisting of 12 plots in each group. Plots in group-A is treated with-out this fertilizer and Plots in group – B is treated with this fertilizer and it is found that mean yield on untreated plots was 4.8 quintals with s.d. of 0.5 quintals. Similarly, mean yield of treated plots is 5.1 quintals and s.d. is 0.36 quintals. Based on this data can we conclude that fertilizer provide significant improvement in rice production? Test at 5% l.o.s.

Solution: First frame hypotheses as follows:

H_0 : There is no significant difference between mean yield of pady in group–A and group-B plots. i.e. $\bar{X}_1 = \bar{X}_2$.

H_1: Fertilizer hah significant effect in increasing the yield of pady.

i.e. $\bar{X}_1 < \bar{X}_2$.

This is a one-tailed test.

From the problem, it is given that $n_1 = 12$ and $n_2 = 12$, $\bar{X}_1 = 4.8$ quintals and $\bar{X}_2 = 5.1$ quintals $s_1 = 0.5$ quintals and $s_2 = 0.36$ quintals.

Substituting these values in equations (9.3.3) and (9.3.5) we have:

$$S = \sqrt{[11\times(0.5)^2 + 11\times(0.36)^2]/(12+12-2)} = \sqrt{[2.75 + 1.4256]/22}$$

$$= \sqrt{4.1756/22} = 0.43566.$$

$$t_{cal} = (4.8 - 5.1)/S\sqrt{(1/12 + 1/12)} = -0.3/0.43566\ (0.408)$$

$$= -0.3/0.17785 = -1.6868.$$

Now *t*-critical value at $\alpha = 0.05$ at d.o.f. $= v = 22$ denoted by $t_{0.05,22} = 1.717$ (from table $A - 3$).

Since $|t_{cal}| < t_{0.05,22}$ we conclude that H_0 is accepted at 5% level of significance and conclude that 'it is not a statistically valid statement that Fertilizer has increased the yield of rice'. This implies that there is no effect of fertilizer to improve the production of rice. This statement is true in 95 cases out of 100 cases.

Example (9.3.5): The following data represents the gain in weights in kgs of cows fed on two diets *X* and *Y*.

Diet X	25	32	30	32	24	14	32			
Diet Y	24	34	22	30	42	31	40	30	32	35

Test at 5% level whether the two diets differ significantly with respect to the mean increase of weight in two samples of cows?

Solution: First frame hypotheses as follows:

H_0: There is no significant difference between the two means of weights of diets *X* and *Y* in increasing mean weights of cows. i.e. $\bar{X} = \bar{Y}$

H_1: There is significant difference between the two means of weights of diets *X* and *Y* in increasing weights of cows. i.e. $\bar{X} \neq \bar{Y}$.

This is a two-tailed test.

Now we calculate the required form the given data.

X	$(x - \bar{x}) = x - 27$	$(x - \bar{x})^2$	Y	$(y - \bar{y}) = y - 32$	$(y - \bar{y})^2$
25	–2	4	24	–8	64
32	5	25	34	2	2
30	3	9	22	–10	100
32	5	25	30	–2	4
24	–3	9	42	10	100
14	–13	169	31	–1	1
32	5	25	40	8	64
			30	–2	4
			32	0	0
			35	3	9
$\Sigma x = 189$	0	$\Sigma(x - \bar{x})^2 = 266$	$\Sigma y = 320$	0	$\Sigma(y - \bar{y})^2 = 350$

$$\bar{X} = 189/7 = 27 \text{ kgs; Sample variance of } x = s_x^2 = \frac{1}{n_1 - 1}\Sigma(x - \bar{x})^2$$

$$= 266/6 = 44.33 \text{ kgs.}$$

$$\bar{Y} = 320/10 = 32 \text{ kgs; Sample variance of } y = s_y^2 - \frac{1}{n_2 - 1}\Sigma(y - \bar{y})^2$$

$$= 350/9 = 38.8889 \text{ kgs.}$$

Substituting these values in (9.33) we have:

$$S = \sqrt{[(n_1 - 1)\, s_1^2 + (n_2 - 1)\, s_2^2]/(n_1 + n_2 - 2)}$$

$= \sqrt{[(6 \times 44.33 + 9 \times 38.8889)]/15} = \sqrt{(265.98 + 350.0001)/15 = 41.06534}$

$= 6.4082$

$$\text{S.E.}(\bar{x} - \bar{y}) = Sx\sqrt{1/n_1 + 1/n_2} = 41.06534 \times \sqrt{(1/7 + 1/10)}$$

$$= \sqrt{41.06534 \times 0.1429 + 0.1} = 6.4082 \times 0.49285 = 3.1582$$

$$t_{cal} = (\bar{x} - \bar{y})/\text{S.E.}(\bar{x} - \bar{y}) = (27 - 32)/3.1582 = -5/3.1582 = -1.5832$$

Now t-critical value at $\alpha = 0.05$ at d.o.f. $= v = 15$ denoted by $t_{0.05,15} = 2.131$ (from table $A - 3$).

Since $|t_{cal}| < t_{0.05,15}$ we conclude that H_0 is accepted at 5% level of significance and conclude that both diets X and Y are equally efficient in increasing weights of cows.

9.4. PAIRED t-TEST

In the student's t-test sample sizes n_1 and n_2 need not be equal. Even if the experimenter starts the experiment with equal sample sizes, due to natural calamities like fire accidents or accidents or floods or death of some experimental units, we may not get the data from all the experimental units. Hence, is left with unequal number of units in the samples. Hence, we have developed student's t-test without putting any restriction on sample sizes. They may be equal or may not be equal. In many clinical experiments, we have to measure the characteristics, at two different time points from each experimental units.

Thus we obtain observations in pairs. In this situation, equal number of observations under each set. In this situation we use a special test called 'Paired t-test' to test the significant difference between the means of two sets of observations which are naturally in pairs and hence this test is called paired t-test, whose procedure is explained as follows:

Let $(x_1, y_1), (x_2, y_2), ..., (x_n, y_n)$ are n pairs of observations measured from n subjects at two different time points about a variable say, B.P. or Sugar levels, or height or temperature and so on.

Step – 1: Frame $H_0 = \mu_1 = \mu_2$ and $H_1 = \mu_1 \neq \mu_2$.

Step – 2: Calculate $D_i = (x_i - y_i), i = 1, 2, ..., n$.

Step – 3: Calculate $\bar{D} = \Sigma D_i/n$ and variance $S^2 = \frac{1}{n-1}[\Sigma D^2 - (\Sigma D)^2/n]$

Step – 4: Calculate S.E. $(\bar{D}) = S/\sqrt{n}$

Step – 5: Calculate test statistic $t_{cal} = \bar{D}/\text{S.E.}(\bar{D})$. (9.4.1)

Step – 6: Determine t critical value at α% level of significance at $v = n - 1$ degrees of freedom from table $A - 3$.

Step – 7: If $t_{cal} \leq t_{v,\alpha}$ we accept H_0 at α% l.o.s. otherwise we reject H_0 and accept H_1 at α% l.o.s.

Example (9.4.1): A drug was administered on 12 patients to reduce the Blood Pressure (systolic) and measured B.P. before and after 30 minutes after using the drug. Differences between these two readings are recorded as : 4, –3, 6, 3, –2, 6, 4, –4, 0, 2, 0 and 2 based on this information can we conclude that the drug has effect in reducing B.P. systolic.

Solution: Frame hypotheses as follows:

H_0: There is no significant difference between the means of B.P. systolic before and after using the drug. i.e. $\bar{D} = 0$.

H_1: There is significant reduction in B.P. systolic after using the medicine. i.e. $\bar{D} > 0$.

This is a one-tailed test. Now calculate the required quantities from the given data:

D:	4	–3	6	3	–2	6	4	–4	0	2	0	4
D^2:	16	9	36	9	4	36	16	16	0	4	0	4

We know that :

$\sum D = 20$ and $\sum D^2 = 150$ thus $\bar{D}$ 20/12 = 1.6667 and

$$S^2 = \frac{1}{n-1}[\Sigma D^2 - (\Sigma D)^2/n] = (1/11)[150 - (20)^2/12]$$

$$= 1/11[150 - 400/12]\ 1/11[150 - 33.3333] = 116.6667/11 = 10.6061.$$

Calculate S.E. $(\bar{D}) = S/\sqrt{n} = \sqrt{10.6061/12} = 0.94012.$

Calculate test statistic $t_{cal} = \bar{D}/\text{S.E.}(\bar{D}) = 1.6667/0.94012 = 1.7728.$

Determine t critical value at 5% level of significance at $v = 11$ is $t_{0.05,11} = 1.796$ (from table $A - 3$).

Since $t_{cal} \le t_{v,\alpha}$ we accept H_0 at 5% l.o.s and conclude that the drug has no significant effect in reducing the B.P. systolic. That is the effect of drug in reducing B.P. systolic is not having statistically valid effect or significant effect.

Example (9.4.2): Two types of yoga exercises is given to 20 housewives to study the effect on their sleep. These 20 subjects are randomly divided into two groups A and B. Additional hours of sleep gained by practicing this yoga exercise-I on group –A and Exercise-II on group-B, is recorded as follows:

Subjects:	1	2	3	4	5	6	7	8	9	10
Group – A:	2.0	0	–1.2	0.7	–1.6	3.4	3.7	0.8	–0.2	–0.1
Group – B:	0.8	1.1	0.1	1.9	1.6	–0.1	5.5	3.6	4.4	4.6

Test at 5% l.o.s., whether the two yoga methods have, same effect on sleep of housewives? Apply (*a*) Paired *t*-test and (*b*) Student's *t*-test procedures and compare your results.

Solution: (*a*) Paired t-test: First calculate differences $D = (x - y)$, where x = Group-A readings and y = Group-B readings. Frame hypotheses as follows:

H_0: There is no significant difference between the means of sleep after practicing yoga exercises I and II. i.e. $\bar{D} = 0$.

H_1: There is significant difference between yoga exercise I and II on the sleep of housewives. i.e. $\bar{D} \neq 0$. This is a two-tailed test.

Now calculate the required quantities from the given data:

Subject No.	Group-A = (x)	Group-B = (y)	D = (x – y)	$D^2 = (x - y)^2$
1	2.0	0.8	1.2	1.44
2	0	1.1	–1.1	1.21
3	–1.2	0.1	–1.3	1.69
4	0.7	0.9	–1.2	1.44
5	–1.6	1.6	–3.2	10.24
6	3.4	–0.1	3.5	12.25
7	3.7	5.5	–1.8	3.24
8	0.8	3.6	–2.8	7.84
9	–0.2	4.4	–4.6	21.16
10	–0.1	4.6	–4.7	22.09
Total			–16	82.6

Hence,

$$\bar{D} = -16/10 = -1.6 \quad \text{and}$$

$$S^2 = \frac{1}{n-1}[\Sigma D^2 - (\Sigma D)^2/n] = (1/9)[82.6 - (-16)^2/10] = 1/9[82.6 - 25.6]$$

$$= 57/9 = 6.3333.$$

Calculate S.E. $(\bar{D}) = S/\sqrt{n} = \sqrt{6.3333/10 = 0.7958}.$

Calculate test statistic $t_{cal} = \bar{D}/\text{ S.E.}(\bar{D}) = -1.6/0.7958 = 2.011.$

Determine t critical value at 5% level of significance at $v = 9$ is $t_{0.05,11} = 2.262$ (from table $A - 3$).

Since $t_{cal} > t_{v,\alpha}$ we reject H_0 at 5% l.o.s and conclude that there exists.

Significant differences between yoga exercises I and II on housewives.

Since the value of is negative, Method-II is having more effect than method-I. This statement is true in 95 times out of 100 times.

(b) Student's t-test.

Let x = Group A readings and y = Group-B readings. Frame hypotheses as follows:

H_0: There is no significant difference between the means of sleep after practicing yoga exercises I and II. i.e. $\bar{x} = \bar{y}$.

H_1 : There is significant difference between Yoga exercise I and II on the sleep of housewives. i.e. $\bar{x} \neq \bar{y}$.

This is a two-tailed test. Now calculate the required quantities from the given data:

Group-A = (x)	Group-B = (y)	x^2	y^2
2.0	0.8	4.0	0.64
0	1.1	0	1.21
–1.2	0.1	1.44	0.01
0.7	1.9	0.79	3.61
–1.6	1.6	2.56	2.56
3.4	–0.1	11.56	0.01
3.7	5.5	13.69	30.25
0.8	3.6	0.64	0.64
–0.2	4.4	0.04	19.36
–0.1	4.6	0.01	21.16
Sum = 7.5	23.5	34.73	79.45

$\bar{x} = 7.5/10 = 0.75$ and $S_x^2 = (1/9)\,[34.73 - (7.5)^2/10]$

$= 1/9[34.73 - 5.625] = 29.105/9 = 3.23$ [putting $D = x$ in (9.3.2)]

$\bar{y} = 23.5/10 = 2.35$ and $S_y^2 = (1/9)\,[79.45 - (23.5)^2/10]$

$= 1/9[79.45 - 55.225] = 24.225/9 = 2.6916.$

$$S = \sqrt{[(n_1-1)\,s_1^2 + (n_2-1)\,s_2^2]/(n_1+n^2-2)}$$

$$= \sqrt{[9\times 3.23 + 9\times 2.6916]/18} = \sqrt{(29.07+24.2244)/18} = \sqrt{2.9608}$$

$$= 1.7206.$$

$$\text{S.E.}\,(\bar{x}-\bar{y}) = Sx\sqrt{1/n_1+1/n_2} = 1.7206x\sqrt{(1/10+1/10)}$$

$$= 1.7206 \times \sqrt{0.2} = 1.7206 \times 0.4472 = 0.76945$$

$$t_{cal} = (\bar{x}-\bar{y})/\text{S.E.}\,(\bar{x}-\bar{y}) = (0.75-2.35)/0.76945 = -1.6/0.7645$$

$$= 2.0929 = 2.01 \text{ (approx.)}$$

Note that we get same value as in paired *t*-test.

Determine *t* critical value at 5% level of significance at $v = 18$ is $t_{0.05,18} = 1.734$ (from table *A* – 3).

Since $t_{cal} > t_{v,\alpha}$ we reject H_0 at 5% l.o.s and conclude that there exists significant differences between yoga exercises I and II on housewives. Since, $\bar{x} < \bar{y}$, it is statistically proved that yoga exercise-I is more effective than exercise-I.

9.5. TESTS OF SAMPLE CORRELATION COEFFICIENTS

Let ρ be the linear correlation coefficient of bi-variate normal population and *r* be the correlation coefficient of a sample of size '*n*' observations (x_i, y_i), $I = 1, 2, .,.,., n$. Then '*r*' be the unbiased estimator of ρ, i.e. $E(r) = \rho$. There are three test procedures available in literature for testing the significance of sample correlation coefficient '*r*', which are explained as follows:

(*a*) Student's t-test for testing of significance of sample correlation coefficient.

When the sample size '*n*' is small, we can use the student's t-test explained in the last section, for testing the significance of sample correlation coefficient. The procedure is explained as follows:

Step – 1: Frame the null hypothesis H_0 : $\rho = 0$, and the alternative hypothesis $H_1 : \rho \neq 0$.

Step – 2: For small samples, standard error of '*r*' denoted by S.E.(*r*) is given by S.E. $(r) = \sqrt{(1-r^2)/(n-2)}$, where *n* is the sample size.

Step – 3: The test statistic '*t*' is given by :

$$t_{cal} = r/\text{S.E. }(r) = r \times \sqrt{(n-2)/(1-r^2)}. \quad (9.5.1)$$

Degrees of freedom for this test is denoted by $v = n - 2$.

Step – 4: The t_{tab} at $(n - 2)$ d.o.f. at α% l.o.s. is denoted by $t_{v,\alpha}$ can be noted from Student's *t*-tables given Appendix table *A* – 3.

Step – 5: If $|t_{cal}| \leq t_{v,\alpha}$, we accept H_0 otherwise we reject H_0.

Example (9.5.1) : In an agricultural study, the correlation between the temperature of the room and the sericulture cocoons formation time of a particular type of sericulture worms is found to be – 0.672 and the sample size if 18. Test whether the observed correlation coefficient is significant or not?

Solution: Frame hypothesis as follows:

Null hypothesis H_0 : $r = 0$. i.e., observed correlation coefficient is insignificant.

Alternative hypothesis H_1 : $r \neq 0$.

This is a two-tailed test. Here d.o.f. $v = 16$.

Test statistic $t_{cal} = r \times \sqrt{(n-2)} / \sqrt{(1-r^2)}$

$= -0.672 \times \sqrt{(18-2)/[1-(-0.672)^2]} = -0.672 \times 4/0.54842$

$= -4.9013.$

From table *A* – 3 (appendix), $t_{16,0.05} = 2.878$. Here, $v = 16$ and $\alpha = 1\%$.

Since $|t_{cal}| > t_{v,\alpha}$, we reject H_0 and conclude that the observed correlation coefficient between room temperature and cocoons formation time by the sericulture worms is significant. This correlation can be considered for prediction or estimation or forecasting of dependent and independent variables as discussed in chapter VII.

Example (9.5.2): A study of ages of 11 pairs of husbands and their wives show that the correlation coefficient is 0.638. Test the significance of *r* at 1% level of significance.

Solution: Frame hypothesis as follows:

Null hypothesis $H_0 : r = 0$. i.e., observed correlation coefficient is insignificant.

Alternative hypothesis H_1 : $r \neq 0$.

This is a two tailed test. Here d.o.f. $v = 16$.

Test statistic $t_{cal} = r \times \sqrt{(n-2)} / \sqrt{(1-r^2)} = 0.638 \times \sqrt{11 - 2/(1 - 0.6832)}$

$= 0.683 \times 3/0.53351 = 3.8406.$

From table *A* – 3 (appendix) $t_{9,0.01} = 3.25$. Here, $v = 9$ and $\alpha = 1\%$.

Since $|t_{cal}| > t_{v,\alpha}$, we reject H_0 and conclude that the observed correlation coefficient between ages of husbands and wives is significant. This correlation can be considered for prediction or estimation or forecasting of dependent and independent variables as discussed in chapter 7.

We can also use the same formula given in (9.5.1) for determining the sample size 'n' which is explained in the following example.

Example (9.5.3): In a study of examining the relationship between intake of food and calories of energy gained, how many pairs of observations must be included in a sample, so that the observed correlation coefficient value 0.42 shall have a calculated value of t greater than 2.72?

Solution: Here we want to calculate the calculated value of t must be more than 2.72. Hence, the test statistic t, i.e.

$$t_{\text{cal}} = r \times \sqrt{(n-2)} / \sqrt{(1-r^2)} > 2.72 \text{ i.e. } 0.42 \times \sqrt{n-2} / \sqrt{1-(2.42)^2} > 2.72$$

or $\quad (0.42/0.908) \times \sqrt{(n-2)} > 2.72$ or $\sqrt{(n-2)} > (2.72 \times 0.908)/0.48 \times 2.272$

or $\quad \sqrt{(n-2)} > 5.145$ or $n - 2 > (5.145)^2$ or $n - 2 > 26.474$ or $n > 28.474$

or $\quad n > 28$ (approx) i.e. the sample size n should the more than or equal to 29 pairs of observations.

(b) Fisher's Z test for significance of sample correlation coefficient

Student's t-test discussed above is to be used when the sample size $n < 30$. i.e., used in small sample case only. When, sample size is large we should not use student's t-statistic given in (9.5.1). Fisher gave a method of testing the significance of the coefficient of correlation for small or large samples. In this method the sample correlation r is transformed into Z. This test is useful when n is small of large i.e., less than or equal to 30 or more than 30. Fisher's Z–transformation is given by:

$$Z = \tfrac{1}{2} \log_e [(1+r)/(1-r)] \qquad (9.5.2)$$

Fisher has shown that the sampling distribution of Z is approximately normal with mean ξ and standard error $1/\sqrt{n} - 3$. Thus $(Z - \xi)\sqrt{(n-3)} \sim N(0, 1)$ i.e. standard normal distribution. Thus

S.E. $(Z) = 1/\sqrt{(n-3)}$. The test statistic for Fisher's Z-test is given by:

$Z = |Z - \xi|/\text{S.E.}(Z)$ follows Standard Normal Distribution.

Note: The values of Z and ξ are defined using the constant 'e'. i.e., natural logarithms, we can convert them to ordinary logarithms i.e., to the base 10 as follows: [we know that $\log_{10} A = \log_e A \times 2.3026$]

$$Z = Z = \tfrac{1}{2} \log_e [(1+r)/(1-r)] = Z = \tfrac{1}{2} \log_{10} [(1+r)/(1-r)] \times \log_e 10$$

Or $\quad Z = \tfrac{1}{2} (2.3026) \times \log_{10} [(1+r)/(1-r)] = 1.1513 \log_{10} [(1+r)/(1-r)]$. (9.5.3)

In calculating problems, we can use ordinary logarithms i.e., $\log_{10}$ instead of Natural logarithms i.e., $\log_e$.

Thus we have $\qquad Z = 1.1513 \log_{10} [(1+r)/(1-r)]$. $\qquad$ (9.5.4)

Application Fisher's Z-test is given in (9.5.4) is used with the following example.

Example (9.5.4): If the correlation of 10 pairs of observations (X, Y) is 0.96, test the hypothesis that the population correlation coefficient is 0.99.

Solution: Null hypothesis: H_0: $\rho = 0.99$.

Alternative hypothesis: H_1: $\rho \neq 0.99$.

This is a two tailed test. Now consider $Z = 1.1513 \log_{10} [(1 + r)/(1 - r)]$
$= 1.1513 \log_{10} [(1 + 0.96)/(1 - 0.96)] = 1.1513 \log_{10} 49 = 1.1513 \times 1.6902$
$= 1.9459$ (using log tables)
Similarly, $\xi = 1.1513 \log_{10} [(1 + r)/(1 - r)]$
$= 1.1513 \log_{10} [(1 + 0.99)/(1 - 0.99)] = 1.1513 \log_{10} 199 = 1.1513 \times 2.2986$
$= 2.6464$. (using log tables)
S.E. (Z) $= 1/\sqrt{n} - 3 = 1/\sqrt{7}$. The test statistic is $Z_{cal} = |Z - \xi|/\text{S.E. }(Z)$
$= |1.9459 - 2.6464| \times \sqrt{7} = 1.8563$.
Table value of Z_α at $\alpha = 5\%$ level of significance = 1.96. [table (8.2.1)]

Since $Z_{cal} < Z_\alpha$, we accept H_0 at 5% l.o.s. and conclude that the population correlation coefficient can be considered as 0.99.

9.6. TESTS FOR SAMPLE VARIANCES

In order to test the significant difference between two sample variances, s_1^2 and s_2^2 , we use F-test. F-test is also known as variance ratio test because, the test statistic F is defined as the ratio of two independent sample variances. That is:

$$F_{cal} = \sigma_1^2/\sigma_2^2 \text{ if } \sigma_1^2 > \sigma_2^2 \qquad (9.6.1).$$

With $(n_1 - 1)$ d.o.f. for numerator and $(n_2 - 1)$ d.o.f. for denominator.

$$F_{cal} = \sigma_2^2/\sigma_1^2 \text{ if } \sigma_1^2 < \sigma_2^2 \qquad (9.6.2)$$

With $(n_2 - 1)$ d.o.f. for numerator and $(n_1 - 1)$ d.o.f. for denominator.

Where, $\sigma_1^2 = n_1 s_1^2/n_1 - 1$ and $\sigma_2^2 = n_2 s_2^2/n_2 - 1$, which are unbiased estimates of population variances.

F-test was first originated by Prof. R.A. Fisher and hence it is also known as Fisher's F–test.

9.6.1. Assumptions of F–test

F–test is mainly based on the following three assumptions. Namely:

1. **Normality assumption:** The values in each group should be normally distributed.
2. **Independence assumption:** The variation of each value around its own group mean, i.e., error should be independent of each value and
3. **Homogeneity assumption:** The variances within each group should be equal for all groups, i.e., $\sigma_1^2 = \sigma_2^2 = .,.,., = \sigma_n^2$. If however, the sample sizes are large enough, we do not require normality assumption because, as n is large (> 30), we use the Z-distribution which itself is a Normal distribution.

9.6.2. Test Procedure for F-test

The following procedure is to be adopted for testing two independent sample variances.

Step – 1: Frame the null hypothesis $H_0 : \sigma_1^2 = \sigma_2^2$ and the alternative hypothesis

$H_1 : \sigma_1^2 \neq \sigma_2^2$. (for two-tailed test)

$H_1 : \sigma_1^2 < \sigma_2^2$ or $\sigma_1^2 > \sigma_2^2$ (for one-tailed test)

Step – 2: Calculate:

$$s_1^2 = \frac{1}{n_1}\Sigma(X_1 - \bar{X}_1)^2 \quad (9.6.3)$$

and

$$s_2^2 = \frac{1}{n_2}\Sigma(X_2 - \bar{X}_2)^2 \quad (9.6.4)$$

from the given data.

Step – 3: The test statistic 'F' is given by :

$$F_{cal} = \sigma_1^2/\sigma_2^2 \text{ if } \sigma_1^2 > \sigma_2^2. \quad (9.6.5)$$

With $(n_1 - 1)$ d.o.f. for numerator and $(n_2 - 1)$ d.o.f. for denominator.

$$F_{cal} = \sigma_2^2/\sigma_1^2 \text{ if } \sigma_1^2 < \sigma_2^2. \quad (9.6.6)$$

With $(n_2 - 1)$ d.o.f. for numerator and $(n_1 - 1)$ d.o.f. for denominator.

Where, $\sigma_1^2 = n_1 s_1^2/n_1 - 1$ and $\sigma_2^2 = n_2 s_2^2/n^2 - 1$, which are unbiased estimates of population variances.

Step – 4: The F_{tab} at $(n - 2)$ d.o.f. at α% l.o.s. is denoted by $F_{v,\alpha}$ can be noted from F - tables given appendix Table A – 4. While noting table values of F, numerator d.o.f is to be read horizontally and denominator d.o.f is to be read vertically in the table A – 4.

Step – 5. If $|F_{cal}| \leq Ft_{v,\alpha}$, we accept H_0 otherwise we reject H_0.

Example (9.6.1): Two independent random samples of fish collected from different ponds of sizes 9 and 13 have the weights with standard deviation 12.1 grams and 11.8 grams. Test whether there exists any significant difference between the two sample standard deviations at 5% level of significance?

Solution: From the data it is given that $n_1 = 9$ and $s_1 = 12.1$ grams

$n_2 = 13$ and $s_2 = 11.8$ grams.

Set hypotheses as follows.

$H_0 : \sigma_1^2 = \sigma_2^2$, and the alternative hypothesis $H_1 : \sigma_1^2 \neq \sigma_2^2$. This is a two tailed test. Un-biased estimates of population variances are calculated as follows:

$$\sigma_1^2 = n_1 s_1^2/n_1 - 1 = 9(12.1)^2/8 = 164.71125$$

and

$$\sigma_2^2 = n_2 s_2^2/n_2 - 1 = 13(11.8)^2/12 = 150.84333$$

The test statistic is given by:

$$F_{cal} = \sigma_1^2/\sigma_2^2 = 164.71125/150.84333$$
$$= 1.0993. \text{ (since } \sigma_1^2 > \sigma_2^2)$$

Here numerator d.o.f is 8 and denominator d.o.f. is 12.

From F-table, A – 4 (appendix) we have $\alpha = 5$% l.o.s., $F_\alpha = 2.9$.

Since $F_{cal} < F_{\alpha}$, we conclude that the null hypothesis H_0 is accepted. This implies that there is no significant difference between the standard deviations of both the sample fish. Thus both ponds collected fish have insignificant variations in weights because there exists insignificant difference between standard deviations. Thus both ponds fish are statistically having similar variance or both pond fish are similar nature of variation.

Example (9.6.2): Two groups of scientists *A* and *B* does similar experiment and the duration to complete the experiment measured in minutes is recorded as follows:

Group-A	29	28	26	35	30	44	46			
Group-B	23	25	41	55	54	41	39	54	54	51

Test whether scientist in both the groups are considered as having statistically, same efficiency in completing the experiment or not?

Solution: To determine whether there exists any significant difference between two groups of scientists, we have to test with respect to the (*a*) means and (*b*) variances of duration of completion for the completion of the experiment. Hence, we have to apply (*a*) Student's t-teat for testing the significant difference between means of duration for the completing the experiment and (*b*) F-test for testing the significant difference between the variances of duration for the completion of the experiment. Thus we have to calculate means and variances for the given data.

Group-A=X	Group-B=Y	x = X – 34	y = Y – 44	x^2	y^2
29	23	–5	–21	25	441
28	25	–6	–19	36	361
26	41	–8	–3	64	9
35	55	1	11	1	121
30	54	–4	10	16	100
44	41	10	–3	100	9
46	39	12	–5	144	25
	54		10		100
	57		13		169
	51		7		49
Total = 238	440	0	0	386	1384

Mean of x = 238/7 = 34 minutes and

mean of y = 440/10 = 44 minutes,

$$\text{Var}(X) = \sigma_1^2 = (n_1\, s_1^2)/n_1 - 1 = [\Sigma(X_1 - \bar{X}_1)^2]/n_1 - 1 = 386/6$$

$$= 64.3333 \text{ minutes and}$$

$$\text{Var}(Y) = \sigma_2^2 = (n_2\, s_2^2)/n_2 - 1 = [\Sigma(X_2 - \bar{X}_2)^2]/n_2 - 1 = 1384/9$$

$$= 153.7778 \text{ minutes.}$$

(a) Student's t-test.

H_0: There is no significant difference between two means i.e. $\bar{X}_1 = \bar{X}_2$.

H_1: There is significant difference between two means i.e. $\bar{X}_1 \neq \bar{X}_2$. This is a two-tailed test.

$$S = \sqrt{[(n_1 - 1)s_1^2 + (n_2 - 1)s_2^2]/(n_1 + n_2 - 2)} = \sqrt{(386 + 1384)/15}$$

$$= \sqrt{1770/15} = \sqrt{118} = 10.8628$$

The test statistic

$$t_{cal} = (\bar{X}_1 = \bar{X}_2)/Sx\sqrt{(1/n_1 + 1/n_2)}$$

$$= (34 - 44)/10.8628\sqrt{(1/7 + 1/10)} = -10/10.8628/10.8628\ (0.4928)$$

$$= -10/5.3532 = -1.86.$$

Here degrees of freedom $v = n_1 + n_2 - 2 = 7 + 10 - 2 = 15$ and $\alpha = 0.05$, i.e. $t_{\alpha,v} = t_{0.05,15} = 2.131$. Here $|t_{cal}| < t_{0.05,15}$. Hence, we accept H_0 at 5% l.o.s., and conclude that there is no significant difference between mean duration for completion of the experiments in group-A and Group-B scientists.

(b) Test for variances: Here the hypotheses are:

H_0: There is no significant difference between two variances i.e. $\sigma_1^2 = \sigma_2^2$

H_1: There is significant difference between two variances i.e. $\sigma_1^2 \neq \sigma_2^2$. This is a two-tailed test.

Here, $s_2^2 > s_1^2$ hence, we have to use the formula given in equation (9.6.6), i.e. we should always consider larger variance in the numerator and smaller variance in the denominator. So that the calculated value of $F > 1$ always.

$$F_{cal} = \sigma_2^2/\sigma_1^2 = 153.7778/64.3333 = 2.3903.$$

F_{tab} at numerator d.o.f. $v_1 = 9$ and and denominator d.o.f. $v_2 = 6$, at $\alpha = 0.05$ is given as 4.10. (from F-table $A - 4$ in appendix).

Thus $F_{cal} < F_{tab}$ hence we accept H_0 at 5% l.o.s., and conclude that the two groups of scientists do not differ significantly with respect to variances of duration for completing the experiment.

Finally, we found that there is no significant difference between two groups of scientists with respect to means and variances in completing their respective experiments. Hence we conclude that there is no statistical significant difference between group-A and group-B scientists. We have statistically proved that both groups of scientists are equally efficient in completing the experiment.

Example (9.6.3): Six guinea pigs injected with 0.5 mg of a medication took an average 15.4 seconds to fall asleep with an unbiased standard deviation 2.2 seconds while six other guinea pigs injected with 1.5 mg of the medication took an average 11.2 seconds; to fall asleep with an unbiased standard deviation of 3.8 seconds. (*a*) Test whether there is any significant difference between the averages of time to fall asleep by guinea pigs? (*b*) Test whether there is any significant difference between the variances of time to fall asleep by guinea pigs?

Solution:

(a) Testing Means

H_0: There is no significant difference between two means i.e. $\bar{X}_1 = \bar{X}_2$.

H_1: There is significant difference between two means i.e. $\bar{X}_1 \neq \bar{X}_2$. This is a two-tailed test.

$$S = \sqrt{[(n_1 - 1)\, s_1^2 + (n_2 - 1)\, s_2^2]/(n_1 + n_2 - 2)}$$

$$= \sqrt{[5(2.2)^2 + 5(3.8)^2]/10}$$

$$= \sqrt{(24.2 + 72.2)/10} = \sqrt{96.4/10} = \sqrt{9.64 = 3.1048}$$

The test statistic $\quad t_{cal} = (\bar{X}_1 - \bar{X}_2)/Sx\sqrt{(1/n_1 + 1/n_2)}$

$= (15.4 - 11.2)/3.1048\sqrt{(1/6 + 1/6)} = 4.2/3.1048(0.5774) = 4.2/1.7926 = 2.34297$

Here degrees of freedom $v = n_1 + n_2 - 2 = 6 + 6 - 2 = 10$ and $\alpha = 0.05$.

$t_{\alpha,v} = t_{0.05,10} = 2.228$. Here $|t_{cal}| > t_{0.05,15}$. Hence, we reject H_0 at 5% l.o.s., and conclude that there is significant difference between mean duration to fall asleep by guinea pigs.

(b) Testing variances

H_0: There is no significant difference between two variances i.e. $\hat{\sigma}_1^2 = \sigma_2^2$

H_1: There is significant difference between two variances i.e. $\sigma_1^2 \neq \sigma_2^2$. This is a two-tailed test. Here $s_1^2 = (2.2)^2 = 4.84$ and $s_2^2 = (3.8)^2 = 14.44$.

Here, $s_2^2 > s_1^2$ hence, we have to use the formula given in equation (9.6.6), i.e. we should always consider larger variance in the numerator and smaller variance in the denominator. So that the calculated value of $F > 1$ always.

$$F_{cal} = \sigma_2^2/\sigma_1^2 = 14.44/4.84 = 2.9835.$$

F_{tab} at numerator d.o.f. $v_1 = 5$ and and denominator d.o.f. $v_2 = 5$, at $\alpha = 0.05$ is given as 5.05. (from F–table $A - 4$ in appendix).

Thus $F_{cal} < F_{tab,}$ hence we accept H_0 at 5% l.o.s., and conclude that the medication has no significant effect on the variances of duration to fall asleep by guinea pigs.

Finally, there is significant difference between dosage differences of medication with respect to means but no significant difference found with respect to variances of duration to fall asleep by guinea pigs. As dosage of medication increases, average duration of times to fall asleep differ significantly. Thus the increased dosage effect to increase duration of asleep is statistically proved at 5% l.o.s.

Example (9.6.4): The chemical presented in medicines produced by two pharmaceutical companies were tested in the laboratory and found the following results:

Pharmaceutical Companies	Sample sizes	Means	Sum squares of deviations from the mean
Alpha	10	15mg	90 mg
Beta	12	12 mg	328 mg

Test whether there exists any statistically significant difference between both company medicines with respect to the content of the chemical.

Solution: We have to test these with respect to both mean and variances by using Student's *t*-test and *f*-test respectively.

(a) Testing means

H_0: There is no significant difference between two means i.e. $\bar{X}_1 = \bar{X}_2$.

H_1: There is significant difference between two means i.e. $\bar{X}_1 \neq \bar{X}_2$. This is a two-tailed test.

$\text{Var}(X) = \sigma_1^2 = (n_1 s_1^2)/n_1 - 1 = [\Sigma(X_1 - \bar{X}_1)^2]/n_1 - 1 = 90/9 = 10 \text{ mg}.$

and

$\text{Var}(Y) = \sigma_2^2 = (n_2 s_2^2)/n_2 - 1 = [\Sigma(X_2 - \bar{X}_2)^2]/n_2 - 1 = 328/11 = 29.812 \text{ mg}.$

$S = \sqrt{[(n_1 - 1)\, s_1^2 + (n_2 - 1)\, s_2^2]/(n_1 + n_2 - 2)} = \sqrt{[90 + 328]/20} = 4.5717.$

The test statistic

$$t_{\text{cal}} = (\bar{X}_1 = \bar{X}_2)/Sx\sqrt{(1/n_2 + 1/n_2)}$$
$$= (15 - 12)/4.5717\sqrt{(1/10 + 1/12)}$$
$$= 3/4.5717(0.4282) = 3/1.9575 = 1.5356.$$

Here degrees of freedom $v = n_1 + n_2 - 2 = 10 + 12 - 2 = 20$ and $\alpha = 0.05$. i.e. $t_{\alpha,v} = t_{0.05,20} = 2.086$. Here $|t_{\text{cal}}| < t_{0.05,15}$. Hence, we accept H_0 at 5% l.o.s., and conclude that there is no significant difference between mean chemical content produced by both pharmaceutical companies.

(b) Testing variances

H_0: There is no significant difference between two variances i.e. $\sigma_1^2 = \sigma_2^2$

H_1: There is significant difference between two variances i.e. $\sigma_1^2 \neq \sigma_2^2$. This is a two-tailed test.

Here, ${s_2}^2 > {s_1}^2$ hence, we have to use the formula given in equation (9.6.6), i.e., we should always consider larger variance in the numerator and smaller variance in the denominator. So that the calculated value of $F > 1$ always.

$$F_{\text{cal}} = \sigma_2^2/\sigma_1^2 = 29.812/10 = 2.9812$$

F_{tab} at numerator d.o.f. $v_1 = 11$ and denominator d.o.f. $v_2 = 9$, at $\alpha = 0.05$ is given as 3.105. (from *F*-table $A - 4$ in appendix).

Note: In the table $A - 4$ for numerator degrees of freedom there is no corresponding column for $v_1 = 11$ d.o.f. To calculate this, we have to calculate the average of column 10 figure and column 12 figure for corresponding denominator degrees of freedom. Thus for $v_2 = 9$, denominator degrees of freedom, 3.14 is for numerator d.o.f. 10 and 3.07 for 12 d.o.f. Thus for 11 we have to calculate (3.14 + 3.07)/2 = 3.105, which is the table value for numerator d.o.f. $v_1 = 11$ and denominator d.o.f. $v_2 = 9$.

Thus $F_{\text{cal}} < F_{\text{tab}}$, hence we accept H_0 at 5% l.o.s., and conclude that the content of chemical in the medicines produced by both pharmaceutical companies are same. There is no statistically valid or significant difference both medicines.

F-test is most popularly used small sample test to test the significant difference between two independent sample variances. This test is also used extensively in Analysis of Variance (ANOVA), which is discussed in detail in the last chapter X.

REVIEW QUESTIONS AND PROBLEMS

A. Objective Questions

1. Student's t-test is used to test --------------------.

   (*a*) proportions (*b*) means
   (*c*) variances (*d*) percentages.

2. Chi-square test is used to test independence of -------------------.

   (*a*) means (*b*) variances
   (*c*) percentages (*d*) attributes.

3. Variance ratio test is also known as -----------------.

   (*a*) F – test (*b*) X^2 – test
   (*c*) Z – test (*d*) t – test.

4. *F*-test is used to test the significant difference between -----------.

   (*a*) proportions (*b*) means
   (*c*) variances (*d*) percentages.

5. Degrees of freedom for student's *t*-test when $n = 15$ and $n = 12$ are -------.

   (*a*) 27 (*b*) 26
   (*c*) 25 (*d*) 24.

6. Degrees of freedom for chi-square test with 3 rows and 5 columns are ----------.

   (*a*) 8 (*b*) 15
   (*c*) 10 (*d*) 12.

7. Degrees of freedom for t-test for testing correlation coefficient with 18 pairs of observations are -----------.

   (*a*) 36 (*b*) 35
   (*c*) 15 (*d*) 16

8. To test the significance of observed sample correlation coefficient we use --------------- test.

   (*a*) F – test (*b*) X^2 – test
   (*c*) Z – test (*d*) t – test.

9. *F*–test was first originated by Prof. --------------------.

   (*a*) S.P. Gupta (*b*) W.S. Gosset
   (*c*) R.A. Fisher (*d*) Spearman

10. We reject the null hypothesis if ---------------------.

    (*a*) $Z_{cal} < Z_{tab}$ (*b*) $F_{cal} < F_{tab}$
    (*c*) $t_{cal} > t_{tab}$ (*d*) $S_1^2 > S_2^2$.

B. Short Answer Questions

1. Write short note on small sample tests.
2. Explain the test procedure of chi-square test.
3. Explain student's t-test procedure.
4. Explain the test procedure of testing sample correlation coefficient.
5. What is *F*-test? Explain with an example.
6. Why *F*-test is called variance ratio test? Explain.
7. Explain the concept of degrees of freedom with suitable examples.
8. What is meant by test statistic? How do you conclude using this test statistic.
9. Define chi-square test statistic and discuss two of it's uses.
10. Explain Fisher's *Z*-test for testing sample correlation coefficients.
11. Explain various assumptions of *F*–test with suitable examples.
12. Explain the test procedure of a *F*-test with an example. Explain the procedure of reading *F*-table values.

C. Essay Type Questions

1. Explain various steps involved in chi-square test procedure for testing independence of two attributes, with an example.
2. Explain various steps involved in paired t-test along with necessary assumptions.
3. What are small sample tests? Explain their applications with suitable examples.
4. A dice is thrown 150 times and obtained the following results:

Number on the die	1	2	3	4	5	6	Total
Frequency	35	30	23	15	27	20	150

   Apply suitable test and test the hypothesis that the dice is unbiased or not? [Ans: $\chi^2_{cal} = 10.32$. Accept H_0]

5. The following figures show the distribution of digits from 0 to 9 in a telephone directory.

Digits:	0	1	2	3	4	5	6	7	8	9
Frequency:	1107	1175	972	966	1107	853	1026	997	964	933

   Test at 5% level of significance, whether the digits occurred with equal probability or not? [Ans: $\chi^2_{cal} = 58.542$. Reject H_0]

6. One thousand girls in a college were measured for their I.Q. and their economic conditions based on their parents income. Apply suitable test and determine whether the I.Q. levels and economic conditions are dependent or independent?

I.Q. levels			
	High	Low	Total
Economic conditions			
Rich	100	300	400
Poor	350	250	600
Total	450	550	1000
			[**Ans:** $\chi^2_{cal} = 107.7$. Reject H_0]

7. From the table given below, determine whether the eye color of daughters has any effect on mother's eye color?

		Daughter's eye color		
		Black	Light green	Total
Mother's eye	Black:	230	148	378
Color	Light green:	151	471	622
	Total:	381	619	1000
				[Ans: $c^2_{cal} = 133.39$. Reject H_0]

8. A child health care centre conducted a survey on the health of 300 children less than 2 completed years of age, along with the hygienic conditions at home. Test whether there exists any relationship between child health and Hygienic conditions of home.

	Conditions of Home		
	Clean	Fairly clean	Dirty
Healthy child condition	80	70	35
Un-healthy	20	45	50

[Ans: $\chi^2_{cal} = 25.636$ Reject H_0]

9. Test the efficiency of a new drug introduced to control lung cancer on 300 patients and 200 other patients were not given this new drug. The patients were monitored and the results recorded are as follows:

	Cured	Condition worsen	No effect	Total
With drug	200	40	60	300
Without drug	120	30	50	200
Total	320	70	110	500

Test whether the drug has any effect in curing lung cancer?

[Ans: $\chi^2_{cal} = 2.434$. Accept H_0]

10. A fertilizer mixing machine is said to give 12 kg of nitrate for every quintal bag of fertilizer. Ten 100 kg bags are selected randomly and verified for percentage of nitrate and are measured as follows: 12, 14, 13, 11, 13, 12, 13, 12, 11, and 14. Is there any reason to believe that the machine is not properly mixing the nitrate? Use appropriate test.

[**Hint:** $|t_{cal}| = 1.464$. Accept H_0]

11. A group of five patients treated with medicine '*A*' weight 39, 41, 60, 48 and 42 kg. Another group of seven patients from the same hospital treated with medicine '*B*' weight 56, 68, 38, 42, 64, 62 and 69 kg based on this data do you agree with the claim that medicine '*B*' increases the weight significantly than medicine '*A*'? Use appropriate test at 5% l.o.s.

[**Ans:** $t_{cal} = -1.72$. Accept H_0]

12. Eight medical students are selected at random and the marks obtained by them (out of 50 maximum marks) in bio-statistics and quantitative reasoning test are as follows:

Student No. :	1	2	3	4	5	6	7	8
Quantitative test:	28	42	35	40	48	46	12	23
Bio-statistics:	40	38	36	32	46	30	28	30

Apply an appropriate test and determine whether there exists any significant difference between mean marks in quantitative test and bio-statistics. [**Hint**: $t_{cal} = 0.153$. Accept H_0]

13. A certain nutritious diet is newly introduced in a hospital and given for 12 patients for a period of 30 days and measured the increased body weights in kgs are recorded as follows:

8, 3, 6, –2, 0, 3, –1, 4, 5, 0, 1 and 6. Can you agree that the newly introduced nutritious diet increase the weights of patients? Use appropriate test.

[**Hint:** paired $t_{cal} = 3.009$. Reject H_0]

14. The increase in weights (in kgs) of 10 patients in the children ward of a hospital, fed with the nourishing food COMPLAN, were recorded as: 14, 11, 12, 13, 13, 12, 14, 13, 11 and 12. Similar type of 12 children from another hospital with another nourishing food BOOST in the same period have increased weights in kgs as: 8, –1, 5, 3, 2, 0, –2, 6, 1, 5, 0 and 4. Use appropriate test to determine whether there exists any statistically valid difference between the average increase of weights in the children fed on two nourished foods, i.e., COMPLAN and BOOST. [**Ans:** Accept H_0]

15. A random sample of 18 pairs of observations representing the relation between intake of food and fasting blood sugar levels, correlation coefficient is found as 0.758. Using appropriate test at 1% l.o.s, examine whether this observed correlation coefficient is significant or not?

[$t_{cal} = 4.6485$. Reject H_0]

16. Two kinds of manure applied to 16 uniform rate of fertility 10 feet × 10 feet plots with sericulture crop, other conditions remaining the same. The yield of sericulture crop measured kgs as follows:

Manure A:	18	20	36	50	36	49	48	34	42
Manure B:	46	44	30	26	35	29	28		

Use appropriate test and examine the significant difference between mean sericulture crop yields due to the application of manures *A* and *B* at 5% level of significance. [**Ans:** $t_{cal} = 0.57$. Accept H_0]

17. The following data gives the weights of gain in rats on two different types of rearing foods. Test whether the difference is significant are not?

Wheat based (gr):	34	28	42	34	44
Ragi based (gr):	36	33	48	38	50

18. In a laboratory two types of rabbits rearing foods are prepared such that type–A food contains high proteins and type–B food contains low proteins. Experiment is conducted on two groups containing 12 and 7 rabbits of similar characteristics. Gain in weights are measured in grams and are recorded as follows:

High protein food	Low protein food
139	10
146	118
104	101
119	55
124	101
161	132
107	44
83	
13	
129	
97	
123	

Test whether there exists any significant effect of proteins in increasing weights of rabbits with respect to means and variances.

19. Two stimulants *A* and *B* were tested on 24 psycho-patients. 24 patients are randomly grouped into two groups of 12 patients each and studied the effect of these two stimulants. The corresponding effects of both stimulants *A* and *B* are measured as *X* and *Y* respectively and resulted the following information:

Stimulant A:	$\Sigma X = 156$	$\Sigma X^2 = 625$
Stimulant B:	$\Sigma Y = 204$	$\Sigma Y = 856$

Does the sample evidence suggest that stimulant *B* is more effective than stimulant *A* on psycho-patients? Test at 5% l.o.s.

[**Ans:** $t_{cal} = 1.19$. Accept H_0]

20. Two labs *A* and *B* carried out independent estimate of fat content in Ice cream made by a firm (or) a company. A sample was taken from each batch and halved. The separated halves were sent to 2 different laboratories to estimate the content of fat in the Ice cream. The laboratory records are as follows:

Batch No.	1	2	3	4	5	6	7	8	9	10
Lab A.	7	8	7	3	8	6	9	4	7	8
Lab B.	9	8	8	4	7	7	9	6	6	6

Test whether any significant differences are there between the estimates given by two laboratories? **[Hint:** paired *t*-test]

21. Two samples are drawn randomly from large consignments of same medicine produced by two pharmaceutical companies. Content of medicine is measured in ml. The data is as follows:

Sample 1:	71	60	65	76	74	87	85	82		
Sample 2:	91	86	88	61	66	67	85	78	63	85

Test whether the above two samples have the same variance or not at 5% l.o.s. **[Ans:** $F_{cal} = 1.467$. Accept H_0]

22. The standard deviations calculated from two random samples of size 9 and 13 are 2 mg and 1.9 mg respectively. Do you agree that both samples came from same population with same standard deviation?

[Ans: $F_{cal} = 1.15$. Accept H_0]

23. Two independent samples of sizes 9 and 8 gave sum of squares 160 and 91 respectively. Can the samples be regarded as drawn from the same population with equal variance? **[Ans:** $F_{cal} = 1.51$. Accept H_0].

References

1. Gupta S.P. 1990 "Statistical Methods". Sultan Chand & Sons, New Delhi.
2. Wayne W. Daniel 2008 "Biostatistics", 9th edition, John Wiley & Sons. Inc. Newyork.
3. P.N. Arora *et al.* 2007 "Comprehensive Statistical Methods" Sultan Chand and company Ltd. First edn. New Delhi.
4. VK. Kapoor 1986 "Problems and solutions in Business statistics" Sultan Chand and sons New Delhi.

Answers to Objective Type Questions

1 – b; 2 – d; 3 – a; 4 – c; 5 – c; 6 – a; 7 – d; 8 – d; 9 – c; 10 – c.

10 ANALYSIS OF VARIANCE OR ANOVA

10.1. INTRODUCTION TO ANALYSIS OF VARIANCE (ANOVA)

Analysis of Variance (ANOVA) is the most popular and powerful statistical tool which is considered as the extension of student's t-test, in the sense that, when we have two sample means and we have to test the significant difference between these two sample means, we use student's t-test. In many real life problems, we come across many situations, where we have to deal more than two variables at a time. For example, heart functioning of a heart patient depends on B.P. both systolic and diastolic, blood sugar, cholesterol levels, age of the patient, gender, LDL, VLDL, serum cretin, temperature of the body and so on. Similarly, in agricultural studies, yield of a crop depend on temperature of the soil, rainfall, seed quality, type of cultivation, manures applied, type of pesticides applied and so on.

In business problems, price of an item depends on its production rate, demand for that produce, availability of the product in the market, Dollar, Rupee conversion rate and so on. Thus there is a need for handling many variables at a time to take right decision. In order to test significant differences among several means or variation among several means (more than two) we have to use Analysis of Variance Technique.

Thus, when we have only two variables to analyze, we use student's t-test and if we have more than two variables to analyze, we use ANOVA technique. In this sense, ANOVA is the generalization of Student's t-test. Thus in ANOVA we consider the null hypothesis as:

H_0 : There is no significant variation among k sample means.

Or $\bar{x}_1 = \bar{x}_2 = ,.,.,. = \bar{x}_k$ Or $V(\bar{x}_i) = 0 \;\; i = 1, 2, .,.,., k.$

Against H_1 : There is significant variation among k sample means.

Or $\bar{x}_1 \neq \bar{x}_2 \neq ,.,.,. \neq \bar{x}_k$ Or $V(\bar{x}_i) > 0 \;\; i = 1, 2, .,.,., k.$

To test above 'k' sample means simultaneously, we use this powerful tool of statistics known as '*Analysis of Variance (ANOVA)*'. ANOVA was first developed by Prof. R.A. Fisher, initially to solve problems which arise in Agriculture. But, now a days, this tool is most popularly used in almost all fields like medical, industrial, marketing, bio-sciences, fields involving laboratory experimentation, meteorology, fisheries, forest research and so on. Basically, ANOVA is a test procedure used for testing '**Homogeneity of several means**'. Analysis of variance is a statistical method with the help of which one can separate the variation assignable to one set of causes from the variation assignable to other set of causes. In other words, total variation present in the sample data will split up into two components as follows:

(*a*) Variation within the subgroups of samples and

(*b*) Variation between the subgroups of the samples.

After obtaining above two variations *A* and *B*, these two variations are tested for their significance using *F*-test. Since, total variation is divided into two orthogonal components and tested for their significance and hence this technique is known as Analysis of Variance (ANOVA).

10.2. OBJECTIVES AND ASSUMPTIONS OF ANOVA

Basic objectives of analysis of variance and assumptions of ANOVA play a very important role, based on which entire statistical analysis rests. Hence they are to be understood clearly:

10.2.1. Objectives of ANOVA

The first objective of analysis of variance is to obtain a measure of the total variation within the given data or sample data collected and the second objective is to find a measure of variation between or among the components. Then the third objective is test the significance of difference between in two or more given series. In other words, with the help of ANOVA we can test the hypothesis that the means of all the *k* components, constituting a population are equal to the mean of the population. This means that we are testing here, whether all the *k* samples, came from the same population or different populations with different means.

10.2.2. Assumptions of ANOVA

The study of analysis of variance has the following underlying assumptions.

1. Each of the samples is a simple random sample.
2. Populations from which the samples are drawn are normally distributed. In large sample case this assumption of normality is not necessary.
3. Each one of the sample is independent of the other samples.
4. Each one of the populations has same variance i.e. $\sigma_1^2 = \sigma_2^2 = .,., = \sigma_k^2$ and are having identical means $\mu_1 = \mu_2 = .,.,., = \mu_k$.
5. The effects of various components are additive. For example, if a person taking one glass of milk, one apple and does an exercise to increase the weight, in total he has milk effect + apple effect + exercise effect = Total increased weight.

10.2.3. Short-cut Method for ANOVA

The analysis of one way or two way, calculations will be reduced by transforming the given data through the change of origin technique. This is because of the fact that if variance of a random *X* i.e. $V(X)$ = '*a*', then $V(X + C) = V(X - C)$ = '*a*' itself. This is because of the fact that calculations of variance is based on the difference between observation and the mean value of the given data. Difference between will not change by adding or subtracting some constant from both numbers. That is difference between 50 – 30 is same as 150 – 130 (by adding a constant 100 to both numbers) or 30 – 10 (by subtracting a constant 20 from both numbers). Thus variance of the given data will not be affected by change of origin.

10.3. ANOVA TABLE AND CLASSIFICATION OF ANOVA

A table showing the (*i*) source of variation, (*ii*) degrees of freedom, (*iii*) sum of squares, (*iv*) Mean sum of squares (variance) and (*v*) the test statistic F_{cal} values is known as 'ANOVA table'. Thus ANOVA table usually consists of 5 columns explaining above five listed components.

General structure of ANOVA table.

Source of variation	Degrees of freedom	Sum of squares	Mean sum of squares or variances	F-Calculated values
S.O.V.	D.O.F.	S.S.	M.S.S.	F_{cal}
Source – 1				
Source – 2				
.				
.				
Error				
Total				

Here the test statistic *F* is calculated as follows:

$$F_{cal} = \left[\frac{\text{Variance between the samples}}{\text{Variance within the samples}}\right] \quad (10.3.1)$$

Variance within the samples is also known as 'error variance' or 'residual variance', which is generally very, very small when compared to the variance between the samples. This is because of the fact that variance between the samples is produced by some cause i.e., because of treatment effect. Nature of random causes is that it is very small and causes for this variation are many in number. Usually random causes of variation is an ignorable variation and we consider that the units are considered as statistically similar. For example, if we put our signature 10 times, the variation among them is very small (almost similar) consider all the signatures are same. But if we do one signature with left hand and others with right hand, then all signatures will not tally usually and variation is large. This is because you have done the signature with hand other than usually used hand. Here the variation is large and we can find a cause for that. Such large variations are known as variations between the samples we can find one or two causes for that variation. Bank manager will ignore small variations and catches variation due to forgery before passing the cheque or a withdrawal.

10.3.1. Classification of ANOVA

The analysis of variance is mainly carried under the following two categories, namely:

(*a*) ANOVA – One way classification and

(*b*) ANOVA – Two way classification.

When all the experimental units are uniform with respect to age, gender, breed and so on, variation is assignable to only one cause i.e., difference in treatments given to these units, then we go for ANOVA-one way classification.

If the experimenter feels that there exists some heterogeneity among experimental units with respect to age or gender, or some character, we have to these heterogeneous experimental units into homogenous sub-groups. In such situations, we use ANOVA-two way classification.

10.4. ANOVA – ONE WAY CLASSIFICATION

Here we assume that all the experimental units are alike in all respects. For example, male children less than 1 year suffering from a viral fever, or agricultural plots of same size say 5ft × 5ft with same fertility rate under the same crop having same climates conditions. All female albino rats less than 8 months in a laboratory, all diabetic mellitus heart patients of age group 30 – 40, male malignant cancer patients in stage-2 above 60 years and so on. Since, all units are assumed uniform, if at all any variation among them is there, that is because of the difference in the treatment adopted or medicine used or fertilizer applied and so on.

Here, if we find significant variation, we can assign the cause for the variation is due to difference among the treatments adopted or difference among the medicine used or difference among the fertilizers applied and so on. Hence this type of analysis is known as ANOVA-one way classification. The data collected or sample observations will be of the following form in one way classification.

Treatments

Units	T_1	T_2	T_3 ,.,.,.,	T_k
1	x_{11}	x_{12}	x_{13} ,.,.,.,	x_{1k}
2	x_{21}	x_{22}	x_{23} ,.,.,.,	x_{2k}
3	x_{31}	x_{32}	x_{33} ,.,.,.,	x_{3k}
.	.	.	.	.
.	.	.	.	.
.				
.				
m	x_{m1}	x_{m2}	x_{m3} ,.,.,.,	x_{mk}
Total	C_1	C_2	C_3 ,.,.,.,	C_k G

In the above table, C_j represents j^{th} column total j = 1, 2, 3 ,.,.,., k and G = grand total = ΣC_j and x_{ji} = i^{th} unit under j^{th} treatment. Here we have $m \times k = N$ experimental units and we assume that all these N units are homogeneous with respect to all characteristics.

Let the treatment means = $\bar{t}_i = \Sigma C_j/m.\ j = 1, 2 ,.,.,., k.$

10.4.1. Test Procedure of ANOVA–One Way Classification

Step – 1: Hypotheses to be framed are:

H_0: There is no significant variation among k sample means.

Or $\bar{t}_1 = \bar{t}_2 = ,.,.,. = \bar{t}_k$ Or $V(\bar{t}_i) = 0 \ i = 1, 2 ,.,.,., k.$

H_1 : There is significant variation among k sample means.

Or $\bar{t}_1 \neq \bar{t}_2 \neq ,.,.,. \neq \bar{t}_k$ Or $V(\bar{t}_i) > 0 \ i = 1, 2 ,.,.,., k.$

Step – 2: Calculate column totals C_j's and grand total G from the given data.

Step – 3: Calculate correction factor = $CF = G^2/N$.

Step – 4: Calculate treatment sum of squares = $TSS = \frac{1}{m}\Sigma C_j^2 - CF = A.$

Step – 5: Calculate total sum of squares = $ToSS = \Sigma x_{ji}^2 - CF = B.$

Step – 6: Prepare ANOVA table as follows:

ANOVA table for one way classification

Source of variation	Degrees of freedom	Sum of squares	Mean sum of squares	Variance ratio
SOV	DOF	SS	MSS	F-statistic
Treatments	k – 1	TSS = A	V_1 = A/k – 1	$F_{cal} = V_1/V_2$
Error	N – k	ESS = B – A = C	V_2 = C/N – k	
Total	N – 1	ToSS = B		

Step – 7: Determine F_{tab} value at α% l.o.s. at $(k - 1, N - k)$ d.o.f. from F-table given appendix A – 4.

Step – 8: If $F_{cal} < F_{tab}$. We accept H_0 at α% level of significance, otherwise reject H_0.

10.4.1. Applications of ANOVA – One-Way Classification

ANOVA one-way classification is most popularly and frequently used in many scientific enquires. This is because of the fact that this is most suitable for laboratory and field experiments. Generally, laboratory experiments are based on small experimental units and one can get homogeneous units in smaller number. Similarly, we can maintain homogeneous climatic conditions and maintain other experimental procedures in a systematic and uniform manner in laboratories. Another basic advantage of ANOVA one-way classification is that without complicating the statistical analysis one can deal with the problem of unequal number of experimental units under each treatment can be dealt easily. The problem of unequal number of units under each treatment is an inevitable problem, which is a natural phenomenon.

Even though the experimenter started the experiment with equal number of subjects or units under each treatment, due to natural calamities like floods or earthquakes or fire accidents in agricultural fields, or death of some animals due to diseases, the experimenter cannot get the data from equal number of units under each treatment. Thus the experimenter is left with un-equal number of observations under each treatment. Sometimes, the experimenter may miss some observations due to forgetfulness or mistakes committed by his subordinates or due to some cause or the other. Thus, the experimenter has no other way to conduct a fresh experiment, and hence the money, time and experimental material will become waste if it is restricted that equal number of units must be there under each treatment.

This problem of unequal number of units under each treatment can be dealt easily in ANOVA one-way classification, without wasting money, material and time. Hence this is most popularly used and frequently applied statistical technique in many scientific studies or enquiries.

Thus without complicating the analysis much, one can delete one or more treatments or data if the experimenter feels that the experiment failed under a particular treatment or in a particular experimental unit. The experimenter has this freedom in ANOVA one way classification and hence, ANOVA one way classification is the most popularly used statistical tool used by many scientists in many laboratory or field experiments.

Example (10.4.1): Three treatments T_1, T_2 and T_3 were given to 15 children less than 5 years, suffering from measles admitted in the children ward of a hospital in the first week of, March 2009. Following data represent the duration of treatment in days to cure the disease.

Treatment – 1:	8	14	10	7	11
Treatment – 2:	7	5	10	9	9
Treatment – 3:	13	9	12	14	12

Determine whether there exists any statistically valid difference with respect to the time taken to cure measles among the three treatments among children less than 5 years. Test at $\alpha = 0.05$ % l.o.s.

Solution:

Step – 1: Hypotheses to be framed are:

H_0: There is no significant variation among 3 treatments means with respect to the duration of the cure of the disease.

Or $\quad \bar{t}_1 = \bar{t}_2 = \bar{t}_3$ Or $V(\bar{t}_i) = 0 \;\; i = 1, 2, 3.$

H_1 : There is significant variation among 3 treatment means.

Or $\quad \bar{t}_1 \neq \bar{t}_2 \neq \bar{t}_3$ Or $V(\bar{t}_i) > 0 \;\; i = 1, 2, 3.$

Step – 2: Calculate sums and sum of squares as follows:

						Total
Treatment – 1:	8	14	10	7	11	50
Treatment – 2:	7	5	10	9	9	40
Treatment – 3:	13	9	12	14	12	60

Grand total = G = 150.

Correction factor = $CF = G^2/N = (150)^2/15 = 1500$

Treatment sum of squares = $TSS = \frac{1}{m}\Sigma C_j^2 - CF$

$= [(50)^2 + (40)^2 + (60)^2]/5 - 1500$

$= [2500 + 1600 + 3600]/5 - 1500$

$= 7700/5 - 1500 = 40 = A.$

Total sum of squares = $\text{ToSS} = \sum x_{ji}^2 - CF = [8^2 + 14^2 + .,.,., + 12^2] - 1500$

$= [64 + 196 + 100 + 49 + 121 + 49 + 25 + 100 + 81$
$+ 81 + 169 + 81 + 144 + 196 + 144] - 1500$

$= [1600] - 1500 = 100 = B.$

Step – 3: Form the ANOVA table as follows:

Source of variation	Degrees of freedom	Sum of squares	Mean sum of squares	Variance ratio
SOV	DOF	SS	MSS	F-statistic
Treatments	3 – 1 = 2	TSS = A = 40	V_1 = A/k – 1 = 40/2 = 20	$F_{cal} = V_1/V_2$ = 25/5 = 4
Error	15 – 3 = 12	B – A = C = 60	V_2 = C/N – k = 60/12 = 5	
Total	15 – 1 = 14	ToSS = B = 100		

Table value of F-statistic denoted by F_{tab} at (2, 12) degrees of freedom at 5% l.o.s. (Table A-4) is given by 3.89. Since $F_{cal} > F_{tab}$, we reject H_0 and conclude that there exists significant difference among 3 treatments in curing the measles in children. That is the three treatments statistically differ from each other in curing the disease. This statement is true in 95 cases out of 100 cases.

Example (10.4.2): The following data represents yield of crops in 15 sample plots each of size 10 feet/10 feet, with uniform fertility rate. Three varieties of cotton crop seeds were sown in these plots. Yield of the cotton crop was measured in kgs in each plot. Test whether there is any significant difference between the cotton seeds variety at 1% l.o.s.

Variety A:	20	21	23	18	20	25
Variety B:	18	22	17	15		
Variety C:	25	28	22	32	29	

Solution:

By applying the change of scale technique, we can reduce the size of each data item. To do this subtract minimum value in the given data from all observations i.e., 15, so that we can avoid negative quantities.

							Total
Variety A:	5	6	8	3	5	10	$37 = R_1$
Variety B:	3	7	2	0			$12 = R_2$
Variety C:	10	13	7	17	14		$61 = R_3$

Grand total = G = 110

Correction factor = $CF = G^2/N = (110)/15 = 806.67$

Null hypothesis H_0 : There is no significant variation among average yield of cotton crop between the 3 varieties of cotton crop seeds or $\bar{x}_1 = \bar{x}_2 = \bar{x}_3$.

Alternative hypothesis $H_1 : \bar{x}_1 \neq \bar{x}_2 \neq \bar{x}_3$.

$$\text{Treatment some of square} = [(37)^2/6 + (12)^2/4 + (61)^2/5] - 806.67$$
$$= [228.167 + 36 + 744.2] - 806.67$$
$$= 1008.367 - 806.67 = 201.697 = A$$

Total some of square

$$= [25 + 36 + 64 + 9 + 25 + 100 + 9 + 49 + 4 + 0 + 100 + 169 + 49 + 289 + 196] - 806.67$$
$$= 1124 - 806.67 = 317.33 = B.$$

ANOVA Table for one way classification

Source of variation	Degrees of freedom	Sum of squares	Mean sum of squares	Variance ratio
SOV	DOF	SS	MSS	F_{cal}
Due to varities	2	A = 201.697	V_1 = 201.697/2 = 100.8485	$F_{cal} = V_1/V_2$ = 10.466
Error	12	C = B – A = 115.633	V_2 = 15.633/12 = 9.636	
Total	14	B = 317.33		

The table value of F_{tab} at 1% l.o.s. with (2, 12) d.o.f. is 6.93 from Table A5.

Since F_{cal} value is larger than F table value at (2, 12) degrees of freedom at 1% l.o.s (level of significance) we reject the null hypothesis at 1% l.o.s. Hence, we conclude that the varieties of cotton seeds not producing same yield of cotton crop. They differ significantly with respect to the average yield of cotton crop. This statement is true 99 times out of 100 times.

Example (10.4.3): Three different treatments are applied on 20 patients suffering from the jaundice disease. The data relating to the reduction of the relevant characteristic in the blood samples are given as follows.

Treatment – 1:	16	8	12	14	10	6	18	
Treatment – 2:	14	10	10	6	12			
Treatment – 3:	4	10	18	20	18	15	6	20

Test whether there is any significant difference between the treatments in the reduction of jaundice in the patients.

Solution:

Frame the hypothesis as follows:

Null hypothesis H_0 : There is no significant variation among average effect among the 3 treatments for reduction of jaundice or $\bar{x}_1 = \bar{x}_2 = \bar{x}_3$.

Alternative hypothesis $H_1 : \bar{x}_1 \neq \bar{x}_2 \neq \bar{x}_3$.

Now calculate various totals as follows:

									Totals
Treatment – 1:	16	8	12	14	10	6	18		$84=R_1$
Treatment – 2:	14	10	10	9	12				$55=R_2$
Treatment – 3:	4	10	18	20	18	15	6	20	$91=R_3$

Grand total = G =230

$$\text{Correction factor} = G^2/N = (230)^2/20 = 2645$$

$$TSS = [(84)^2/7 + (55)^2/5 + (91)^2/8] - 2645$$
$$= [1008 + 605 + 1035.125] - 2645$$
$$= 2648.125 - 2645 = 3.125 = A.$$

$$ToSS = [256 + 64 + 144 + 196 + 100 + 36 + 324 + 196 + 100 + 100 + 81 + 144 + 16 + 100 + 324 + 400 + 324 + 225 + 36 + 400] - 2645$$
$$= 3313 - 2645 = 668 = B.$$

ANOVA Table for one way classification

Source of variation	Degrees of freedom	Sum of squares	Mean sum of squares	
SOV	DOF	SS	MSS	F_{cal}
Due to varieties	2	A = 3.125	$V_1 = 3.125/2 = 1.5625$	$F_{cal} = V_1/V_2$ Not possible to calculate
Error	17	C = B – A = 664.875	$V_2 = 664.875/17 = 39.11$	
Total	19	B = 668		

Since $F_{cal} < 1$, we conclude the data is not suitable for statistical analysis. It is suggested that a fresh experiment is to be conducted.

Important note : In any case, if F_{cal} value is less than 1, which means that error variance is larger than treatment variance and this situation is impossible. This situation is similar to the incidence that without treatment, we can get much better yield. This is not true in general. This is similar situation that a student can get marks more better than the concerned teacher teaching the subject. Hence, in any case error variance is larger than treatment variance we have to suspect the data and suggest for a fresh experiment.

10.5. ANOVA – TWO WAY CLASSIFICATION

In one way classification, the basic assumption is that, all the N experimental units must be uniform with respect to all other characteristics except in treatment effects. When N is large, getting such homogeneous units is not possible and without our knowledge, heterogeneity will enter with respect some characteristic and affect our experimental results. That is experimental error will increase enormously, because of heterogeneity prevailed among these experimental units. To reduce the experimental error, we have to divide these heterogeneous units into homogeneous groups. This technique of dividing the heterogeneous experimental units into homogeneous sub-groups is known as '*Local control*' by Prof. R.A. Fisher. Such homogeneous sub-groups are called Blocks and variation due to blocks can be separated from total variation so that error variance will be automatically reduced. That is here, along with the treatment variance, we are separating block variance also from total variance present in the experimental data.

Hence, this technique is known as 'ANOVA – two way classification'. Error variance in ANOVA two way classification will generally be less than or equal to the error variance of ANOVA one way classification. If there is no effect of 'Local control' i.e., all experimental units are uniform, then both variances i.e., ANOVA one way or two way variances will be equal to each other.

The experimental data under two-way classification is tabulated as follows:

Treatments

Blocks	T_1	T_2	T_3 ,.,.,.,	T_k	Total.
1	x_{11}	x_{12}	x_{13} ,.,.,.,	x_{1k}	R_1
2	x_{21}	x_{22}	x_{23} ,.,.,.,	x_{2k}	R_2
3	x_{31}	x_{32}	x_{33} ,.,.,.,	x_{3k}	R_3
.	.	.	.	.	.
.	.	.	.	.	.
.					
.					
m	x_{m1}	x_{m2}	x_{m3} ,.,.,.,	x_{mk}	R_m
Total	C_1	C_2	C_3 ,.,.,.,	C_k	G

In the above table, R_i represents i^{th} row total i =1, 2, 3 ,.,.,., m; C_j represents j^{th} column total j = 1, 2, 3 ,.,.,., k and G = grand total = $\sum R_i = \sum C_j$ and $x_{ji} = i^{th}$ unit under j^{th} treatment. Here we have $m \times k = N$ experimental units. We assume that all the units in each Block are homogeneous with respect to all characteristics.

Let $\bar{t}_i = \Sigma C_j/m$ and $\bar{b}_i = \Sigma R_i/k$.

In two way analysis we have to separate out block variance and treatment variance from total variance which is explained as follows:

10.5.1. Test Procedure of ANOVA – Two Way Classification

Step – 1: Hypotheses to be framed are:

H_{01} : There is no significant variation among k sample means.

Or $\bar{t}_1 = t_2 = ,.,.,., = t_k$ Or $V(\bar{t}_i) = 0 \; i = 1, 2 ,.,.,., k.$

H_{02} : There is no significant variation among m block means.

Or $\bar{b}_1 = \bar{b}_2 = ,.,.,., = b_m$ Or $V(\bar{b}_i) = 0 \; i = 1, 2 ,.,.,., m.$

H_{11} : There is significant variation among k sample means.

Or $\bar{t}_1 \neq t_2 \neq ,.,.,., \neq t_k$ Or $V(\bar{t}_i) > 0 \; i = 1, 2 ,.,.,., k.$

H_{12} : There is significant variation among b block means.

Or $\bar{b}_1 \neq b_2 \neq ,.,.,., \neq b_m$ Or $V(\bar{b}_i) > 0 \; i = 1, 2 ,.,.,., m.$

Step – 2: Calculate column totals C_j's, row totals R_i's and grand total G from the given data.

Step – 3: Calculate correction factor = $CF = G^2/N$.

Step – 4: Calculate treatment sum of squares = $TSS = \frac{1}{m}\Sigma C_j^2 - CF = A.$

Step – 5: Calculate block sum of squares = $BSS = \frac{1}{k}\Sigma R_i^2 - CF = B.$

Step – 6: Calculate total sum of squares = $ToSS = \Sigma x_{ji}{}^2 - CF = C.$

Step – 7: Prepare ANOVA table as follows:

ANOVA table for one way classification.

Source of variation	Degrees of freedom	Sum of squares	Mean sum of squares	Variance ratio
SOV	DOF	SS	MSS	F-statistic
Treatments	k – 1	TSS = A	V_1 = A/k – 1	$F_{cal} = V_1/V_3$
Blocks	m – 1	BSS = B	V_2 = B/m – 1	$F_{cal} = V_2/V_3$
Error (Residual)	(k – 1) (m – 1) = E	ESS = C–(A+B) = D	V_3 = D/E	
Total	N – 1	ToSS = C		

Step – 8: Determine F_{tab} values at α% l.o.s. at (k – 1, E) d.o.f. and at $(m - 1E)$, from F-table given appendix A– 4. (Here we get two F values one for treatments and one for Blocks)

Step – 9: (*a*) For treatments: If $F_{cal} < F_{tab}$. We accept H_{01} at α% level of significance, otherwise reject H_{01}.

***(b)* For blocks:** If $F_{cal} < F_{tab}$. We accept H_{02} at α% level of significance. Otherwise reject H_{02}.

Thus we can observe that in the analysis we have to calculate additional calculations on rows also along with column totals and corresponding sum of squares, variances and F-statistic. Thus we get two F_{cal} values one for treatments and the other one for blocks. Based on the table values, for treatments and blocks conclusions are drawn separately for treatments and blocks as explained in step–9.

10.5.1. Applications of ANOVA Two-Way Classification

ANOVA two-way classification is suitable in agricultural and industrial research. This is popularly used in forest, animal husbandry, fisheries, clinical trials, business, medical and market researches. In such studies experimenter need to study on many experimental units and it is very difficult to get uniform experimental units for the study.

For example, in animal husbandry, we can consider lactating belonging to a particular age group can be considered as one block, such that all animals in that block are uniform.

Similarly, in fisheries, a particular breed or type of fish in a separate tank can be considered one block so that, fish in that block are uniform with respect to breed or type. In forest studies, trees of different type like sandalwood trees or rosewood trees or teak trees having similar trunk diameter can be considered as one block.

In clinical trials, we can consider all children one block, all adults as one block and all aged or old people as one block. We can consider all patients suffering from one disease as one block. For example, heart patients block/ward, casualty block/ward, maternity block/ward, or neurology block/ward, emergency block/ward and so on.

In market research, markets in different cities or districts can be considered as one block. Similarly, market of different commodities can be considered as one block. For example, stock market, bullion market, grocery items market, fish market and vegetable market and so on. Each market can be considered as one block.

In agricultural studies, it is very difficult to get uniform fields with respect to climatic conditions and having uniform fertility rate, and so on. Usually within the same plots, the fertility rate changes and hence we may not divide such plots into homogeneous sub-plots for the experiment.

Hence, before applying local control, the experimenter must have an idea how this fertility rate of the plot is varying? If the fertility rate varies horizontally, experimenter has to divide blocks horizontally and sub-group those plots as 'blocks' so that plots within the block have same fertility rate. This is shown in the figure as follows:

Fig. (10.5.1) Picture showing the division of blocks when fertility rate is changing horizontally.

Fertility rate: High Medium Low

Block - 1	Block - 2	Block - 3
Plot - 1	Plot - 1	Plot - 1
Plot - 2	Plot - 2	Plot - 2
Plot - 3	Plot - 3	Plot - 3
Plot - 4	Plot - 4	Plot - 4

Similarly, if the fertility rate is varying vertically, then blocks are to be formed horizontally, so that sub-plots within each block have uniform fertility rate or climatic conditions. This concept is explained clearly, in the following figure (10.5.2).

Fig. (10.5.2): Picture showing the division of blocks when fertility rate is varying horizontally.

Fertility rate

Very High	Block A	Plot - 1	Plot - 2	Plot - 3
High	Block B	Plot - 1	Plot - 2	Plot - 3
Medium	Block C	Plot - 1	Plot - 2	Plot - 3
Low	Block D	Plot - 1	Plot - 2	Plot - 3
Very low	Block E	Plot - 1	Plot - 2	Plot - 3

Because of above explained procedure of making block, one can apply ANOVA in many scientific studies, where one can study the effect of treatments along with block effects and can test for their respective significant effects.

Example (10.5.1): To study the performance of three detergent soaps and three different water temperatures, the following specially designed experiment is conducted to measure brightness of washed cloths. The measured data is as follows:

Water temperature	Detergent soap A	Detergent soap B	Detergent soap C
Cold water	57	55	67
Warm water	49	52	60
Hot water	54	46	58

Test whether there exists any significance variation among different detergent soaps and also test whether there exists any significance difference with different temperature levels of water in bringing brightness among washed cloths. Test at 5% l.o.s.

Solution:

We can reduce the volume of the given data by subtracting each figure from a value *A*. In the analysis the answer will not be affected by change of origin of the given data. From the given data, subtract a constant $A = 46$ (The number 46 is selected because one can avoid negative numbers). Thus the given data is transformed as follows:

Water temperature	Detergent soap A	Detergent soap B	Detergent soap C
Cold water	57 – 46 = 11	55 – 46 = 9	67 – 46 = 21
Warm water	49 – 46 = 3	52 – 46 = 6	60 – 46 = 14
Hot water	54 – 46 = 8	46 – 46 = 0	58 – 46 = 12

Frame hypothesis as follows:

H_{01} : There is no significant difference between detergent soaps in bringing brightness in washed cloths.

H_{02} : There is no significant effect of temperature of water in bringing brightness in washed cloths.

H_{11} : There is significant difference between detergent soaps in bringing brightness in washed cloths.

H_{12} : There is significant effect of temperature of water in bringing brightness in washed cloths.

Now calculate various totals as follows:

Soaps:	A	B	C	Total
Cold water	11	9	21	$41 = R_1$
Warm water	3	6	14	$23 = R_2$
Hot water	8	0	12	$20 = R_3$
Total	$C_1 = 22$	$C_2 = 15$	$C_3 = 47$	$G = 84$

Correction factor $= CF = G^2/N = (84)^2/9 = 7056/9 = 784.$

$$\text{Treatment sum of squares} = TSS = \frac{1}{m}\Sigma C_j^2 - CF$$

$$= [(22)^2 + (15)^2 + (47)^2]\ /3\ - CF$$

$$= [484 + 225 + 2209]/3 - 784 = 2918/3 - 784$$

$$= 972.6667 - 784 = 188.6667 = A.$$

$$\text{Block sum of squares} = BSS = \frac{1}{k}\Sigma R_i^2 - CF = [(41)^2 + (23)^2 + (20)^2]/3 - 784$$

$$= [1681 + 529 + 400]/3 - 784$$

$$= 2610/3 - 784 = 870 - 784 = 86 = B.$$

$$\text{Total sum of squares} = ToSS = \Sigma x_{ji}^2 - CF = [11^2 + 9^2 + .,., + 12^2] - 784$$

$$= [121 + 81 + 441 + 9 + 36 + 196 + 64 + 0 + 144]$$

$$- 784 = 1092 - 784 = 308 = C.$$

Now prepare ANOVA table as follows:

ANOVA table for two way classification.

Source of variation	Degrees of freedom	Sum of squares	Mean sum of squares	Variance ratio
SOV	DOF	SS	MSS	F-statistic
Treatments/ soaps	3 – 1 = 2	A = 188.6667	V_1 = 188.6667/2 = 94.3335	$F_{cal} = V_1/V_3$ = 4.6667/8.3333 = 11.36
Blocks/water	3 – 1 = 2	B = 86	V_2 = 86/2 = 43	$F_{cal} = V_2/V_3$ = 43/8.3333=5.16
Error (Residual)	(3 – 1) (3 – 1) = 4 = E	ESS = C–(A+B) = D = 33.3333	V_3 = D/E = 33.3333/4 = 8.3333	
Total	9 – 1 = 8	TSS = C = 308		

F_{tab} at 5% l.o.s. at (2, 4) d.o.f. is 6.59. (Table A4)

For Soaps: Since $F_{cal} > F_{tab}$, we reject H_{01} at 5% l.o.s. and conclude that: There exists significance variation among the effects of detergent soaps *A, B* and *C* in bringing brightness in washed cloths.

For Water: Since $F_{cal} > F_{tab}$, we reject H_{01} at 5% l.o.s. and conclude that: There exists significance variation among the effects of temperature of water in bringing brightness in washed cloths.

Thus, there exist statistically significant effects of soaps as well as temperature of waters in bringing of brightness in washed cloths.

Example (10.5.2): There are 4 salesmen in a T.V. shop sold T.V. sets in 3 different towns. The following data represents the total amount of rupees of gain measured in 1000's for the shop keeper by these salesmen.

	Salesmen			
	1	2	3	4
Town A	6	5	3	8
Town B	8	9	6	5
Town C	10	7	8	7

Test whether there exists any statistical difference among 4 salesmen in selling T.V. sets. Also test whether there exists any statistically valid difference in usage of T.V. sets in the 3 towns *A, B* and *C*.

Solution: Frame hypotheses as follows:

H_{01} : There is no significant difference between salesmen in selling the T.V. sets.

H_{02} : There is no significant difference of usage of T.V. sets in these 3 towns *A, B* and *C*.

H_{11} : There is significant difference between the salesmen in selling T.V. sets.

H_{12} : There is significant difference in the usage of T.V. sets in the 3 towns *A, B* and *C*.

Calculate various totals as follows:

	Salesmen				
	1	2	3	4	Total
Town A	4	5	3	8	20
Town B	8	9	8	5	30
Town C	10	15	8	7	40
Totals:	22	29	19	20	G = 90

$$\text{Correction factor} = CF = (90)^2/12 = 675.$$

$$\text{Salesmen sum of squares} = [400 + 900 + 1600]/4 - 675 = 2900/4 - 675$$
$$= 725 - 675 = 50 = A$$

$$\text{Town sum of squares} = [484 + 841 + 361 + 400]/3 - 675 = 2086/3 - 675$$
$$= 695.3333 - 675 = 20.3333 = B$$

$$\text{Total sum of squares} = [16 + 25 + 9 + 64 + 64 + 81 + 64 + 25 + 100$$
$$+ 225 + 64 + 49] - 675 = 786 - 675 = 111 = C$$

ANOVA table for two way classification.

Source of variation	Degrees of freedom	Sum of squares	Mean sum of squares	Variance ratio
SOV	DOF	SS	MSS	F-statistic
Salesmen	$4 - 1 = 3$	$A = 50$	$V_1 = 50/3$ $= 16.6667$	$F_{cal} = V_1/V_3$ $= 16.6667/$ $6.7778 = 2.459$
Blocks/Towns	$3 - 1 = 2$	$B = 20.3333$	$V_2 = 20.333/2$ $= 10.1667$	$F_{cal} = V_2/V_3 =$ $10.1667/6.7778$ 1.4999
Error (Residual)	$(4 - 1)(3 - 1)$ $= 6 = E$	$ESS = C-(A+B)$ $= D = 40.667$	$V_3 = D/E$ $= 40.667/6$ $= 6.7778$	
Total	$12 - 1 = 11$	$C = 111$		

For salesmen: Table value of F_{tab} at 5% l.o.s at (3, 6) d.o.f is 4.35. Similarly, for towns: F_{tab} at 5% l.o.s at (2, 6) d.o.f. is 5.14 (Table A4).

Comparing corresponding calculated values of F with the corresponding table values of F, we accept both H_{01} and H_{02} at 5% l.o.s. This implies that all salesmen are equally efficient in selling T.V. sets. There is no statistical evidence that one salesman is superior or inferior to other salesmen. Similarly, there is no statistical evidence that demand for T.V. sets are different in different towns. That is the demand for T.V. sets is similar in all the three towns.

10.6. FURTHER STATISTICAL ANALYSIS – DMR-TEST

When we accept the Null-hypothesis in ANOVA there is no need for further statistical analysis, because there is no significant difference between the treatments under consideration and hence one can use any one of the treatments which he desires. When we reject the Null-hypothesis, that is, if there is significant difference between the treatments, automatically raises an immediate question that "which treatment is the best one and which treatment is most suitable?" Unless otherwise we answer this question, the analysis is not complete. To do this we need to apply "Further Statistical Analysis". For example, we have rejected null hypotheses in example (10.4.1) at 5% l.o.s.; in example (10.4.2) at 1% l.o.s.; and in example (10.5.1) at 5% l.o.s. If we simply say that there exists significant difference between treatments under consideration, the analysis is not complete, unless we say that which treatment is the best one or which of the two are having same effect or which of them have last preferable. In order to answer such questions, we have to go for further statistical analysis. In this analysis, we have three tests, namely:

1. Least Significant Difference test (LSD-test)

   or Critical Difference test (CD – test).

   This test is based on student's t-tables. (table *A* – 3 in appendix)
2. **Tukey's Test:** Tukey prepared special tables useful for comparing multiple comparisons of means (which are available in a very few books).
3. **Duncan's Multiple Range Test (DMR-test):** DMR test is popularly used by many biological researchers in their investigations. This test is based on the tables prepared by Duncan considering order statistics of the means arranged in an increasing order. To apply this test, first treatment means are to be calculated and then they are to be arranged in an increasing order. These arranged means are to be compared with DMR table values given in table *A*- 7 in appendix.

If the calculated difference 'D_{cal}' is less than or equal to the Duncan's table value 'D_{tab}' we accept that there is no difference between the treatments under consideration. These treatments are put under the same bar. Otherwise we conclude that there is significant difference between the two treatments. In this case we put them under different bars.

For example, there are five treatments *A, B, C, D* and *E* and these five treatments are arranged after DMR-test as: (*A, E*) (*B, C, D*).

This implies that :

1. There is no significant difference between treatments *A* and *E*.
2. There is no significant difference between treatments *B* and *C*.
3. There is no significant difference between treatments *B* and *D*.
4. There is no significant difference between treatments *C* and *D*. This is because they are under the same bar.
5. There exists significant difference between the treatments *A* and *B*.
6. There exists significant difference between treatments *A* and *C*.
7. There exists significant difference between treatments *A* and *D*.
8. There exists significant difference between treatments *E* and *B*.
9. There exists significant difference between treatments *E* and *C*. and
10. There exists significant difference between treatments *E* and *D*.

This is because, that these treatments under different bars.

In the above explained manner, we can analyze pair wise and one can take decisions accordingly. Thus DMR test helps the experimenter to subgroup the treatments under consideration. Among above mentioned tests, DMR test is the most appropriate one and most popularly used in almost all Scientific enquiries to take most appropriate decisions. Hence this test is discussed in a more detailed fashion in this book because this book is meant for biology, zoology, bio-technology, sericulture and medical students. We can apply in other fields also like market research, fisheries, forest research, agricultural research, industry and so on.

10.6.1. Duncan's Multiple Range (DMR) Test Procedure

Various steps involved in Duncan's Multiple range test are explained as follows:

Step – 1: First calculate treatment means from the given data.

Step – 2: Arrange these means in an ascending (increasing) order.

Step – 3: Maximum difference that is maximum treatment mean – minimum treatment difference mean = D_1.

Step – 4 : Note down DMR table value D_{tab} from table A – 6 (appendix). While noting the table values, we have to see the degrees of freedom as in F-tables explained earlier.

Step – 5 : If $D_1 \leq D_{tab}$ the difference is insignificant. Otherwise the difference D_1 is significant.

Step – 6 : On similar lines, calculate other differences and compare with D_{tab} value and conclusions are drawn accordingly.

Application of DMR test is discussed with some examples as follows:

Example (10.6.1): Apply DMR test in example (10.4.1) draw your conclusions accordingly.

Solution:

Step – 1: First calculate treatment means from the given data. We know that treatment sums are: $T_1 = 50$, $T_2 = 40$ and $T_3 = 60$. Thus $\bar{t}_1 = 50/5 = 10$; $\bar{t}_2 = 40/5 = 8$ and $\bar{t}_3 = 60/5 = 12$.

Step – 2: Arrange these means in an ascending (increasing) order as follows: $\bar{t}_2 = 8$, $\bar{t}_1 = 10$, and $\bar{t}_3 = 12$.

Step – 3: Maximum difference is $\bar{t}_3 - \bar{t}_2 = D_1 = 12 - 8 = 4$.

Step – 4: Note down DMR table value from table A-6 (appendix). While noting the table values, we have to see the degrees of freedom as on F-tables explained earlier. Thus D_{tab} value at 5% l.o.s at (2, 12) is 3.081.

Step – 5: If $D_{cal} \leq D_{tab}$ the difference is insignificant. Otherwise the difference is significant.

1. Since $D_1 > D_{tab}$, the difference between treatment – 3 and treatment – 2 is significant.

Similarly, difference between $\bar{t}_3 - \bar{t}_1 = D_2 = 12 - 10 = 2$ and $\bar{t}_1 - \bar{t}_2 = D_3 = 10 - 8 = 2$.

Since, $D_2 < D_{tab}$ and $D_3 < D_{tab}$ we conclude that there is no significant difference between treatment–1 and treatment–3; treatment–1 and treatment–2, thus we conclude that :

1. Between treatment – 1 and treatment – 2: No significant difference.
2. Between treatment – 1 and treatment – 3: No significant difference.
3. Between treatment – 2 and treatment – 3: There is significant difference.

Example (10.6.2): Apply DMR test for the data in example (10.4.2) and draw your conclusions.

Solution: From the given data in the problem (10.4.2) we have varieties totals are 127, 72 and 136 for varieties 1, 2 and 3 respectively. DMR test procedure is as follows:

Step – 1: First calculate treatment means from the given data. We know that treatment sums are: $T_1 = 127$, $T_2 = 72$ and

$$T_3 = 136.$$

Thus

$$\bar{v}_1 = 127/6 = 21.1667; \; \bar{v}_2 = 72/4 = 18 \text{ and}$$

$$\bar{v}_3 = 136/5 = 27.2.$$

Step – 2: Arrange these means in an ascending (increasing) order as follows:

$$\bar{v}_2 = 18, \; \bar{v}_1 = 21.1667, \text{ and } \bar{v}_3 = 27.2.$$

Step – 3: Maximum difference is $\bar{t}_3 - \bar{t}_2 = D_1 = 27.2 - 18 = 9.2$.

Step – 4: Note down DMR table value from table $A - 6$ (appendix) . While noting the table values, we have to see the degrees of freedom as in F-tables explained earlier. Thus D_{tab} value at 5% l.o.s at (2, 12) is 3.081.

Step – 5: If $D_{cal} \leq D_{tab}$ the difference is insignificant. Otherwise the difference is significant.

1. Since $D_1 > D_{tab}$, the difference between variety – 3 and variety – 2 is significant.

Similarly, difference between $\bar{v}_3 - \bar{v}_1 = D_2 = 27.2 - 21.1667 = 6.0338$ and $v_1 - \bar{v}_2 = D_3 = 21.1667 - 18 = 3.1667$.

Since, $D_2 > D_{tab}$ and $D_3 > D_{tab}$ we conclude that there is significant difference between variety – 1 and variety – 3; variety – 1 and variety – 2, thus we conclude that :

1. Between treatment – 1 and treatment – 2: Significant difference.
2. Between treatment – 1 and treatment – 3: Significant difference.
3. Between treatment – 2 and treatment – 3: Significant difference.

REVIEW QUESTIONS AND PROBLEMS

A. Objective Questions

1. In ANOVA we test the significance difference between ------------.

   (*a*) variances (*b*) correlations
   (*c*) means (*d*) standard deviations

2. In ANOVA one way classification with 5 treatments and 25 observations, degrees of freedom for error is ---------.

   (*a*) 20 (*b*) 21
   (*c*) 19 (*d*) 24.

3. In ANOVA if sum of squares is divided by the corresponding degrees of freedom we obtain ----------------------.

   (*a*) mean (*b*) mean sum of squares
   (*c*) *F*–value (*d*) error

4. In ANOVA two way classification total variation split into ----------- components.

   (*a*) two (*b*) four
   (*c*) three (*d*) six.

5. If $F_{cal} > F_{tab}$ we ----------------------- .

   (*a*) accept H_0 (*b*) reject H_0
   (*c*) reject H_1 (*d*) take no decision.

6. If $F_{cal} \leq F_{tab}$ we ----------------------- .

   (*a*) accept H_0 (*b*) reject H_0
   (*c*) reject H_1 (*d*) take no decision.

7. Further statistical analysis is required when we ---------------.

   (*a*) accept H_0 (*b*) reject H_0
   (*c*) reject H_1 (*d*) take no decision.

8. In ANOVA G^2/N is known as -------------------------.

   (*a*) sum of squares (*b*) degrees freedom
   (*c*) error (*d*) correction factor.

9. DMR test is to be used when we -------------------------.

   (*a*) accept H_0 (*b*) reject H_0
   (*c*) reject H_1 (*d*) take no decision.

10. In ANOVA we assume the treatment effectives are -----------------.

    (*a*) additive (*b*) multiplicative
    (*c*) significant (*d*) not significant.

B. Short Answers Questions

1. Explain the need for analysis of variance.
2. ANOVA is the generalization of student's t-test – comment on it.
3. Explain various assumptions of ANOVA.
4. Distinguish between ANOVA one-way and two-way classifications.
5. Write down ANOVA table for one way classification.
6. Write down ANOVA table for two-way classification.
7. Explain the need for further statistical analysis.
8. Explain briefly about ANOVA one-way test procedure.

9. Explain briefly about ANOVA two-way test procedure.
10. Explain DMR test procedure.

C. Essay Type Questions

1. Explain various test procedures of ANOVA.
2. Explain the need of ANOVA with suitable examples.
3. Explain the need of further statistical analysis with suitable examples.
4. A pharmaceutical company has purchased three new medicines manufacturing machines of different makes and wishes to determine which machine is producing faster medicines. The following data represents 5 hours random output from each machine. Determine whether all the machines are equally efficient in producing medicines or not? If not, which machine can produce faster the medicines?

Observations	Machine – A	Machine – B	Machine – C
1st hour	25	30	24
2nd hour	30	39	30
3rd hour	36	38	28
4th hour	38	42	25
5th hour	31	35	28

[**Hint:** use ANOVA one-way, F_{cal} = 7.5 reject H_0. Machine-2 is faster than other machines]

5. The following table gives the yield of wheat on 15 sample plots of equal size and fertility rate under three different seed qualities.

Quality A:	20	21	23	16	20
Quality B:	18	20	17	15	25
Quality C:	25	28	22	28	32

Test whether there exists any difference between seed qualities with respect to average yield of wheat production.

[**Hint:** Use ANOVA one way. Reject H_0]

6. A pharmaceutical company has four medical representatives *A, B, C* and *D*. Their sales (in lakhs of rupees) is given as follows in different seasons. Test whether there exists any statistical difference among medical representatives and sale of medicine in different seasons.

Medical representatives	A	B	C	D
Summer	36	36	21	35
Winter	28	29	31	32
Rainy	26	28	29	29

[**Hint:** Use ANOVA two-way. F_1 = 0.71 and F_2 = 0.62. No significant difference among medical representatives and sale of medicine in different seasons]

7. Four varieties of rice were grown on each of the four beds of three identical plots. The output in quintals are given as follows:

	Varieties of Rice			
Plots	A	B	C	D
1.	9	7	6	5
2.	7	4	5	4
3.	6	5	6	7

Test whether there exists any significant difference between

(*a*) Varieties of rice (*b*) different sample plots.

[**Hint:** Use ANOVA two-way. $F_1 = 1.68$ and $F_2 = 2.82$]

8. Five types of fertilisers are applied to four varieties of potatoes, each planted on five plots of land of same size and fertility rate. The yields in quintals are as follows:

		Potatoes		
Fertilisers	A	B	C	D
1	34	50	42	38
2	38	38	36	44
3	44	46	50	52
4	40	52	46	36
5	42	44	48	42

[Use two-way ANOVA. $F_1 = 1.67$ and $F_2 = 2.03$]

9. Explain DMR test with a suitable example.

10. Apply DMR test for the treatment means 35, 22, 46 and 38.

References

1. Gupta S.P. 1990 "Statistical Methods". Sultan Chand & Sons, New Delhi.
2. Wayne W. Daniel 2008 Biostatistics, 9th edition, John Wiley & Sons. Inc. Newyork.
3. P.N. Arora *et al.* 2007 "Comprehensive Statistical Methods" Sultan Chand and company Ltd. First edn. New Delhi.
4. VK. Kapoor 1986 "Problems and solutions in Business statistics" Sultan Chand and sons New Delhi.

Answers to Objective Questions

1 – c; 2 – a; 3 – b; 4 – c; 5 – b; 6 – a; 7 – b; 8 – d; 9 – b; 10 – a.

APPENDIX

TABLE – A-1: CUMULATIVE STANDARD NORMAL DISTRIBUTION

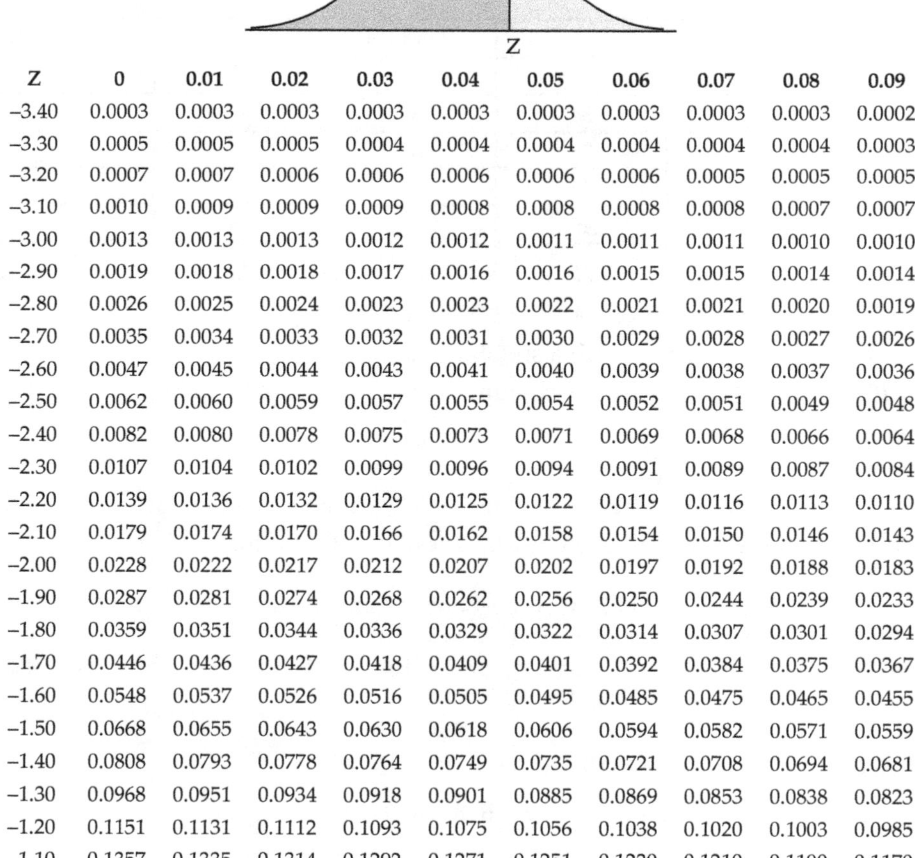

Z	0	0.01	0.02	0.03	0.04	0.05	0.06	0.07	0.08	0.09
–3.40	0.0003	0.0003	0.0003	0.0003	0.0003	0.0003	0.0003	0.0003	0.0003	0.0002
–3.30	0.0005	0.0005	0.0005	0.0004	0.0004	0.0004	0.0004	0.0004	0.0004	0.0003
–3.20	0.0007	0.0007	0.0006	0.0006	0.0006	0.0006	0.0006	0.0005	0.0005	0.0005
–3.10	0.0010	0.0009	0.0009	0.0009	0.0008	0.0008	0.0008	0.0008	0.0007	0.0007
–3.00	0.0013	0.0013	0.0013	0.0012	0.0012	0.0011	0.0011	0.0011	0.0010	0.0010
–2.90	0.0019	0.0018	0.0018	0.0017	0.0016	0.0016	0.0015	0.0015	0.0014	0.0014
–2.80	0.0026	0.0025	0.0024	0.0023	0.0023	0.0022	0.0021	0.0021	0.0020	0.0019
–2.70	0.0035	0.0034	0.0033	0.0032	0.0031	0.0030	0.0029	0.0028	0.0027	0.0026
–2.60	0.0047	0.0045	0.0044	0.0043	0.0041	0.0040	0.0039	0.0038	0.0037	0.0036
–2.50	0.0062	0.0060	0.0059	0.0057	0.0055	0.0054	0.0052	0.0051	0.0049	0.0048
–2.40	0.0082	0.0080	0.0078	0.0075	0.0073	0.0071	0.0069	0.0068	0.0066	0.0064
–2.30	0.0107	0.0104	0.0102	0.0099	0.0096	0.0094	0.0091	0.0089	0.0087	0.0084
–2.20	0.0139	0.0136	0.0132	0.0129	0.0125	0.0122	0.0119	0.0116	0.0113	0.0110
–2.10	0.0179	0.0174	0.0170	0.0166	0.0162	0.0158	0.0154	0.0150	0.0146	0.0143
–2.00	0.0228	0.0222	0.0217	0.0212	0.0207	0.0202	0.0197	0.0192	0.0188	0.0183
–1.90	0.0287	0.0281	0.0274	0.0268	0.0262	0.0256	0.0250	0.0244	0.0239	0.0233
–1.80	0.0359	0.0351	0.0344	0.0336	0.0329	0.0322	0.0314	0.0307	0.0301	0.0294
–1.70	0.0446	0.0436	0.0427	0.0418	0.0409	0.0401	0.0392	0.0384	0.0375	0.0367
–1.60	0.0548	0.0537	0.0526	0.0516	0.0505	0.0495	0.0485	0.0475	0.0465	0.0455
–1.50	0.0668	0.0655	0.0643	0.0630	0.0618	0.0606	0.0594	0.0582	0.0571	0.0559
–1.40	0.0808	0.0793	0.0778	0.0764	0.0749	0.0735	0.0721	0.0708	0.0694	0.0681
–1.30	0.0968	0.0951	0.0934	0.0918	0.0901	0.0885	0.0869	0.0853	0.0838	0.0823
–1.20	0.1151	0.1131	0.1112	0.1093	0.1075	0.1056	0.1038	0.1020	0.1003	0.0985
–1.10	0.1357	0.1335	0.1314	0.1292	0.1271	0.1251	0.1230	0.1210	0.1190	0.1170
–1.00	0.1587	0.1562	0.1539	0.1515	0.1492	0.1469	0.1446	0.1423	0.1401	0.1379
–0.90	0.1841	0.1814	0.1788	0.1762	0.1736	0.1711	0.1685	0.1660	0.1635	0.1611
–0.80	0.2119	0.2090	0.2061	0.2033	0.2005	0.1977	0.1949	0.1922	0.1894	0.1867

–0.70	0.2420	0.2389	0.2358	0.2327	0.2296	0.2266	0.2236	0.2206	0.2177	0.2148
–0.60	0.2743	0.2709	0.2676	0.2643	0.2611	0.2578	0.2546	0.2514	0.2483	0.2451
–0.50	0.3085	0.3050	0.3015	0.2981	0.2946	0.2912	0.2877	0.2843	0.2810	0.2776
–0.40	0.3446	0.3409	0.3372	0.3336	0.3300	0.3264	0.3228	0.3192	0.3156	0.3121
–0.30	0.3821	0.3783	0.3745	0.3707	0.3669	0.3632	0.3594	0.3557	0.3520	0.3483
–0.20	0.4207	0.4168	0.4129	0.4090	0.4052	0.4013	0.3974	0.3936	0.3897	0.3859
–0.10	0.4602	0.4562	0.4522	0.4483	0.4443	0.4404	0.4364	0.4325	0.4286	0.4247
0.00	0.5000	0.4960	0.4920	0.4880	0.4840	0.4801	0.4761	0.4721	0.4681	0.4641

Z	**0**	**0.01**	**0.02**	**0.03**	**0.04**	**0.05**	**0.06**	**0.07**	**0.08**	**0.09**
0.00	0.5000	0.5040	0.5080	0.5120	0.5160	0.5199	0.5239	0.5279	0.5319	0.5359
0.10	0.5398	0.5438	0.5478	0.5517	0.5557	0.5596	0.5636	0.5675	0.5714	0.5753
0.20	0.5793	0.5832	0.5871	0.5910	0.5948	0.5987	0.6026	0.6064	0.6103	0.6141
0.30	0.6179	0.6217	0.6255	0.6293	0.6331	0.6368	0.6406	0.6443	0.6480	0.6517
0.40	0.6554	0.6591	0.6628	0.6664	0.6700	0.6736	0.6772	0.6808	0.6844	0.6879
0.50	0.6915	0.6950	0.6985	0.7019	0.7054	0.7088	0.7123	0.7157	0.7190	0.7224
0.60	0.7257	0.7291	0.7324	0.7357	0.7389	0.7422	0.7454	0.7486	0.7517	0.7549
0.70	0.7580	0.7611	0.7642	0.7673	0.7704	0.7734	0.7764	0.7794	0.7823	0.7852
0.80	0.7881	0.7910	0.7939	0.7967	0.7995	0.8023	0.8051	0.8078	0.8106	0.8133
0.90	0.8159	0.8186	0.8212	0.8238	0.8264	0.8289	0.8315	0.8340	0.8365	0.8389
1.00	0.8413	0.8438	0.8461	0.8485	0.8508	0.8531	0.8554	0.8577	0.8599	0.8621
1.10	0.8643	0.8665	0.8686	0.8708	0.8729	0.8749	0.8770	0.8790	0.8810	0.8830
1.20	0.8849	0.8869	0.8888	0.8907	0.8925	0.8944	0.8962	0.8980	0.8997	0.9015
1.30	0.9032	0.9049	0.9066	0.9082	0.9099	0.9115	0.9131	0.9147	0.9162	0.9177
1.40	0.9192	0.9207	0.9222	0.9236	0.9251	0.9265	0.9279	0.9292	0.9306	0.9319
1.50	0.9332	0.9345	0.9357	0.9370	0.9382	0.9394	0.9406	0.9418	0.9429	0.9441
1.60	0.9452	0.9463	0.9474	0.9484	0.9495	0.9505	0.9515	0.9525	0.9535	0.9545
1.70	0.9554	0.9564	0.9573	0.9582	0.9591	0.9599	0.9608	0.9616	0.9625	0.9633
1.80	0.9641	0.9649	0.9656	0.9664	0.9671	0.9678	0.9686	0.9693	0.9699	0.9706
1.90	0.9713	0.9719	0.9726	0.9732	0.9738	0.9744	0.9750	0.9756	0.9761	0.9767
2.00	0.9772	0.9778	0.9783	0.9788	0.9793	0.9798	0.9803	0.9808	0.9812	0.9817
2.10	0.9821	0.9826	0.9830	0.9834	0.9838	0.9842	0.9846	0.9850	0.9854	0.9857
2.20	0.9861	0.9864	0.9868	0.9871	0.9875	0.9878	0.9881	0.9884	0.9887	0.9890
2.30	0.9893	0.9896	0.9898	0.9901	0.9904	0.9906	0.9909	0.9911	0.9913	0.9916
2.40	0.9918	0.9920	0.9922	0.9925	0.9927	0.9929	0.9931	0.9932	0.9934	0.9936
2.50	0.9938	0.9940	0.9941	0.9943	0.9945	0.9946	0.9948	0.9949	0.9951	0.9952
2.60	0.9953	0.9955	0.9956	0.9957	0.9959	0.9960	0.9961	0.9962	0.9963	0.9964
2.70	0.9965	0.9966	0.9967	0.9968	0.9969	0.9970	0.9971	0.9972	0.9973	0.9974
2.80	0.9974	0.9975	0.9976	0.9977	0.9977	0.9978	0.9979	0.9979	0.9980	0.9981
2.90	0.9981	0.9982	0.9982	0.9983	0.9984	0.9984	0.9985	0.9985	0.9986	0.9986
3.00	0.9987	0.9987	0.9987	0.9988	0.9988	0.9989	0.9989	0.9989	0.9990	0.9990
3.10	0.9990	0.9991	0.9991	0.9991	0.9992	0.9992	0.9992	0.9992	0.9993	0.9993
3.20	0.9993	0.9993	0.9994	0.9994	0.9994	0.9994	0.9994	0.9995	0.9995	0.9995
3.30	0.9995	0.9995	0.9995	0.9996	0.9996	0.9996	0.9996	0.9996	0.9996	0.9997
3.40	0.9997	0.9997	0.9997	0.9997	0.9997	0.9997	0.9997	0.9997	0.9997	0.9998

TABLE A–2 : CHI-SQUARE RIGHT HAND TAIL AREA

α = Right Hand Tail Area

ν	**0.999**	**0.995**	**0.99**	**0.975**	**0.95**	**0.9**	**0.1**	**0.05**	**0.025**	**0.01**	**0.005**	**0.001**
1	0.00	0.00	0.00	0.00	0.00	0.02	2.71	3.84	5.02	6.63	7.88	10.83
2	0.00	0.01	0.02	0.05	0.10	0.21	4.61	5.99	7.38	9.21	10.60	13.82
3	0.02	0.07	0.11	0.22	0.35	0.58	6.25	7.81	9.35	11.34	12.84	16.27
4	0.09	0.21	0.30	0.48	0.71	1.06	7.78	9.49	11.14	13.28	14.86	18.47
5	0.21	0.41	0.55	0.83	1.15	1.61	9.24	11.07	12.83	15.09	16.75	20.51
6	0.38	0.68	0.87	1.24	1.64	2.20	10.64	12.59	14.45	16.81	18.55	22.46
7	0.60	0.99	1.24	1.69	2.17	2.83	12.02	14.07	16.01	18.48	20.28	24.32
8	0.86	1.34	1.65	2.18	2.73	3.49	13.36	15.51	17.53	20.09	21.95	26.12
9	1.15	1.73	2.09	2.70	3.33	4.17	14.68	16.92	19.02	21.67	23.59	27.88
10	1.48	2.16	2.56	3.25	3.94	4.87	15.99	18.31	20.48	23.21	25.19	29.59
11	1.83	2.60	3.05	3.82	4.57	5.58	17.28	19.68	21.92	24.73	26.76	31.26
12	2.21	3.07	3.57	4.40	5.23	6.30	18.55	21.03	23.34	26.22	28.30	32.91
13	2.62	3.57	4.11	5.01	5.89	7.04	19.81	22.36	24.74	27.69	29.82	34.53
14	3.04	4.07	4.66	5.63	6.57	7.79	21.06	23.68	26.12	29.14	31.32	36.12
15	3.48	4.60	5.23	6.26	7.26	8.55	22.31	25.00	27.49	30.58	32.80	37.70
16	3.94	5.14	5.81	6.91	7.96	9.31	23.54	26.30	28.85	32.00	34.27	39.25
17	4.42	5.70	6.41	7.56	8.67	10.09	24.77	27.59	30.19	33.41	35.72	40.79
18	4.90	6.26	7.01	8.23	9.39	10.86	25.99	28.87	31.53	34.81	37.16	42.31
19	5.41	6.84	7.63	8.91	10.12	11.65	27.20	30.14	32.85	36.19	38.58	43.82
20	5.92	7.43	8.26	9.59	10.85	12.44	28.41	31.41	34.17	37.57	40.00	45.31
21	6.45	8.03	8.90	10.28	11.59	13.24	29.62	32.67	35.48	38.93	41.40	46.80
22	6.98	8.64	9.54	10.98	12.34	14.04	30.81	33.92	36.78	40.29	42.80	48.27
23	7.53	9.26	10.20	11.69	13.09	14.85	32.01	35.17	38.08	41.64	44.18	49.73
24	8.08	9.89	10.86	12.40	13.85	15.66	33.20	36.42	39.36	42.98	45.56	51.18
25	8.65	10.52	11.52	13.12	14.61	16.47	34.38	37.65	40.65	44.31	46.93	52.62
26	9.22	11.16	12.20	13.84	15.38	17.29	35.56	38.89	41.92	45.64	48.29	54.05
27	9.80	11.81	12.88	14.57	16.15	18.11	36.74	40.11	43.19	46.96	49.65	55.48
28	10.39	12.46	13.56	15.31	16.93	18.94	37.92	41.34	44.46	48.28	50.99	56.89
29	10.99	13.12	14.26	16.05	17.71	19.77	39.09	42.56	45.72	49.59	52.34	58.30
30	11.59	13.79	14.95	16.79	18.49	20.60	40.26	43.77	46.98	50.89	53.67	59.70
32	12.81	15.13	16.36	18.29	20.07	22.27	42.58	46.19	49.48	53.49	56.33	62.49
34	14.06	16.50	17.79	19.81	21.66	23.95	44.90	48.60	51.97	56.06	58.96	65.25
36	15.32	17.89	19.23	21.34	23.27	25.64	47.21	51.00	54.44	58.62	61.58	67.98
38	16.61	19.29	20.69	22.88	24.88	27.34	49.51	53.38	56.90	61.16	64.18	70.70
40	17.92	20.71	22.16	24.43	26.51	29.05	51.81	55.76	59.34	63.69	66.77	73.40
42	19.24	22.14	23.65	26.00	28.14	30.77	54.09	58.12	61.78	66.21	69.34	76.08
44	20.58	23.58	25.15	27.57	29.79	32.49	56.37	60.48	64.20	68.71	71.89	78.75
46	21.93	25.04	26.66	29.16	31.44	34.22	58.64	62.83	66.62	71.20	74.44	81.40
48	23.29	26.51	28.18	30.75	33.10	35.95	60.91	65.17	69.02	73.68	76.97	84.04
50	24.67	27.99	29.71	32.36	34.76	37.69	63.17	67.50	71.42	76.15	79.49	86.66
55	28.17	31.73	33.57	36.40	38.96	42.06	68.80	73.31	77.38	82.29	85.75	93.17
60	31.74	35.53	37.48	40.48	43.19	46.46	74.40	79.08	83.30	88.38	91.95	99.61

TABLE A-3: VALUES OF *T* FOR A SPECIFIED RIGHT TAIL AREA

Percentage Points of the t Distribution

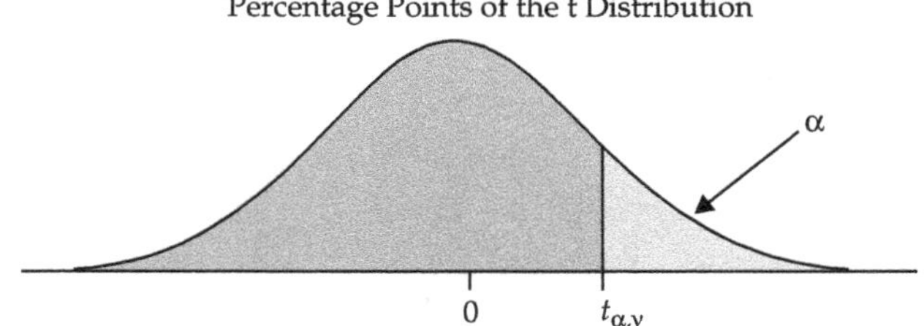

Level of Significance α

ν	**0.4**	**0.25**	**0.1**	**0.05**	**0.025**	**0.01**	**0.005**	**0.0025**	**0.001**	**0.0005**
1	0.325	1.000	3.078	6.314	12.706	31.821	63.656	127.321	318.289	636.578
2	0.289	0.816	1.886	2.920	4.303	6.965	9.925	14.089	22.328	31.600
3	0.277	0.765	1.638	2.353	3.182	4.541	5.841	7.453	10.214	12.924
4	0.271	0.741	1.533	2.132	2.776	3.747	4.604	5.598	7.173	8.610
5	0.267	0.727	1.476	2.015	2.571	3.365	4.032	4.773	5.894	6.869
6	0.265	0.718	1.440	1.943	2.447	3.143	3.707	4.317	5.208	5.959
7	0.263	0.711	1.415	1.895	2.365	2.998	3.499	4.029	4.785	5.408
8	0.262	0.706	1.397	1.860	2.306	2.896	3.355	3.833	4.501	5.041
9	0.261	0.703	1.383	1.833	2.262	2.821	3.250	3.690	4.297	4.781
10	0.260	0.700	1.372	1.812	2.228	2.764	3.169	3.581	4.144	4.587
11	0.260	0.697	1.363	1.796	2.201	2.718	3.106	3.497	4.025	4.437
12	0.259	0.695	1.356	1.782	2.179	2.681	3.055	3.428	3.930	4.318
13	0.259	0.694	1.350	1.771	2.160	2.650	3.012	3.372	3.852	4.221
14	0.258	0.692	1.345	1.761	2.145	2.624	2.977	3.326	3.787	4.140
15	0.258	0.691	1.341	1.753	2.131	2.602	2.947	3.286	3.733	4.073
16	0.258	0.690	1.337	1.746	2.120	2.583	2.921	3.252	3.686	4.015
17	0.257	0.689	1.333	1.740	2.110	2.567	2.898	3.222	3.646	3.965
18	0.257	0.688	1.330	1.734	2.101	2.552	2.878	3.197	3.610	3.922
19	0.257	0.688	1.328	1.729	2.093	2.539	2.861	3.174	3.579	3.883
20	0.257	0.687	1.325	1.725	2.086	2.528	2.845	3.153	3.552	3.850
21	0.257	0.686	1.323	1.721	2.080	2.518	2.831	3.135	3.527	3.819
22	0.256	0.686	1.321	1.717	2.074	2.508	2.819	3.119	3.505	3.792
23	0.256	0.685	1.319	1.714	2.069	2.500	2.807	3.104	3.485	3.768
24	0.256	0.685	1.318	1.711	2.064	2.492	2.797	3.091	3.467	3.745
25	0.256	0.684	1.316	1.708	2.060	2.485	2.787	3.078	3.450	3.725
26	0.256	0.684	1.315	1.706	2.056	2.479	2.779	3.067	3.435	3.707
27	0.256	0.684	1.314	1.703	2.052	2.473	2.771	3.057	3.421	3.689
28	0.256	0.683	1.313	1.701	2.048	2.467	2.763	3.047	3.408	3.674
29	0.256	0.683	1.311	1.699	2.045	2.462	2.756	3.038	3.396	3.660
30	0.256	0.683	1.310	1.697	2.042	2.457	2.750	3.030	3.385	3.646
40	0.255	0.681	1.303	1.684	2.021	2.423	2.704	2.971	3.307	3.551
60	0.254	0.679	1.296	1.671	2.000	2.390	2.660	2.915	3.232	3.460
120	0.254	0.677	1.289	1.658	1.980	2.358	2.617	2.860	3.160	3.373
∞	0.253	0.674	1.282	1.645	1.960	2.326	2.576	2.807	3.090	3.291

TABLE A – 4

Values of F for a Specified Right Tail Area $F_{0.05\ \nu_1, \nu_2}$

ν_2 DOF for Denominator

Degrees of Freedom for Numerator (ν_1)

(ν_2)	1	2	3	4	5	6	7	8	9	10	12	15	20	24	30	40	60	120	∝
1	161	199	216	225	230	234	237	239	241	242	244	246	248	249	250	251	252	253	254
2	18.5	19.0	19.2	19.2	19.3	19.3	19.4	19.4	19.4	19.4	19.4	19.4	19.4	19.5	19.5	19.5	19.5	19.5	19.5
3	10.1	9.55	9.28	9.12	9.01	8.94	8.89	8.85	8.81	8.79	8.74	8.70	8.66	8.64	8.62	8.59	8.57	8.55	8.53
4	7.71	6.94	6.59	6.39	6.26	6.16	6.09	6.04	6.00	5.96	5.91	5.86	5.80	5.77	5.75	5.72	5.69	5.66	5.63
5	6.61	5.79	5.41	5.19	5.05	4.95	4.88	4.82	4.77	4.74	4.68	4.62	4.56	4.53	4.50	4.46	4.43	4.40	4.37
6	5.99	5.14	4.76	4.53	4.39	4.28	4.21	4.15	4.10	4.06	4.00	3.94	3.87	3.84	3.81	3.77	3.74	3.70	3.67
7	5.59	4.74	4.35	4.12	3.97	3.87	3.79	3.73	3.68	3.64	3.57	3.51	3.44	3.41	3.38	3.34	3.30	3.27	3.23
8	5.32	4.46	4.07	3.84	3.69	3.58	3.50	3.44	3.39	3.35	3.28	3.22	3.15	3.12	3.08	3.04	3.01	2.97	2.93
9	5.12	4.26	3.86	3.63	3.48	3.37	3.29	3.23	3.18	3.14	3.07	3.01	2.94	2.90	2.86	2.83	2.79	2.75	2.71
10	4.96	4.10	3.71	3.48	3.33	3.22	3.14	3.07	3.02	2.98	2.91	2.85	2.77	2.74	2.70	2.66	2.62	2.58	2.54
11	4.84	3.98	3.59	3.36	3.20	3.09	3.01	2.95	2.90	2.85	2.79	2.72	2.65	2.61	2.57	2.53	2.49	2.45	2.40
12	4.75	3.89	3.49	3.26	3.11	3.00	2.91	2.85	2.80	2.75	2.69	2.62	2.54	2.51	2.47	2.43	2.38	2.34	2.30
13	4.67	3.81	3.41	3.18	3.03	2.92	2.83	2.77	2.71	2.67	2.60	2.53	2.46	2.42	2.38	2.34	2.30	2.25	2.21
14	4.60	3.74	3.34	3.11	2.96	2.85	2.76	2.70	2.65	2.60	2.53	2.46	2.39	2.35	2.31	2.27	2.22	2.18	2.13
15	4.54	3.68	3.29	3.06	2.90	2.79	2.71	2.64	2.59	2.54	2.48	2.40	2.33	2.29	2.25	2.20	2.16	2.11	2.07
16	4.49	3.63	3.24	3.01	2.85	2.74	2.66	2.59	2.54	2.49	2.42	2.35	2.28	2.24	2.19	2.15	2.11	2.06	2.01
17	4.45	3.59	3.20	2.96	2.81	2.70	2.61	2.55	2.49	2.45	2.38	2.31	2.23	2.19	2.15	2.10	2.06	2.01	1.96
18	4.41	3.55	3.16	2.93	2.77	2.66	2.58	2.51	2.46	2.41	2.34	2.27	2.19	2.15	2.11	2.06	2.02	1.97	1.92
19	4.38	3.52	3.13	2.90	2.74	2.63	2.54	2.48	2.42	2.38	2.31	2.23	2.16	2.11	2.07	2.03	1.98	1.93	1.88
20	4.35	3.49	3.10	2.87	2.71	2.60	2.51	2.45	2.39	2.35	2.28	2.20	2.12	2.08	2.04	1.99	1.95	1.90	1.84
21	4.32	3.47	3.07	2.84	2.68	2.57	2.49	2.42	2.37	2.32	2.25	2.18	2.10	2.05	2.01	1.96	1.92	1.87	1.81
22	4.30	3.44	3.05	2.82	2.66	2.55	2.46	2.40	2.34	2.30	2.23	2.15	2.07	2.03	1.98	1.94	1.89	1.84	1.78
23	4.28	3.42	3.03	2.80	2.64	2.53	2.44	2.37	2.32	2.27	2.20	2.13	2.05	2.01	1.96	1.91	1.86	1.81	1.76
24	4.26	3.40	3.01	2.78	2.62	2.51	2.42	2.36	2.30	2.25	2.18	2.11	2.03	1.98	1.94	1.89	1.84	1.79	1.73
25	4.24	3.39	2.99	2.76	2.60	2.49	2.40	2.34	2.28	2.24	2.16	2.09	2.01	1.96	1.92	1.87	1.82	1.77	1.71
26	4.23	3.37	2.98	2.74	2.59	2.47	2.39	2.32	2.27	2.22	2.15	2.07	1.99	1.95	1.90	1.85	1.80	1.75	1.69
27	4.21	3.35	2.96	2.73	2.57	2.46	2.37	2.31	2.25	2.20	2.13	2.06	1.97	1.93	1.88	1.84	1.79	1.73	1.67
28	4.20	3.34	2.95	2.71	2.56	2.45	2.36	2.29	2.24	2.19	2.12	2.04	1.96	1.91	1.87	1.82	1.77	1.71	1.65
29	4.18	3.33	2.93	2.70	2.55	2.43	2.35	2.28	2.22	2.18	2.10	2.03	1.94	1.90	1.85	1.81	1.75	1.70	1.64
30	4.17	3.32	2.92	2.69	2.53	2.42	2.33	2.27	2.21	2.16	2.09	2.01	1.93	1.89	1.84	1.79	1.74	1.68	1.62
40	4.08	3.23	2.84	2.61	2.45	2.34	2.25	2.18	2.12	2.08	2.00	1.92	1.84	1.79	1.74	1.69	1.64	1.58	1.51
60	4.00	3.15	2.76	2.53	2.37	2.25	2.17	2.10	2.04	1.99	1.92	1.84	1.75	1.70	1.65	1.59	1.53	1.47	1.39
120	3.92	3.07	2.68	2.45	2.29	2.18	2.09	2.02	1.96	1.91	1.83	1.75	1.66	1.61	1.55	1.50	1.43	1.35	1.25
∝	3.84	3.00	2.60	2.37	2.21	2.10	2.01	1.94	1.88	1.83	1.75	1.67	1.57	1.52	1.46	1.39	1.32	1.22	1.00

Table A-5: Values of F for a Specified Right Tail Area $F_{0.01\ \nu_1,\nu_2}$

(V_2) degrees of freedom for denominator.

Degrees of Freedom for Numerator (ν_1)

(ν_2)	1	2	3	4	5	6	7	8	9	10	12	15	20	24	30	40	60	120	∞
1	4052	4999	5404	5624	5764	5859	5928	5981	6022	6056	6107	6157	6209	6234	6260	6286	6313	6340	6366
2	98.5	99.0	99.2	99.3	99.3	99.3	99.4	99.4	99.4	99.4	99.4	99.4	99.4	99.5	99.5	99.5	99.5	99.5	99.5
3	34.1	30.8	29.5	28.7	28.2	27.9	27.7	27.5	27.3	27.2	27.1	26.9	26.7	26.6	26.5	26.4	26.3	26.2	26.1
4	21.2	18.0	16.7	16.0	15.5	15.2	15.0	14.8	14.7	14.5	14.4	14.2	14.0	13.9	13.8	13.7	13.7	13.6	13.5
5	16.3	13.3	12.1	11.4	11.0	10.7	10.5	10.3	10.2	10.1	9.89	9.72	9.55	9.47	9.38	9.29	9.20	9.11	9.02
6	13.7	10.9	9.78	9.15	8.75	8.47	8.26	8.10	7.98	7.87	7.72	7.56	7.40	7.31	7.23	7.14	7.06	6.97	6.88
7	12.2	9.55	8.45	7.85	7.46	7.19	6.99	6.84	6.72	6.62	6.47	6.31	6.16	6.07	5.99	5.91	5.82	5.74	5.65
8	11.3	8.65	7.59	7.01	6.63	6.37	6.18	6.03	5.91	5.81	5.67	5.52	5.36	5.28	5.20	5.12	5.03	4.95	4.86
9	10.6	8.02	6.99	6.42	6.06	5.80	5.61	5.47	5.35	5.26	5.11	4.96	4.81	4.73	4.65	4.57	4.48	4.40	4.31
10	10.0	7.56	6.55	5.99	5.64	5.39	5.20	5.06	4.94	4.85	4.71	4.56	4.41	4.33	4.25	4.17	4.08	4.00	3.91
11	9.65	7.21	6.22	5.67	5.32	5.07	4.89	4.74	4.63	4.54	4.40	4.25	4.10	4.02	3.94	3.86	3.78	3.69	3.60
12	9.33	6.93	5.95	5.41	5.06	4.82	4.64	4.50	4.39	4.30	4.16	4.01	3.86	3.78	3.70	3.62	3.54	3.45	3.36
13	9.07	6.70	5.74	5.21	4.86	4.62	4.44	4.30	4.19	4.10	3.96	3.82	3.66	3.59	3.51	3.43	3.34	3.25	3.17
14	8.86	6.51	5.56	5.04	4.69	4.46	4.28	4.14	4.03	3.94	3.80	3.66	3.51	3.43	3.35	3.27	3.18	3.09	3.00
15	8.68	6.36	5.42	4.89	4.56	4.32	4.14	4.00	3.89	3.80	3.67	3.52	3.37	3.29	3.21	3.13	3.05	2.96	2.87
16	8.53	6.23	5.29	4.77	4.44	4.20	4.03	3.89	3.78	3.69	3.55	3.41	3.26	3.18	3.10	3.02	2.93	2.84	2.75
17	8.40	6.11	5.19	4.67	4.34	4.10	3.93	3.79	3.68	3.59	3.46	3.31	3.16	3.08	3.00	2.92	2.83	2.75	2.65
18	8.29	6.01	5.09	4.58	4.25	4.01	3.84	3.71	3.60	3.51	3.37	3.23	3.08	3.00	2.92	2.84	2.75	2.66	2.57
19	8.18	5.93	5.01	4.50	4.17	3.94	3.77	3.63	3.52	3.43	3.30	3.15	3.00	2.92	2.84	2.76	2.67	2.58	2.49
20	8.10	5.85	4.94	4.43	4.10	3.87	3.70	3.56	3.46	3.37	3.23	3.09	2.94	2.86	2.78	2.69	2.61	2.52	2.42
21	8.02	5.78	4.87	4.37	4.04	3.81	3.64	3.51	3.40	3.31	3.17	3.03	2.88	2.80	2.72	2.64	2.55	2.46	2.36
22	7.95	5.72	4.82	4.31	3.99	3.76	3.59	3.45	3.35	3.26	3.12	2.98	2.83	2.75	2.67	2.58	2.50	2.40	2.31
23	7.88	5.66	4.76	4.26	3.94	3.71	3.54	3.41	3.30	3.21	3.07	2.93	2.78	2.70	2.62	2.54	2.45	2.35	2.26
24	7.82	5.61	4.72	4.22	3.90	3.67	3.50	3.36	3.26	3.17	3.03	2.89	2.74	2.66	2.58	2.49	2.40	2.31	2.21
25	7.77	5.57	4.68	4.18	3.85	3.63	3.46	3.32	3.22	3.13	2.99	2.85	2.70	2.62	2.54	2.45	2.36	2.27	2.17
26	7.72	5.53	4.64	4.14	3.82	3.59	3.42	3.29	3.18	3.09	2.96	2.81	2.66	2.58	2.50	2.42	2.33	2.23	2.13
27	7.68	5.49	4.60	4.11	3.78	3.56	3.39	3.26	3.15	3.06	2.93	2.78	2.63	2.55	2.47	2.38	2.29	2.20	2.10
28	7.64	5.45	4.57	4.07	3.75	3.53	3.36	3.23	3.12	3.03	2.90	2.75	2.60	2.52	2.44	2.35	2.26	2.17	2.06
29	7.60	5.42	4.54	4.04	3.73	3.50	3.33	3.20	3.09	3.00	2.87	2.73	2.57	2.49	2.41	2.33	2.23	2.14	2.03
30	7.56	5.39	4.51	4.02	3.70	3.47	3.30	3.17	3.07	2.98	2.84	2.70	2.55	2.47	2.39	2.30	2.21	2.11	2.01
40	7.31	5.18	4.31	3.83	3.51	3.29	3.12	2.99	2.89	2.80	2.66	2.52	2.37	2.29	2.20	2.11	2.02	1.92	1.80
60	7.08	4.98	4.13	3.65	3.34	3.12	2.95	2.82	2.72	2.63	2.50	2.35	2.20	2.12	2.03	1.94	1.84	1.73	1.60
120	6.85	4.79	3.95	3.48	3.17	2.96	2.79	2.66	2.56	2.47	2.34	2.19	2.03	1.95	1.86	1.76	1.66	1.53	1.38
∞	6.64	4.61	3.78	3.32	3.02	2.80	2.64	2.51	2.41	2.32	2.18	2.04	1.88	1.79	1.70	1.59	1.47	1.32	1.00

TABLE A-6. DUNCAN'S MULTIPLE RANGE TABLES

Critical values q'(p, df, 0.05) for Duncan's multiple range tests

df	p= 2	3	4	5	6	7	8	9	10	11	12	13	14	15	16	17	18	19	20
1	17.969	17.969	17.969	17.969	17.969	17.969	17.969	17.969	17.969	17.969	17.969	17.969	17.969	17.969	17.969	17.969	17.969	17.969	17.969
2	6.085	6.085	6.085	6.085	6.085	6.085	6.085	6.085	6.085	6.085	6.085	6.085	6.085	6.085	6.085	6.085	6.085	6.085	6.085
3	4.501	4.516	4.516	4.516	4.516	4.516	4.516	4.516	4.516	4.516	4.516	4.516	4.516	4.516	4.516	4.516	4.516	4.516	4.516
4	3.926	4.013	4.033	4.033	4.033	4.033	4.033	4.033	4.033	4.033	4.033	4.033	4.033	4.033	4.033	4.033	4.033	4.033	4.033
5	3.635	3.748	3.796	3.814	3.814	3.814	3.814	3.814	3.814	3.814	3.814	3.814	3.814	3.814	3.814	3.814	3.814	3.814	3.814
6	3.46	3.586	3.648	3.68	3.694	3.697	3.697	3.697	3.697	3.697	3.697	3.697	3.697	3.697	3.697	3.697	3.697	3.697	3.697
7	3.344	3.477	3.548	3.588	3.611	3.622	3.625	3.625	3.625	3.625	3.625	3.625	3.625	3.625	3.625	3.625	3.625	3.625	3.625
8	3.261	3.398	3.475	3.521	3.549	3.566	3.575	3.579	3.579	3.579	3.579	3.579	3.579	3.579	3.579	3.579	3.579	3.579	3.579
9	3.199	3.339	3.42	3.47	3.502	3.523	3.536	3.544	3.547	3.547	3.547	3.547	3.547	3.547	3.547	3.547	3.547	3.547	3.547
10	3.151	3.293	3.376	3.43	3.465	3.489	3.505	3.516	3.522	3.525	3.525	3.525	3.525	3.525	3.525	3.525	3.525	3.525	3.525
11	3.113	3.256	3.341	3.397	3.435	3.462	3.48	3.493	3.501	3.506	3.509	3.51	3.51	3.51	3.51	3.51	3.51	3.51	3.51
12	3.081	3.225	3.312	3.37	3.41	3.439	3.459	3.474	3.484	3.491	3.495	3.498	3.498	3.498	3.498	3.498	3.498	3.498	3.498
13	3.055	3.2	3.288	3.348	3.389	3.419	3.441	3.458	3.47	3.478	3.484	3.488	3.49	3.49	3.49	3.49	3.49	3.49	3.49
14	3.033	3.178	3.268	3.328	3.371	3.403	3.426	3.444	3.457	3.467	3.474	3.479	3.482	3.484	3.484	3.484	3.484	3.484	3.484
15	3.014	3.16	3.25	3.312	3.356	3.389	3.413	3.432	3.446	3.457	3.465	3.471	3.476	3.478	3.48	3.48	3.48	3.48	3.48
16	2.998	3.144	3.235	3.297	3.343	3.376	3.402	3.422	3.437	3.449	3.458	3.465	3.47	3.473	3.476	3.477	3.477	3.477	3.477
17	2.984	3.13	3.222	3.285	3.331	3.365	3.392	3.412	3.429	3.441	3.451	3.459	3.465	3.469	3.472	3.474	3.475	3.475	3.475
18	2.971	3.117	3.21	3.274	3.32	3.356	3.383	3.404	3.421	3.435	3.445	3.454	3.46	3.465	3.469	3.472	3.473	3.474	3.474
19	2.96	3.106	3.199	3.264	3.311	3.347	3.375	3.397	3.415	3.429	3.44	3.449	3.456	3.462	3.466	3.469	3.472	3.473	3.474
20	2.95	3.097	3.19	3.255	3.303	3.339	3.368	3.39	3.409	3.423	3.435	3.445	3.452	3.459	3.463	3.467	3.47	3.472	3.473
21	2.941	3.088	3.181	3.247	3.295	3.332	3.361	3.385	3.403	3.418	3.431	3.441	3.449	3.456	3.461	3.465	3.469	3.471	3.473
22	2.933	3.08	3.173	3.239	3.288	3.326	3.355	3.379	3.398	3.414	3.427	3.437	3.446	3.453	3.459	3.464	3.467	3.47	3.472
23	2.926	3.072	3.166	3.233	3.282	3.32	3.35	3.374	3.394	3.41	3.423	3.434	3.443	3.451	3.457	3.462	3.466	3.469	3.472
24	2.919	3.066	3.16	3.226	3.276	3.315	3.345	3.37	3.39	3.406	3.42	3.431	3.441	3.449	3.455	3.461	3.465	3.469	3.472
25	2.913	3.059	3.154	3.221	3.271	3.31	3.341	3.366	3.386	3.403	3.417	3.429	3.439	3.447	3.454	3.459	3.464	3.468	3.471
26	2.907	3.054	3.149	3.216	3.266	3.305	3.336	3.362	3.382	3.4	3.414	3.426	3.436	3.445	3.452	3.458	3.463	3.468	3.471
27	2.902	3.048	3.144	3.211	3.262	3.301	3.332	3.358	3.379	3.397	3.412	3.424	3.434	3.443	3.451	3.457	3.463	3.467	3.471
28	2.897	3.044	3.139	3.206	3.257	3.297	3.329	3.355	3.376	3.394	3.409	3.422	3.433	3.442	3.45	3.456	3.462	3.467	3.47
29	2.892	3.039	3.135	3.202	3.253	3.293	3.326	3.352	3.373	3.392	3.407	3.42	3.431	3.44	3.448	3.455	3.461	3.466	3.47
30	2.888	3.035	3.131	3.199	3.25	3.29	3.322	3.349	3.371	3.389	3.405	3.418	3.429	3.439	3.447	3.454	3.46	3.466	3.47
31	2.884	3.031	3.127	3.195	3.246	3.287	3.319	3.346	3.368	3.387	3.403	3.416	3.428	3.438	3.446	3.454	3.46	3.465	3.47
32	2.881	3.028	3.123	3.192	3.243	3.284	3.317	3.344	3.366	3.385	3.401	3.415	3.426	3.436	3.445	3.453	3.459	3.465	3.47
33	2.877	3.024	3.12	3.188	3.24	3.281	3.314	3.341	3.364	3.383	3.399	3.413	3.425	3.435	3.444	3.452	3.459	3.465	3.47
34	2.874	3.021	3.117	3.185	3.238	3.279	3.312	3.339	3.362	3.381	3.398	3.412	3.424	3.434	3.443	3.451	3.458	3.464	3.469
35	2.871	3.018	3.114	3.183	3.235	3.276	3.309	3.337	3.36	3.379	3.396	3.41	3.423	3.433	3.443	3.451	3.458	3.464	3.469
36	2.868	3.015	3.111	3.18	3.232	3.274	3.307	3.335	3.358	3.378	3.395	3.409	3.421	3.432	3.442	3.45	3.457	3.464	3.469
37	2.865	3.013	3.108	3.178	3.23	3.272	3.305	3.333	3.356	3.376	3.393	3.408	3.42	3.431	3.441	3.449	3.457	3.463	3.469
38	2.863	3.01	3.106	3.175	3.228	3.27	3.303	3.331	3.355	3.375	3.392	3.407	3.419	3.431	3.44	3.449	3.456	3.463	3.469
39	2.861	3.008	3.104	3.173	3.226	3.268	3.301	3.33	3.353	3.373	3.391	3.406	3.418	3.43	3.44	3.448	3.456	3.463	3.469
40	2.858	3.005	3.102	3.171	3.224	3.266	3.3	3.328	3.352	3.372	3.389	3.404	3.418	3.429	3.439	3.448	3.456	3.463	3.469
48	2.843	2.991	3.087	3.157	3.211	3.253	3.288	3.318	3.342	3.363	3.382	3.398	3.412	3.424	3.435	3.445	3.453	3.461	3.468
60	2.829	2.976	3.073	3.143	3.198	3.241	3.277	3.307	3.333	3.355	3.374	3.391	3.406	3.419	3.431	3.441	3.451	3.46	3.468
80	2.814	2.961	3.059	3.13	3.185	3.229	3.266	3.297	3.323	3.346	3.366	3.384	3.4	3.414	3.427	3.438	3.448	3.458	3.467
120	2.8	2.947	3.045	3.116	3.172	3.217	3.254	3.286	3.313	3.337	3.358	3.377	3.394	3.409	3.423	3.435	3.446	3.457	3.466
240	2.786	2.933	3.031	3.103	3.159	3.205	3.243	3.276	3.304	3.329	3.35	3.37	3.388	3.404	3.418	3.432	3.444	3.455	3.466
Inf	2.772	2.918	3.017	3.089	3.146	3.193	3.232	3.265	3.294	3.32	3.343	3.363	3.382	3.399	3.414	3.428	3.442	3.454	3.466

INDEX

www.ingramcontent.com/pod-product-compliance
Lightning Source LLC
Chambersburg PA
CBHW021435180326
41458CB00001B/283
9789351301189